Recent Advances in

Critical Care Medicine

2025

AF473844

Recent Advances in Critical Care Medicine 2025

Volume 2

Editors

Atul Prabhakar Kulkarni
MD (Anesthesiology)
Professor and Head
Division of Critical Care
Department of Anesthesiology, Critical Care, and Pain
Tata Memorial Hospital
Homi Bhabha National Institute
Mumbai, Maharashtra, India

Kushal Rajeev Kalvit
MD DM EDIC EDEC PGDMT
Senior Consultant
Department of Critical Care Medicine
Sir HN Reliance Foundation Hospital
Mumbai, Maharashtra, India

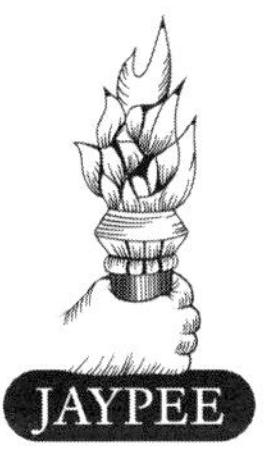

JAYPEE BROTHERS MEDICAL PUBLISHERS
The Health Sciences Publisher
New Delhi | London

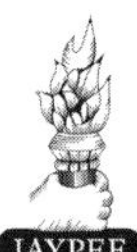

Jaypee Brothers Medical Publishers (P) Ltd

Headquarters
EMCA House, 23/23-B
Ansari Road, Daryaganj
New Delhi 110 002, India
Landline: +91-11-23272143, +91-11-23272703
+91-11-23282021, +91-11-23245672
e-mail: jaypee@jaypeebrothers.com

Corporate Office
4838/24, Ansari Road, Daryaganj
New Delhi 110 002, India
Phone: +91-11-43574357
Fax: +91-11-43574314
e-mail: jaypee@jaypeebrothers.com

Overseas Office
JP Medical Ltd.
83, Victoria Street, London
SW1H 0HW (UK)
Phone: +44-20 3170 8910
e-mail: info@jpmedpub.com

EU GPSR Authorised Representative
Logos Europe, 9 rue Nicolas Poussin
17000, La Rochelle, France
Phone: +33 (0) 6 67 93 73 78
e-mail: contact@logoseurope.eu

Website: www.jaypeebrothers.com
Website: www.jaypeedigital.com

© 2026, Jaypee Brothers Medical Publishers

The views and opinions expressed in this book are solely those of the original contributor(s)/author(s) and do not necessarily represent those of editor(s) or publisher of the book.

All rights reserved. No part of this publication may be reproduced, stored or transmitted in any form or by any means, electronic, mechanical, photocopying, recording or otherwise, without the prior permission in writing of the publishers.

All brand names and product names used in this book are trade names, service marks, trademarks or registered trademarks of their respective owners. The publisher is not associated with any product or vendor mentioned in this book.

Medical knowledge and practice change constantly. This book is designed to provide accurate, authoritative information about the subject matter in question. However, readers are advised to check the most current information available on procedures included and check information from the manufacturer of each product to be administered, to verify the recommended dose, formula, method and duration of administration, adverse effects and contraindications. It is the responsibility of the practitioner to take all appropriate safety precautions. Neither the publisher nor the author(s)/editor(s) assume any liability for any injury and/or damage to persons or property arising from or related to use of material in this book.

This book is sold on the understanding that the publisher is not engaged in providing professional medical services. If such advice or services are required, the services of a competent medical professional should be sought.

Every effort has been made where necessary to contact holders of copyright to obtain permission to reproduce copyright material. If any have been inadvertently overlooked, the publisher will be pleased to make the necessary arrangements at the first opportunity.

Inquiries for bulk sales may be solicited at: jaypee@jaypeebrothers.com

Recent Advances in Critical Care Medicine 2025 (Vol 2)

First Edition: **2026**

ISBN: 978-93-7202-966-6

Printed at: Samrat Offset Pvt. Ltd.

Dedicated to

The newer, more aware and assertive doctors,
the practitioners of critical care medicine.

Contributors

Abhishek Pratap Singh
MBBS DNB DrNB
Associate Consultant
Department of Critical Care Medicine
Medanta—The Medicity
Gurugram, Haryana, India

Abhishek Rajput
DM (Critical Care Medicine)
Assistant Professor (Critical Care Medicine)
Department of Anesthesiology, Critical Care, and Pain
Tata Memorial Hospital
Homi Bhabha National Institute
Navi Mumbai, Maharashtra, India

Afzal Azim MD
Professor
Department of Critical Care Medicine
Sanjay Gandhi Postgraduate Institute of Medical Sciences
Lucknow, Uttar Pradesh, India

Ambuj Yadav MD (Medicine) PDCC (Critical Care Medicine)
Associate Professor
Department of General Medicine
King George's Medical University
Lucknow, Uttar Pradesh, India

Amit Srivastava MD FNB DM
Assistant Professor
Department of Critical Care Medicine
Sanjay Gandhi Postgraduate Institute of Medical Sciences
Lucknow, Uttar Pradesh, India

Amol Trimbakrao Kothekar
MD IDCCM
Professor (Intensive Care Medicine)
Department of Anesthesiology, Critical Care, and Pain
Advanced Centre for Treatment, Research and Education in Cancer
Tata Memorial Centre
Homi Bhabha National Institute
Navi Mumbai, Maharashtra, India

Anirban Som MD FRCA
Consultant in Anesthetics
Department of Anesthetics and Critical Care
Hull University Teaching Hospitals NHS Trust
Hull, England, UK

Anjali Mishra MD FNB
Consultant
Department of Critical Care Medicine
Holy Family Hospital
New Delhi, India

Ashish Khanna
MD MS FCCP FCCM FASA
Professor and Vice-Chair of Research
Department of Anesthesiology, Division of Critical Care Medicine
Wake Forest University School of Medicine, Atrium Health
Wake Forest Baptist Medical Center
Medical Center Boulevard
Winston-Salem, North Caolina, USA

Atul Prabhakar Kulkarni
MD (Anesthesiology)
Professor and Head
Division of Critical Care
Department of Anesthesiology, Critical Care, and Pain
Tata Memorial Hospital
Homi Bhabha National Institute
Mumbai, Maharashtra, India

Balkrishna Nimavat
MD DNB IDCCM FNB EDIC EDIAC
Consultant (Critical Care)
Department of Critical Acre
Heartland Hospital
Birmingham, UK

Bhuvana Krishna
MD (General Medicine) IDCCM IFCCM
Professor and Head
Department of Critical Care Medicine
St John's Medical College and Hospital
Bengaluru, Karnataka, India

Binila Chacko MD (Med) DNB FCICM (Australia) DM (Critical Care) FICCM
Professor and Head
Department of Critical Care
Christian Medical College
Vellore, Tamil Nadu, India

Dalim Kumar Baidya MD EDIC
Professor and Head
Department of Anesthesiology, Critical Care, and Pain Medicine
All India Institute of Medical Sciences
Guwahati, Assam, India

Deepak Govil MD EDIC FCCM
Vice Chairman
Department of Critical Care Medicine
Medanta—The Medicity
Gurugram, Haryana, India

Devansh Gupta MD
Senior Resident
Department of Critical Care Medicine
Sanjay Gandhi Postgraduate Institute of Medical Sciences
Lucknow, Uttar Pradesh, India

Deven Juneja DNB FNB EDIC
Director
Department of Institute of Critical Care Medicine
Max Super Specialty Hospital
New Delhi, India

Jacob George Pulinilkunnathil
MD DM DrNB MNAMS IDCCM IFCCM EDIC
Medical Superintendent and Senior Consultant and Head
Department of Critical Care
Caritas Hospital
Kottayam, Kerala, India

John Victor Peter MD DNB FRACP FJFICM FCICM FICCM FAMS FRCP (Edin) MPhil
Professor
Department of Critical Care Medicine
Christian Medical College
Vellore, Tamil Nadu, India

Kapil Gangadhar Zirpe
MD (Chest) FICCM FCCM FSNCC
Head
Department of Neuro-Intensive Care Unit
Grant Medical Foundation
Ruby Hall Clinic
Pune, Maharashtra, India

Keyur Shah DM (Critical Care Medicine)
Assistant Professor (Critical Care Medicine)
Department of Anesthesiology, Critical Care, and Pain
Tata Memorial Hospital
Homi Bhabha National Institute
Navi Mumbai, Maharashtra, India

Kushal Rajeev Kalvit
MD DM EDIC EDEC PGDMT
Senior Consultant
Department of Critical Care Medicine
Sir HN Reliance Foundation Hospital
Mumbai, Maharashtra, India

Malini Premkumar Joshi
MD (Anesthesia)
Professor
Department of Anesthesiology, Critical Care, and Pain
Advanced Centre for Treatment, Research and Education in Cancer
Tata Memorial Centre
Homi Bhabha National Institute
Navi Mumbai, Maharashtra, India

Nagalakshmi Swaminathan
MD PDCC (Critical Care) DNB
Assistant Professor
Department of Anesthesiology, Critical Care, and Pain
Advanced Centre for Treatment, Research and Education in Cancer
Tata Memorial Centre
Homi Bhabha National Institute
Navi Mumbai, Maharashtra, India

Nishanth Baliga
MD DM (Critical Care Medicine)
Assistant Professor
Department of Critical Care Medicine
Father Muller Medical College
Mangaluru, Karnataka, India

Palepu B Gopal MD FRCA FICCM FCCM
Senior Consultant and Head
Department of Critical Care Medicine
Citizens Specialty Hospital
Hyderabad, Telangana, India

Prabhat Kumar MD
Attending Consultant
Department of Pulmonology and Sleep Medicine
Fortis Memorial Research Institute
Gurugram, Haryana, India

Prashant Nasa MD FNB (Critical Care Medicine) EDIC MSc (Healthcare Management) CESR Fellow
Department of Integrated Critical Care Unit
New Cross Hospital, The Royal Wolverhampton NHS Trust
Wolverhampton, UK

Prashant Saxena
MD FRCP (Edin) EDIC FCCP FICM EDARM
Senior Director and Head
Department of Pulmonology, Critical Care and Sleep Medicine
Fortis Hospital
New Delhi, India

Prem Prakeerth P MD (Internal medicine) DNB (Internal medicine) DM (Critical Care) EDIC
Consultant and Head
Department of Critical Care Medicine
Lisie Medicity
Kochi, Kerala, India

Rahul Harne MBBS DA IDCCM
Associate Director
Department of Critical Care Medicine
Medanta—The Medicity
Gurugram, Haryana, India

Roshni Sharma
MD (Med) DrNB (Critical Care)
Assistant Professor
Department of Critical Care
Christian Medical College
Vellore, Tamil Nadu, India

Ruchi Gupta MD FNB (Critical Care Medicine)
Senior Consultant
Department of Critical Care Medicine
Holy family Hospital
New Delhi, India

Sahil Kataria
MD DrNB (Critical Care Medicine)
Consultant
Department of Critical Care Medicine
Holy Family Hospital
New Delhi, India

Santosh Kumar Paiualla
MD FNB (CCM)
Senior Consultant
Department of Critical Care Medicine
Citizens Specialty Hospital
Hyderabad, Telangana, India

Shaveta Devesar MSc (A) FICM
Advanced Critical Care Practitioner
Department of Integrated Critical Care Unit
New Cross Hospital
The Royal Wolverhampton NHS Trust
Wolverhampton, UK

Sheila Nainan Myatra
MD FCCM FICCM
Professor (Critical Care Medicine)
Department of Anesthesiology, Critical Care, and Pain
Tata Memorial Hospital
Mumbai, Maharashtra, India

Shilpushp Jagannath Bhosale
DM (Critical Care)
Professor and Head ICU
Department of Critical Care
Advanced Centre for Treatment, Research and Education in Cancer
Tata Memorial Centre
Homi Bhabha National Institute
Navi Mumbai, Maharashtra, India

Shobhit Jadhav MD (Anesthesiology)
DM 2nd year, Critical Care Medicine
Division of Critical Care
Department of Anesthesiology, Critical Care, and Pain
Advanced Centre for Treatment, Research and Education in Cancer
Tata Memorial Centre
Homi Bhabha National Institute
Navi Mumbai, Maharashtra, India

Srinivas Samavedam MD DNB FRCP FNBE EDIC FICCM DME MBA
Consultant and Head (Critical Care)
Sindhu Hospital
Hyderabad, Telangana, India

Sudivya Sharma MD (Anesthesiology) DNB EPIC PGDHHM
Professor (Critical Care Medicine)
Division of Critical Care
Department of Anesthesiology, Critical Care, and Pain
Advanced Centre for Treatment, Research and Education in Cancer
Tata Memorial Centre
Homi Bhabha National Institute
Navi Mumbai, Maharashtra, India

Suhail Sarwar Siddiqui MD DM (Critical Care Medicine) Fellowship in Critical Care EDIC
Additional Professor
Department of Critical Care Medicine
King George's Medical University
Lucknow, Uttar Pradesh, India

Sumit Ray MD
Senior Consultant and Chief
Department of Critical Care Medicine
Holy Family Hospital
New Delhi, India

Swagata Tripathy
MD DNB IDCC EDIC FSNCC (Hon) FICCM
Professor
Department of Anesthesia and Critical Care
All India Institute of Medical Sciences
Bhubaneswar, Odisha, India

Tejasree Rajoli MD DrNB
Consultant
Department of Critical Care Medicine
Sindhu Hospitals
Hyderabad, Telangana, India

Theresa Grace Daily MD DESAR
Consultant Intensivist
Department of Critical Care
King Hamad American Mission Hospital
Ali, Bahrain

Preface

परिवर्तनमेव स्थिरमस्ति ।।
(*Meaning:* Change is constant)

The frontiers of critical care medicine are expanding due to manifold changes simultaneously occurring in all directions, all fields 360°. A busy student and the busier practitioner are likely to find it difficult to track all these innovations and put them into practice. This, the second volume of *Recent Advances in Critical Care Medicine 2025,* is an attempt to help these colleagues to stay abreast of the way CCM is moving at a break-neck speed. Within 1 year, we have a new collection of topics; just confirming how fast the horizons of critical care medicine are exploding. The topics tackled in the current book range from the physiologically difficult airway, something which critical care physicians are getting familiar with and used to in daily practice, to the completely of the left field, and new monoclonal antibodies (mAbs) in bacterial infections in the critically ill, something yet to reach common practice. We hope that the myriad fields the topics in the book touch, some areas will become routine practice soon and we will say the future is now, while some may remain a dream for a few more years. A long list of experts has been involved in the writing of this book, and hopefully this book will open new vistas for the readers. Some of these may appear magic to our colleagues from past, but as Arthur C Clarke said, *"Any sufficiently advanced technology is indistinguishable from magic".* Lastly back to the old saying, all technology and therapies apart, the true worker of miracles (advanced science) is that *Man behind the Machine.*

We hope you enjoy reading it as much as we enjoyed the process of putting this together for you.

We are thankful to the Adiyogi Mahadev for his blessings and to our families for their support. We await as usual the honest opinion and constructive criticism from all our readers. Suggestions about topics for the next version of the book are most welcome.

Atul Prabhakar Kulkarni
Kushal Rajeev Kalvit

Acknowledgments

We wish to thank the experienced and senior practitioners of the art of critical care medicine for making a scholarly contribution to this book, to make it impactful. They have given valuable time, a very precious commodity, which does not come back and dealt very patiently with our impatient pestering worked within the limits of timeframe. We hope that we get critical, constructive, and positive feedback from discerning and learned practitioners and the new entrants in the specialty.

Many thanks to our families, who stood by us to support us in these time-consuming endeavors tolerate our mental and sometimes physical absence and eccentric behavior, which may have nothing to do with our work on the book, anyway.

We are especially thankful to Shri Jitendar P Vij (Group Chairman), Mr Ankit Vij (Managing Director), Ms Pooja Bhandari [Director-Production (Books and Journals)], Mr Sabyasachi Hazra (Director—PG and PNR Content), Ms Kajal Keshri (Development Editor), and the team of M/s Jaypee Brothers Medical Publishers (P) Ltd, New Delhi, India, for helping us in every way possible to bring out this book.

Last but not the least, our prayers and thanks to the *Adiyogi Mahadev* for blessing us in this task.

Atul Prabhakar Kulkarni
Kushal Rajeev Kalvit

Contents

CHAPTER

Green ICU: Hurdles for Developing Nations

John Victor Peter, Theresa Grace Daily, Swagata Tripathy

INTRODUCTION

Climate change is a major topic in today's world. According to a survey conducted by the United Nations Development Program in 2024, 56% of people worldwide think about it daily or weekly, and 80% want their country to increase their climate action.[1]

In addition to being a preoccupying topic for many, climate change has negative repercussions for global health, both directly and indirectly. This includes heat-related illnesses, an increased risk of drought (resulting in food and water insecurity, malnutrition, and famine) and a greater frequency of severe extreme weather events (tropical storms, floods, etc.). In addition, changes in weather patterns make larger areas suitable for certain pathogens (such as *Plasmodium falciparum* and *Vibrio cholerae*) to thrive. Climate changes can also cause increased migration and poverty, that contribute to the spread of infectious diseases (including drug-resistant organisms). These consequences, in turn, place additional strain on healthcare systems, requiring an increased use of finite resources.[2,3]

At the same time, healthcare itself has environmental impact, evaluated to be between 1 and 5% of the global impact depending on the indicator used, including 4.4% of the emission of greenhouse gases.[4] This paradox causes a vicious cycle, where climate change increases the demand for healthcare, and this increased demand leads to a larger carbon footprint, which makes climate change worse **(Fig. 1)**.

Within healthcare, intensive care units (ICUs) contribute significantly to the environmental footprint. A study done in 2018 showed that the daily carbon footprint of a patient treated for septic shock was 3.5 times the daily footprint of an average American, and 1.5 that of an average Australian.[5] The above observations have led to efforts to make ICUs more sustainable. The term "green ICU" is used to refer to this process.

More recently, "GREEN ICUs" have been defined as "GREater ENvironmental sustainability in intensive care units" by a multidisciplinary team working on providing an evidence-based guide on how to reduce the environmental footprint of the ICU.[6] However, to reduce this footprint, it is first necessary to understand the ways in which healthcare in general, and ICUs in particular, affect the environment.

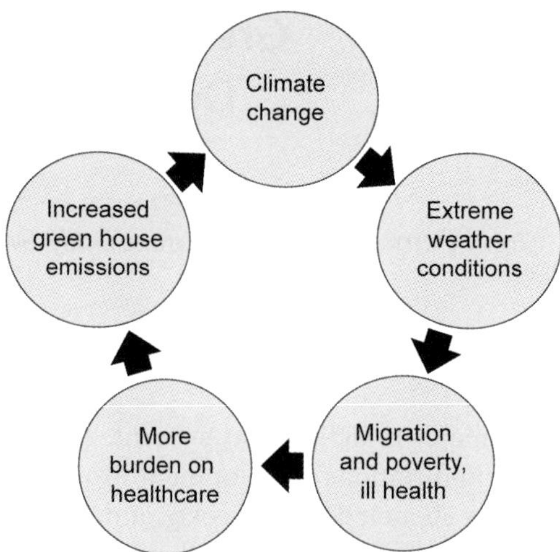

Fig. 1: The vicious cycle of climate change and healthcare.
Note: Climate change is characterized by extreme weather conditions. This results in migration and poverty with families moving to more habitable areas. The ill-health associated with climate change and poverty results in an added burden on healthcare. This, in turn, causes increased greenhouse emissions which perpetuates the vicious cycle of climate change and healthcare.

THE FOOTPRINTS

In addition to the resources (energy, water, and materials) needed to provide healthcare services, waste is produced at every step of the process. Plastic, soiled water, and biodegradable waste contribute to environmental impact. In order to evaluate this impact, different standpoints are used, known as footprints.

The *carbon footprint* refers to the total amount of greenhouse gases (such as carbon dioxide and methane) generated by the action, product or process being evaluated. These greenhouse gases trap heat in the atmosphere and directly contribute to global warming.[7] In the same way, the *water footprint* is the amount of water used to produce the goods and services required,[8] and the *plastic footprint* is the weight of plastic used or produced by the person, action or process in question over a defined time.[9]

Beyond these material requirements, since energy is also needed to perform a service, the *energy footprint* refers to the amount of energy required, including that which is necessary to produce the requisite equipment.[10] Finally, any production or service will lead to a *waste footprint,* which is the amount of waste produced over a given period of time.[11]

GREEN HEALTHCARE

Green healthcare refers to the attempt to make healthcare environmentally sustainable, to maximize outcomes for individual patients and for the population, while minimizing its environmental impact. The term "green ICU" is the application of the same principle specifically to the ICU.

Healthcare in general and ICUs in particular have specific constraints related to patient's outcomes that need to be taken into consideration. However, the basic concepts of "Reduce, Reuse, Recycle" still apply.[3,6]

Reduce

The first step in sustainability is to avoid unnecessary use of resources. In a healthcare setting, such an approach can range from turning off the lights in an unused room to an ethical discussion about the futility on certain interventions in an end-of-life setting. It is important to note that reducing resource consumption does not mean compromising care. Instead, as the increasingly popular concept of "less is more" suggests, in certain situations, the same (or better) results can be achieved with fewer interventions, meaning the patient is less exposed to intervention-related risks.[12,13] Some examples include restrictive blood transfusion strategies in critically ill patients, which has been shown to be associated with reduced morbidity and mortality,[13] or delayed initiation of parenteral feeding in patients who are not meeting their caloric targets enterally, which was associated with a shorter length of stay and fewer ICU infections.[13]

Reuse

The second principle is what must be used should be reused. Of course, hygiene constraints can limit the applicability of this idea in healthcare, but there are numerous examples where reusing is feasible without risk (such as nondisposable tableware) or with minimal precautions (tourniquets and BP cuffs). In addition, cleaning and sterilization procedures make it possible to reuse many tools, though of course the energy, water, and chemical use that is required to facilitate reuse can limit the benefits of choosing reusable equipment. Finally, repairing rather than repurchasing equipment is usually better for the environment, and can save money as well.[14]

Recycle

When reusing is no longer possible, resources should be transformed rather than discarded. Another way of looking at this idea is the "cradle-to-cradle" approach, rather than the "cradle-to-grave" one. Products should be designed with a view to their whole lifecycle, not just one part of it, so that their components can be creatively transformed to support other processes and products, just as in nature dead biological matter is biodegraded to provide nourishment for new growth.[15,16]

WHAT DOES A GREEN ICU LOOK LIKE?

While the three principles of "reduce, reuse, and recycle" may seem basic, their impact can be far-reaching and extensive. Some of the steps that can be undertaken to promote a green ICU are given below.

Prevention

The very first step in environmental sustainability in healthcare is to promote healthy lifestyle choices, such as exercise, diet, and limiting exposure to harmful chemicals, to prevent disease and mitigate its severity, so as to limit the demand for more intensive care.[17] Such an approach requires that both patients and practitioners are actively involved and that they approach health from a preventative perspective, rather than a curative one.

Architecture

Location, orientation, layout, and type of materials impact the carbon footprint of any structure. For example, orientation relative to the sun impacts heating and cooling requirements, as will layout (open vs. closed floor plan, high vs. low ceiling, wall thickness, and number of windows and doors). Using local materials as opposed to ones from other locations will also have a bearing on the building's carbon footprint initially (type and length of transport to the construction site). The type of material used will influence energy requirements for heating and cooling as well as repair options and structural durability. In addition, as extreme weather events become more frequent, building norms will evolve, placing new constraints on the construction of hospital buildings.[14]

The most sustainable architectural choices will vary from place to place (type of climate, available materials, etc.) and will be influenced by cultural preferences and taboos, budget concerns, practicality, and availability. It is important to note that decisions made in the initial stages of a new hospital or unit will affect its environmental impact for decades to come.

Energy and Power Sources

Electricity is required for many aspects of patient's care in ICUs, including monitors, infusion pumps, ventilators, and dialysis machines. It is also needed for other functions, such as lighting, computer systems, and temperature control. Many of these systems are required 24/7 and are, therefore, constantly using energy. Even when they are not actively in use, they are often in standby mode, where they continue to consume electricity. One study in Germany showed that they could save 2,707 kW/year, or 1.2 tons of CO_2-equivalent per year, just by switching off devices rather than leaving them in standby mode.[18] The energy saving is more than the yearly consumption of a single-person household (1,943 kW/year in 2018).[19] Switching off lights and shutting down computers (and other machines) when not in use is a simple way to reduce energy consumption.

The ambient temperatures recommended for hospitals in high-income countries (HICs) is 20–23°C. The National Building Code of Government of India suggests temperatures up to 26°C in wards and 24°C in critical areas

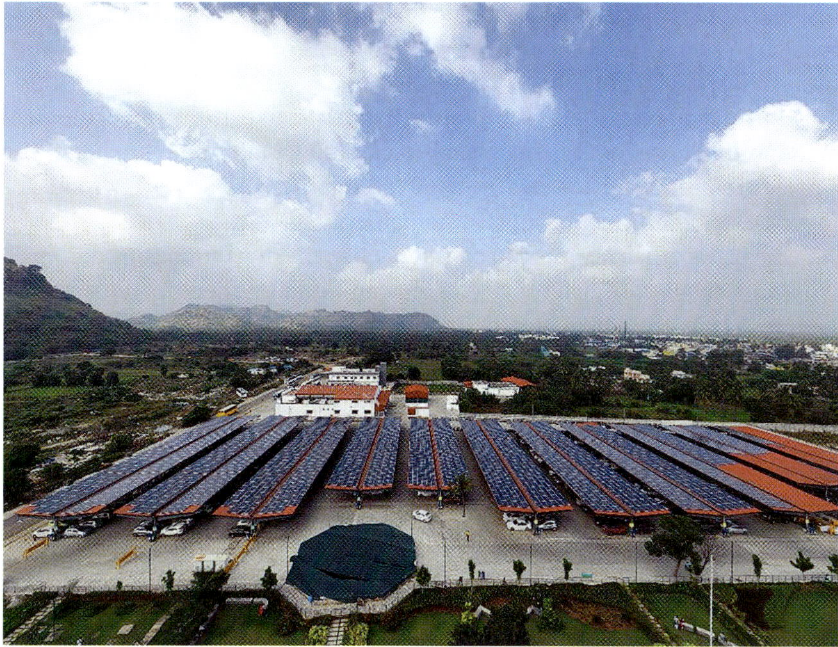

Fig. 2: Parking lot with solar panels.
Note: Solar paneling of the car parking area of a newly constructed hospital that generates around 1,000 kW of power during peak hours.

and operation theaters. Even a 1°C increase in the set ambient temperature lowers energy expenditure by 6%.[20] Many low- and middle-income countries' (LMIC) hospitals utilize naturally ventilated and lit open-room ICUs, reducing dependency on artificial lighting and cooling systems. Research suggests that this model may also lower hospital-acquired infection risks.[21]

Another way for ICUs to be more sustainable is to use renewable energy sources such as solar panels **(Fig. 2)** to complement and replace nonrenewable energy sources. Such initiatives also reduce costs in the mid- to long-term, despite the initial investment. Beyond local initiatives, infrastructure choices made by public authorities will influence the production of greenhouse gases and emissions by ICU energy consumption. Within the EU, in 2023, the amount of energy produced by fossil fuels varied from 1.3% in Sweden to 87.0% in Malta,[22] meaning that the same amount of electricity consumption in different countries does not have the same ecological impact. This observation underscores the importance of decisions made on a higher scale than just the ICU or even the institution.

Equipment

Medical equipment has an ecological impact through its production, delivery, use (particularly for electrical devices or those requiring sterilization), disposal, and replacement. Reducing this impact requires the cooperation of those intervening at every stage of its lifecycle, from manufacturers to end-users to disposal teams.[15]

Multiuse devices are preferable to single-use from an ecological standpoint. However, it is necessary to carefully analyze the impact of the procedures required for safe re-use (the energy cost of sterilization, for instance) to determine the most sustainable choice.[23]

One of the other key areas to consider when making purchasing decisions is the repairability of a given device, as this can reduce the need for replacement and, thus, the ecological impact. In the same way, how recyclable a device will be when it must be disposed of should also be taken into account.[15]

Drugs

Environmental aspects often take a backseat to efficacy and tolerance when it comes to medication choices. However, there are ways to improve their ecological effect without compromising patient care. For example, Choosing Wisely Canada, an initiative supported by the Canadian Medical Association, recommends switching to enteral alternatives when they are equally safe and effective. Examples in the ICU could include paracetamol, certain antibiotics like linezolid, and proton-pump inhibitors (PPIs).[24]

In HICs, policies dictate the use of single-dose vials, dispensing full blister packs, having sufficient drug quantities in stock, and discarding expired drugs. These practices, while enhancing patient's safety, result in increased cost and wastage. Studies have shown that many drugs retain their potency well beyond the expiry date with some drugs retaining 90% of their potency for at least 5 years after the labeled expiry date.[25] The move by the Food and Drug Administration (FDA) to launch several programs for shelf-life extension to defer replacement costs and to prevent drug shortages due to supply disruption is a step toward minimizing drug wastage.[26] LMICs have long been using strategies for optimizing drug use, sharing surplus medications and repurposing drugs when safe and effective.[27] However, concerns regarding expired and counterfeit drugs, which are quite prevalent in some LMICs, are valid.

Medical Gases

Anesthesia gases such as desflurane and sevoflurane are known to have a direct greenhouse gas effect.[28] However, even "basic" medical gases, such as oxygen, have an environmental footprint linked to their production. It is estimated that the 100-year global warming potential (GWP_{100}) value associated with the production of 1 kg of medical oxygen (approximately 700 L) is between 0.62 and 1.17 kg CO_2 equivalent.[29] As such, titrating oxygen levels to patients' actual needs is not only the best practice,[30] but also ecologically beneficial.

Laboratories and Imaging

In the ICU, some tests are routinely done at regular intervals with little justification, to the point that the Critical Care Societies Collaborative (the four major critical care societies in the United States) made avoiding ordering diagnostic tests at regular intervals their first recommendation in their Choosing Wisely campaign. Instead, they recommend that tests should be ordered based on a specific clinical question.[31]

That being said, defensive medicine research has shown that suboptimal choices are made for a variety of reasons, including perceived pressure from patients, healthcare system working conditions, fear of litigation and physician's tolerance of uncertainty.[32,33] As such, while the first step in this process is to make healthcare providers aware of the lack of benefit of certain tests, reducing unnecessary testing will likely require addressing underlying root causes as well.

Dialysis

Dialysis is a resource-intensive therapy, with specific challenges, one of which is reverse osmosis (RO) water. This water is usually prepared from municipal water, which is additionally purified before use in dialysis machines. The remaining water, about 350–400 L per hemodialysis session[34] is often discarded. This can be repurposed for various uses such as cleaning, laundry, agriculture, and steam production for sterilization.[35,36]

It is also possible to decrease water consumption by choosing a lower dialysis flow rate, without any repercussions for the patient.[35] Another area to consider is the type of dialysis fluid used: Solid, semi-solid, and liquid forms exist. Solid forms are reconstituted on location, which decreases the amount of weight that needs to be transported and, therefore, reduces the carbon footprint. It also makes storage easier, though it does require staff training and some dedicated time for preparation.[37]

Plastic Use and Waste Management

Plastic usage in hospitals is a major contributor to its ecological footprint. For example, each session of dialysis produces 1.5–8 kg of plastic waste, of which a significant amount is recyclable, though it is often mixed with nonrecyclables.[15] By segregating plastics on-site, recycling options can be increased. In addition, while some plastic is contaminated and requires specific management, a significant portion is not and can be recycled without further treatment. LMICs have practiced innovative ways to do this,[38] including making cement,[39] or constructing roads.[40] Additionally, some work has been done on recycling contaminated plastic (via steam sterilization, shredding, and integrating into concrete),[9] so this type of approach may also be further developed in the years to come.

Finally, one way in which plastic use can be reduced, for example, in dialysis, is through the re-use of patient circuits, with appropriate identification and sterilization procedures. Many countries, particularly HICs, have abandoned this practice for fear of the risks associated (improper labeling, contamination, and allergic reaction through improper rinsing), but it is widespread in others, and significantly reduces plastic waste, and especially contaminated plastic waste, which is beneficial from an ecological perspective. As such, it may become more globally acceptable in the future.[34]

Water

The same principles that apply in the home also apply at the hospital and in the ICU (using only what is needed, ensuring the tap is turned off when not in use, installing dual flush toilets, promptly identifying and repairing leaks, etc.). In addition, it is also possible to decrease water usage by repurposing rainwater and sewage water (after appropriate treatment) for gardening, lavatories and laundry. A significant amount of wastewater in hospitals can be recycled for the above purposes.[41,42] Such an approach is ecologically sustainable and can also allow institutions to save money once the infrastructure is in place **(Fig. 3)**.

Waste Management

As previously mentioned, the first step in sustainable waste management is to reduce waste production. For instance, only using personal protective equipment (such as gowns and single-use gloves), when required, could significantly reduce the ICU's waste footprint: In one study, disposable gloves were the most used items (108 per patient/day) in the ICU, and had

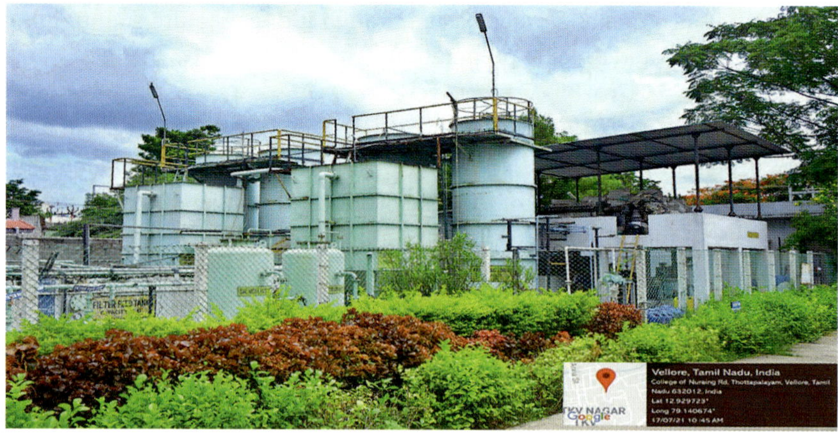

Fig. 3: Sewage treatment plant.

Note: Sewage treatment plant enables a significant proportion of the wastewater to be treated and used for various purposes such as gardening, laundry, etc.

the highest carbon footprint.[43] The remaining waste should be recycled and repurposed as much as possible. For instance, food waste can be transformed into biomass for energy production.[44]

One of the challenges in hospital waste management is the specific treatment required for contaminated waste, which is often managed through incineration, but requires greater temperatures and, therefore, consumes more energy. As such, appropriate point-of-care segregation is crucial in reducing the burden of contaminated waste, which requires staff education and information.[16]

Finally, it is important to note that discarded waste can contaminate the air, water, and soil, whether through landfills, incineration or even sewage, with potential negative consequences for the health of those exposed. While waste disposal according to established guidelines cannot completely remove this risk, it does minimize it, which underlines the importance of adhering to the appropriate protocols.[15,45]

Travel

Critical patients may need to be transported to institutions with higher levels of care. In some situations, telemedicine can reduce the number of transfers required, thus removing the carbon footprint of the patient's travel, as well as allowing them to be evaluated in a timelier fashion. Studies on this topic have not evaluated the carbon footprint of the equipment needed to make telemedicine possible.[14] However, it does seem to hold promise, both for quality of care and sustainability.

In addition, the way patients, bystanders, and staff travel to the hospital can significantly contribute to the overall carbon footprint of an ICU. If public transportation is available, or if there are walking or cycling options, encouraging people to utilize these methods when it is safe for them to do so can help to reduce this footprint.[3]

WHAT ARE THE HURDLES TO IMPLEMENTING A GREEN STRATEGY?

As seen above, sustainable choices can be made at various levels. However, there are various challenges to implementing a green strategy, some of which are particularly relevant in LMICs.

High Upfront Cost versus Budget Constraints

Low- and middle-income countries' health systems often operate with limited capital budgets, prioritizing essential equipment and staffing over sustainability upgrades.[46] Retrofitting ICUs with energy-efficient heating, ventilation, and air-conditioning (HVAC) systems or renewable energy sources (like solar) may be technically feasible but unaffordable without external grants. However, once present, these systems can reduce energy costs as well as energy and carbon footprints.

Budget constraints are a major hurdle, but they can also be a strong incentive. LMICs have already incorporated many sustainable practices into their way of functioning for decades, out of frugality and necessity.[47]

Infrastructure and Technology Gaps

Many LMIC ICUs face unreliable electricity supply, inadequate waste segregation facilities, and limited access to suppliers of sustainable materials.[46] Without stable power or proper biomedical waste systems, integrating green tech (e.g., automated energy management and closed-loop anesthesia systems) becomes difficult.

Lack of Policy Incentives and Awareness

As seen above, many simple and every-day improvements can be made at a grass-roots level and increase sustainability. For instance, merely conveniently positioning containers for recyclables have been shown to increase their appropriate use.[48]

However, doing so requires staff, patients and bystanders to become actively engaged in such a strategy. Some may be reluctant to change their daily habits, particularly if they feel it requires extra effort and time, especially if there is no policy incentive.[3] Currently, few national healthcare guidelines in LMICs mandate environmental performance standards for ICUs, which does not encourage institutions to prioritize sustainable initiatives.[46] In addition, clinicians and administrators may be aware of sustainability in principle but lack specific training or benchmarks for ICU greening.[46]

Competing Public Health Priorities

ICU greening competes for attention with urgent challenges such as infectious disease control, maternal health, and malnutrition, which makes sustainability goals vulnerable to de-prioritization during crises.[16,49]

CONCLUSION

By being mindful of the impact of ICU care, and implementing strategies to reduce its environmental footprint, we position ourselves to continue to provide high-quality care to those who need it for generations to come. Doing so will clearly be a step-by-step process, building on what is already in place at each level. The longest journey begins with the first step, so it is important not to overlook the benefits of starting small, but rather to make strategical changes that will be sustainable over time, and that can be expanded as awareness and engagement increase.

REFERENCES

1. United Nations Development Program. (2025). Peoples' Climate Vote. Retrieved July 19, 2025. [online] Available from https://peoplesclimate.vote/. [Last accessed Jan., 2025].
2. Romanello M, McGushin A, Di Napoli C, Drummond P, Hughes N, Jamart L, et al. The 2021 report of the Lancet Countdown on health and climate change: code red for a healthy future. Lancet (London, England). 2021;398(10311): 1619-62.
3. De Waele JJ, Hunfeld N, Baid H, Ferrer R, Iliopoulou K, Ioan AM, et al. Environmental sustainability in intensive care: the path forward. An ESICM Green Paper. Intensive Care Med. 2025;50(11):1729-39.
4. Lenzen M, Malik A, Li M, Fry J, Weisz H, Pichler PP, et al. The environmental footprint of health care: a global assessment. Lancet. Planetary Health. 2020;4(7):e271-9.
5. McGain F, Burnham JP, Lau R, Aye L, Kollef MH, McAlister S. The carbon footprint of treating patients with septic shock in the intensive care unit. Crit Care Resuscitat: J Austral Acad Crit Care Med. 2018;20(4):304-12.
6. Gabiña IS, José Pita López M. GREEN ICU: responsible and sustainable ICU. Med Intensiva (Engl Ed). 2024;48(4):231-4.
7. Selin NE. Carbon footprint. Encyclopedia Britannica. 2025.
8. Hoekstra AY, Chapagain AK. The water footprints of Morocco and the Netherlands: Global water use as a result of domestic consumption of agricultural commodities. Ecolog Econom. 2007;64:143-51.
9. Cambridge Dictionary. (2025). Plastic footprint. In Cambridge Dictionary. [online] Available from https://dictionary.cambridge.org/dictionary/english/plastic-footprint [Last accessed Jan., 2026].
10. Eurostat. (2025). Glossary: Energy footprint. European Union, Eurostat. [online] Available from https://ec.europa.eu/eurostat/statistics-explained/index.php?title=Glossary:Energy-footprint [Last accessed Jan., 2026].
11. Towa E, Zeller V, Merciai S, Achten WMJ. Regional waste footprint and waste treatments analysis. Waste management (New York, N.Y.). 2021;124:172-84.
12. Kox M, Pickkers P. "Less is more" in critically ill patients: not too intensive. JAMA Internal Med. 2013;173(14):1369-72.
13. Auriemma CL, Van den Berghe G, Halpern SD. Less is more in critical care is supported by evidence-based medicine. Intensive Care Med. 2019;45(12): 1806-9.
14. Masud FN, Sasangohar F, Ratnani I, Fatima S, Hernandez MA, Riley T, et al. Past, present, and future of sustainable intensive care: narrative review and a large hospital system experience. Crit Care (London, England). 2024;28(1):154.
15. Piccoli GB, Cupisti A, Aucella F, Regolisti G, Lomonte C, Ferraresi M, et al.; and On the Behalf of Conservative treatment, Physical activity and Peritoneal dialysis project groups of the Italian Society of Nephrology. Green nephrology and eco-dialysis: a position statement by the Italian Society of Nephrology. J Nephrol. 2020;33(4):681-98.
16. Smale E, Baid H, Balan M, McGain F, McAlistar S, de Waele JJ, et al. The green ICU: how to interpret green? A multiple perspective approach. Crit Care (London, England). 2025;29(1):80.

17. Barraclough KA, Agar JWM. Green nephrology. Nat Rev Nephrol. 2020;16(5):257-68.
18. Drinhaus H, Schumacher C, Drinhaus J, Wetsch WA. W(h)at(t) counts in electricity consumption in the intensive care unit. Intensive Care Med. 2023;49(4):437-9.
19. Statistisches Bundesamt. (2020, Sept 9). Energy consumption. Statistisches Bundesamt, Destatis. [online] Available from https://www.destatis.de/EN/Society-Environment/Environment/Material-Energy-Flows/Tables/elextricity-consumption.households.html [Last accessed Jan., 2026].
20. Bureau of Energy Efficiency. (2025). BEE: Raising AC setting by 1° can save 6% power. Bureau of Energy Efficiency, Urja Dakshata Information Tool. Retrieved on Aug 7th, 2025. [online] Available from https://udit.beeindia.gov.in/bee-raising-ac-setting-by-1-can-save-6-power/ [Last accessed Jan., 2026].
21. Atkinson J, Chartier Y, Pessoa-Silva CL, Jensen P, Li Y, Seto WH. Natural ventilation for infection control in health-care settings. World Health Organization. 2009.
22. Council of the European Union. (2025). How is EU electricity produced and sold? European Council. [online] Available from https://www.consilium.europa.eu/en/infographics/how-is-eu-electricity-produced-and-sold/ [Last accessed Jan., 2026].
23. McGain F, McAlister S. Reusable versus single-use ICU equipment: what's the environmental footprint? Intensive Care Med. 2023;49(12)1523-5.
24. Canadian Critical Care Society, Canadian Association of Critical are Nurses, Canadian Society of Respiratory Therapists. (2024). Twelve Tests and Treatments to Question. Choosing Wisely Canada. [online] Available from https://choosingwiselycanada.org/recommendation/critical-care/ [Last accessed Jan., 2026].
25. Gikonyo D, Gikonyo A, Luvayo D, Ponoth P. Drug expiry debate: the myth and the reality. African Health Sci. 2019;19(3):2737-9.
26. Zilker M, Sörgel F, Holzgrabe U. A systematic review of the stability of finished pharmaceutical products and drug substances beyond their labeled expiry dates. J Pharmaceut Biomed Anal. 2019;166:222-35.
27. Kamba PF, Nambatya W, Aguma HB, Charani E, Rajab K. Gaps and opportunities in sustainable medicines use in resource limited settings: a situational analysis of Uganda. Br J Clin Pharmacol. 2022;88(9):3936-42.
28. Wang J, DasSarma S. Contributions of Medical Greenhouse Gases to Climate Change and Their Possible Alternatives. Int J Environ Res Public Health. 2024;21(12):1548.https://doi.org/10.3390/ijerph21121548
29. Seglenieks R, McAlister S, McGain F. Environmental impact of medical oxygen production in Australia. Comment on Br J Anaesth. 2020;125:773-8. Br J Anaesth. 2020;127(3):e104-5.
30. Semler MW, Casey JD, Lloyd BD, Hastings PG, Hays MA, Stollings JL, et al.; PILOT Investigators and the Pragmatic Critical Care Research Group. Oxygen-saturation targets for critically ill adults receiving mechanical ventilation. N Engl J Med. 2022;387(19):1759-69.
31. Kleinpell RM, Farmer JC, Pastores SM. Reducing unnecessary testing in the intensive care unit by choosing wisely. Acute Crit Care. 2018;33(1):1-6.
32. Baungaard N, Skovvang PL, Assing Hvidt E, Gerbild H, Kirstine Andersen M, Lykkegaard J. How defensive medicine is defined in European medical literature: a systematic review. BMJ Open. 2022;12(1):e057169.

33. Strobel CJ, Oldenburg D, Steinhäuser J. Factors influencing defensive medicine-based decision-making in primary care: a scoping review. J Evaluat Clin Pract. 2023;29(3):529-38.
34. Rathore SS, Nirja K, Choudhary S, Jeswani G. Green dialysis from the indian perspective: a systematic review. Cureus. 2024;16(6):e62876.
35. Vanholder R, Agar J, Braks M, Gallego D, Gerritsen KGF, Harber M, et al. The European Green Deal and nephrology: a call for action by the European Kidney Health Alliance. Nephrol Dialysis Transplantation: Eur Dialysis Transplant Assoc Eur Renal Assoc. 2023;38(5):1080-8.
36. Chang E, Lim JA, Low CL, Kassim A. Reuse of dialysis reverse osmosis reject water for aquaponics and horticulture. J Nephrol. 2021;34(1):97-104.
37. Zawierucha J, Marcinkowski W, Prystacki T, Malyszko JS, Pyrza M, Zebrowski P, et al. Green dialysis: let us talk about dialysis fluid. Kidney Blood Press Res. 2023;48(1):385-91.
38. Ravichandran P. A model for plastic neutrality in dialysis: converting surrogate plastic waste to sinkable pebbles. Med Res Arch. 2023;11(9).
39. Plastics Technology. (2019). Costa Rican Startup Makes Cement Blocks with Recycled Ocean-Bound Plastic. Plastics Technology. [online] Available from https://www.ptonline.com/blog/post/costa-rican-startup-makes-cement-blocks-with-recycled-ocean-bound-plastic [Last accessed Jan., 2026].
40. Sisodia K. (2023). Innovative Solutions: Plastic for Road Construction in India. See positive. [online] available from https://seepositive.in/environment-and-%20sustainability/plastic-for-road-construction-in-india/#google_vignette [Last accessed Jan., 2026].
41. Haddad S, Kittner N, Flythe JE. Thinking globally, acting locally: water use in a hospital hemodialysis unit. Kidney. 2024;360;5(11):1747-9.
42. Tarrass F, Benjelloun M, Benjelloun O. Recycling wastewater after hemodialysis: an environmental analysis for alternative water sources in arid regions. Am J Kidney Dis Official J Nat Kid Foundation. 2008;52(1):154-8.
43. Hunfeld N, Diehl JC, Timmermann M, van Exter P, Bouwens J, Browne-Wilkinson S, et al. Circular material flow in the intensive care unit-environmental effects and identification of hotspots. Intensive Care Med. 2023;49(1):65-74.
44. Dhakal N, Kumar A, Nakari M. Waste to energy: management of biodegradable healthcare waste through anaerobic digestion. Nepal J Sci Technol. 2015;16(1):41-8.
45. Gabiña IS, Martinez SP, Vidal FG. Green ICU-4Ps: it is not an option to not accomplish it. ICU Manage Pract. 2023;23(3):114-20.
46. Rasheed FN, Baddley J, Prabhakaran P, De Barros EF, Reddy KS, Vianna NA, et al. Decarbonising healthcare in low and middle income countries: potential pathways to net zero emissions. BMJ (Clin Res ed.). 2021;375:n1284.
47. Tripathy S, Nasa P, Ramakrishnan N, Schultz MJ, Peter JV. Green intensive care: reimplementing what LMICs have long practised. Lancet Global Health. 2025;13(7):e1166-167.
48. Pruijm M, Rho E, Woywodt A, Segerer S. Ten tips from the Swiss Working Group on Sustainable Nephrology on how to go green in your dialysis unit. Clin Kidney J. 2024;17(6):sfae144.
49. Yau A, Agar JWM, Barraclough KA. Addressing the environmental impact of kidney care. Am J Kidney Dis: Official J Nat Kidney Found. 2021;77(3):406-9.

CHAPTER 2

Ultrasound for the Nutritional Assessment of Critically Ill Patients

Amol Trimbakrao Kothekar, Nagalakshmi Swaminathan

INTRODUCTION

Nutritional status at the time of admission to the intensive care unit (ICU) and throughout its course is a key factor in determining outcomes in critically ill patients. The prevalence of malnutrition among ICU patients has been variably reported to be as high as 40–50% and is known to be associated with poor outcomes.[1] While some patients present to the ICU with malnutrition, others develop significant loss of lean body mass (LBM) during the acute phase of critical illness.

The initial phase of critical illness is categorized as the catabolic phase, due to a surge in adrenergic hormones and an increase in circulating proinflammatory markers. Loss of muscle mass, also referred to as sarcopenia, has been reported in mechanically ventilated patients[2] and is independently associated with increased mortality.

Nutritional screening involves the "identification of patients who are already malnourished or at risk for malnutrition to determine if a detailed nutritional assessment is indicated" as defined by the American Society for Parenteral and Enteral Nutrition (ASPEN).[3] This process should aim to identify the subset of patients who will benefit most from nutritional interventions. The NRS-2002 (Nutrition Risk Screening 2002) or mNUTRIC (modified Nutrition Risk in the Critically Ill) score may be used for this purpose. The modified NUTRIC score is particularly suited and validated for critically ill patients to assess nutritional risk. It integrates key clinical parameters such as age, APACHE II (Acute Physiology, Age and Chronic Health Evaluation II) score, SOFA (Sequential Organ Failure Assessment) score, number of comorbidities, and days from hospital to ICU admission to stratify patients based on their likelihood of adverse outcomes. A higher mNUTRIC score (≥5) correlates with increased mortality and morbidity, emphasizing the importance of early and targeted nutritional intervention to improve outcomes in the ICU setting.[4,5]

Nutritional assessment is a structured and formal evaluation of nutritional status, typically conducted by a dietitian or other trained healthcare professional. For this, the Subjective Global Assessment (SGA) tool or the Academy of Nutrition and Dietetics (AND)–ASPEN criteria may be used.

The AND-ASPEN criteria require two or more of the following: Insufficient energy intake, weight loss, loss of muscle mass, loss of subcutaneous fat, fluid accumulation, or diminished functional status (evidenced by handgrip strength). The SGA also incorporates recent food intake and gastrointestinal symptoms.[4]

LIMITATIONS OF TRADITIONAL NUTRITION ASSESSMENT TOOLS

Skeletal muscle mass, or LBM, is an important indicator of body protein stores, and its loss during critical illness is significantly associated with increased morbidity, manifested as higher infection rates, prolonged ICU stays, and increased mortality.[2,6] Traditional nutritional screening and assessment tools rely on anthropometric measures such as body weight, body mass index (BMI), mid-arm circumference, and tests like handgrip strength as surrogates for muscle mass (LBM) and indirect markers of nutritional status. However, these tools do not reliably estimate LBM due to the following pitfalls.

Weight does not always correlate well with LBM and may be elevated due to factors such as fluid retention in critically ill patients. Patients with sarcopenic obesity (the coexistence of sarcopenia and obesity) may have high body weight due to excess fat, despite minimal muscle mass. Therefore, weight alone may not accurately reflect a patient's nutritional status, protein reserves, or nutritional requirements.

Body mass index presents similar limitations, as it cannot distinguish between LBM and adipose tissue. Other parameters, such as mid-arm circumference and calf muscle circumference, may also fail to reliably detect malnutrition in all patients.[7] Additionally, measurement of volitional parameters like handgrip strength may not be feasible in all ICU patients.

Hence, there is a pressing need for tools that can reliably assess LBM, as anthropometric and other traditional parameters may not consistently detect the presence or progression of malnutrition and sarcopenia in critically ill individuals.[1]

EMERGING ROLE OF ULTRASONOGRAPHY IN NUTRITIONAL ASSESSMENT

Ultrasound is rapidly emerging as a promising tool for noninvasive, serial, bedside, and objective nutritional assessment in critically ill patients. In addition to its portability and ease of use, ultrasound possesses the advantages of avoiding exposure to ionizing radiation and is applicable across a wide range of patient populations.

Fundamentals of Ultrasound for Nutritional Assessment as Part of Body Composition Assessment

Principles of operation: Ultrasonography utilizes high-frequency sound waves to produce real-time images of tissues and internal structures. These sound waves are emitted by piezoelectric crystals located within the transducer. As the waves encounter interfaces between tissues, some reflect back to the transducer. The ultrasound machine then generates a real-time image by measuring the amplitude of the reflected waves and the time taken for them to return.[8]

Ultrasonography can be used to assess both muscle mass and muscle quality. Skeletal muscle ultrasound has been studied extensively in critically ill patients across numerous prospective studies.[9,10] While various muscles—including those of the lower and upper limbs (e.g., biceps brachii, flexor carpi radialis), diaphragm, and rectus abdominis—have been evaluated using sonography, the lower-limb muscles are most frequently studied in this population. These muscles are easily accessible and tend to undergo atrophy earlier than upper-limb muscles.[11-13]

The quadriceps femoris group of the anterior thigh, particularly the rectus femoris (RF) and vastus intermedius (VI), is preferred for assessment due to their well-delineated fascial layers and ease of access in critically ill patients. **Figure 1** illustrates the sonoanatomy of this muscle group.

Skeletal muscle ultrasonography in the critically ill has been used to assess five parameters: (1) *muscle thickness (MT),* (2) *cross-sectional area (CSA),* (3) *echogenicity,* (4) *pennation angle (PA), and* (5) *fascicle length (FL).*

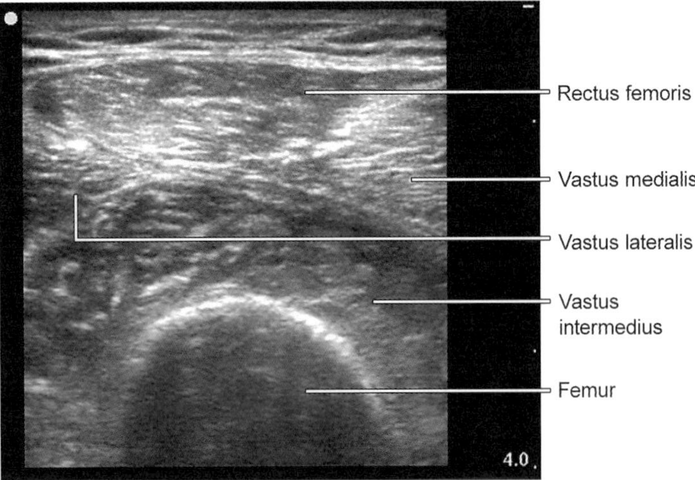

Fig. 1: Sonoanatomy of the quadriceps femoris muscle group in short axis (cross-sectional image), captured at the junction of the upper two-thirds and lower one-third of a line *joining the anterior superior iliac spine (ASIS) and the superior patellar border (SPB).*

MT and CSA are quantitative measurements of muscle mass (quantity), whereas echogenicity, PA, and FL are tools to assess muscle quality.[10]

Parameters pertaining to muscle quantity:

- Quadriceps muscle layer thickness (QMLT)
- Rectus femoris muscle thickness (RFMT)
- Rectus femoris muscle cross-sectional area (RF CSA).

Methodological considerations: Although these parameters have been widely studied, systematic reviews and meta-analyses have revealed significant heterogeneity across trials. Variations exist in the anatomical landmarks used for measurement, patient positioning, and the degree of probe compression (maximal vs. minimal).[13-15] This lack of standardization complicates comparisons and limits the generalizability of findings.

Currently, there is no universally accepted cutoff or reference range to define normal muscle mass, reduced muscle mass, or "muscle wasting" in critically ill patients. This is largely due to the heterogeneous nature of ICU populations and the diversity of clinical pathologies represented in various studies.

The ultrasound protocol for measuring these parameters is generally based on the most commonly adopted methods, as reported in meta-analyses by Venco et al. and Weinel et al.[14,15] For all three parameters, patient positioning and probe type are consistent. Measurements are ideally taken as the average of three readings to enhance reliability and reduce variability.

The patient is positioned supine, with the leg in passive extension and neutral rotation, and toes pointing upward. A linear probe is placed in a transverse orientation, perpendicular to the skin surface. Although a linear probe is suitable for CSA assessment in pediatric patients, a curvilinear probe may be considered in adults and larger children when the muscle of interest cannot be captured in its entirety using a linear probe **(Figs. 2A and B)**.

The anatomical landmarks and degree of probe compression are described separately for each parameter to ensure consistency and accuracy in measurement.

Quadriceps muscle layer thickness: The quadriceps muscle group is readily accessible and reliably visualized using ultrasound, owing to distinct fascial layers delineating its anatomy. QMLT is defined as the combined thickness of the *RF* and *VI* muscles. It is measured as the vertical distance between the deep fascial layer enveloping the RF and the upper margin of the femoral bone, upon which the VI rests.

For probe placement, a high-frequency linear transducer is positioned at the midpoint of a line connecting the anterior superior iliac spine (ASIS) and the superior border of the patella (SPB). Alternatively, some protocols use the junction of the upper two-thirds and lower one-third of this line as the measurement site.

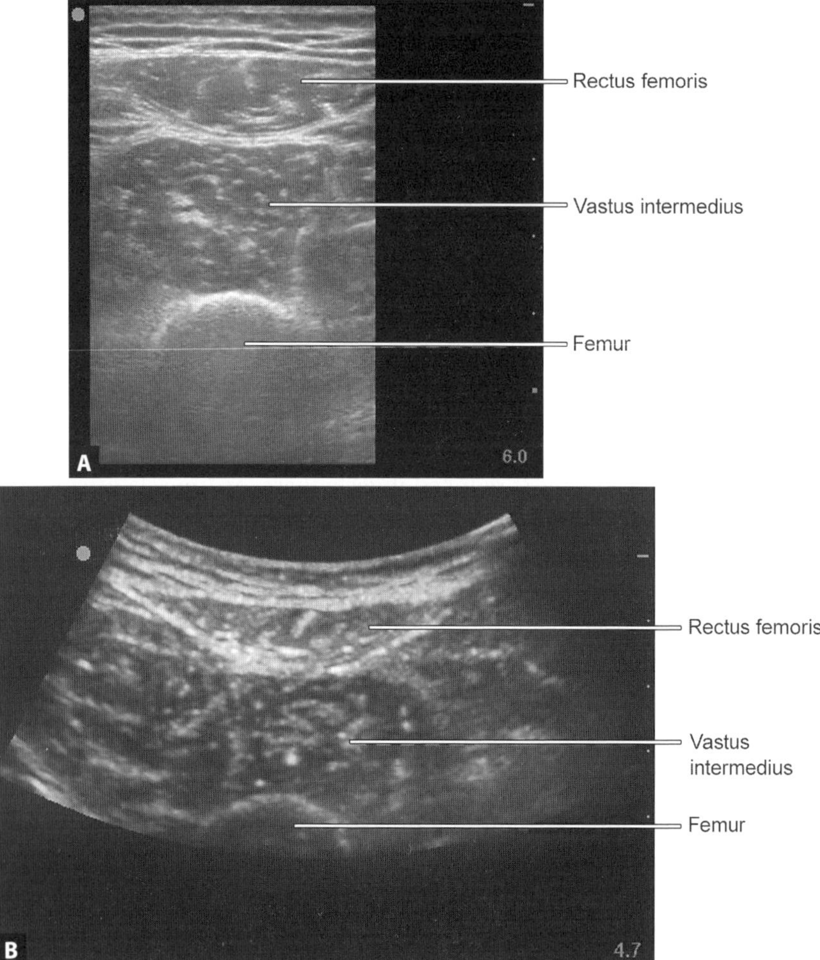

Figs. 2A and B: (A) The rectus femoris (RF) muscle is partially visualized and not captured in its entirety using a linear probe; (B) The RF muscle is fully visualized using a curvilinear probe.

Regarding probe pressure, most studies advocate for minimal or no compression during QMLT assessment. This approach enhances reproducibility and avoids artifactual thinning, as excessive compression can reduce measured thickness by nearly 50%.[14] However, some investigators have employed maximal compression to improve image quality and standardization, particularly in critically ill patients with tissue edema.[16] The optimal degree of probe pressure remains unresolved. Therefore, it is advisable to record QMLT under both minimal and maximal compression, especially when performing serial measurements in critically ill populations.

Rectus femoris muscle thickness: Rectus femoris muscle thickness is measured using ultrasound at the junction of the upper two-thirds and lower one-third

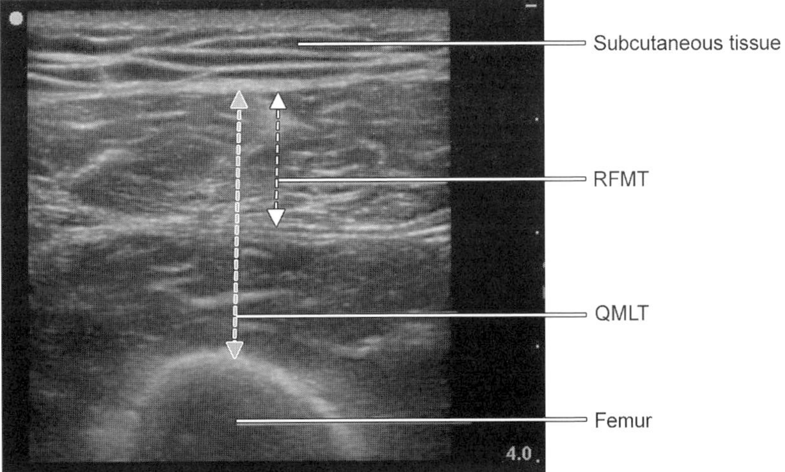

Fig. 3: Cross-sectional image of quadriceps muscle layer thickness (QMLT) and rectus femoris muscle thickness (RFMT), obtained at the junction of the upper two-thirds and lower one-third of a line *joining the anterior superior iliac spine (ASIS) and the superior patellar border (SPB)*, with minimal compression by the transducer.

of the line connecting the ASIS and SPB. Alternatively, some protocols use the midpoint of this line. The measurement is taken as the vertical distance from the fat–muscle interface (superficial fascia overlying the RF) to the muscle–muscle interface between the RF and VI **(Fig. 3)**. Minimal compression is preferred to avoid underestimation of thickness and to maintain consistency across serial assessments.

Rectus femoris cross-sectional area: The optimal anatomical landmark for transducer placement to visualize the RF in its entirety lies at a point located three-fifths of the distance from the ASIS to SPB, along the lower thigh.[17] At this site, the RF CSA is measured by manually tracing the inner surface of its hyperechoic border on ultrasound **(Figs. 4A and B)**.

Most studies have performed RF-CSA measurements using minimal probe compression to preserve anatomical fidelity and ensure consistency across assessments. Notably, RF CSA is less susceptible to compression-related variability compared to MT. A threshold value of 2.39 cm^2 has been identified as a critical cutoff, beyond which there is a significantly increased association with adverse outcomes, including ICU mortality.[14,18]

PARAMETERS RELATED TO MUSCLE QUALITY

Pennation Angle and Fascicle Length

The PA is an indirect marker of muscle strength, defined as the angle between the orientation of muscle fascicles and the lower aponeurosis. It reflects the

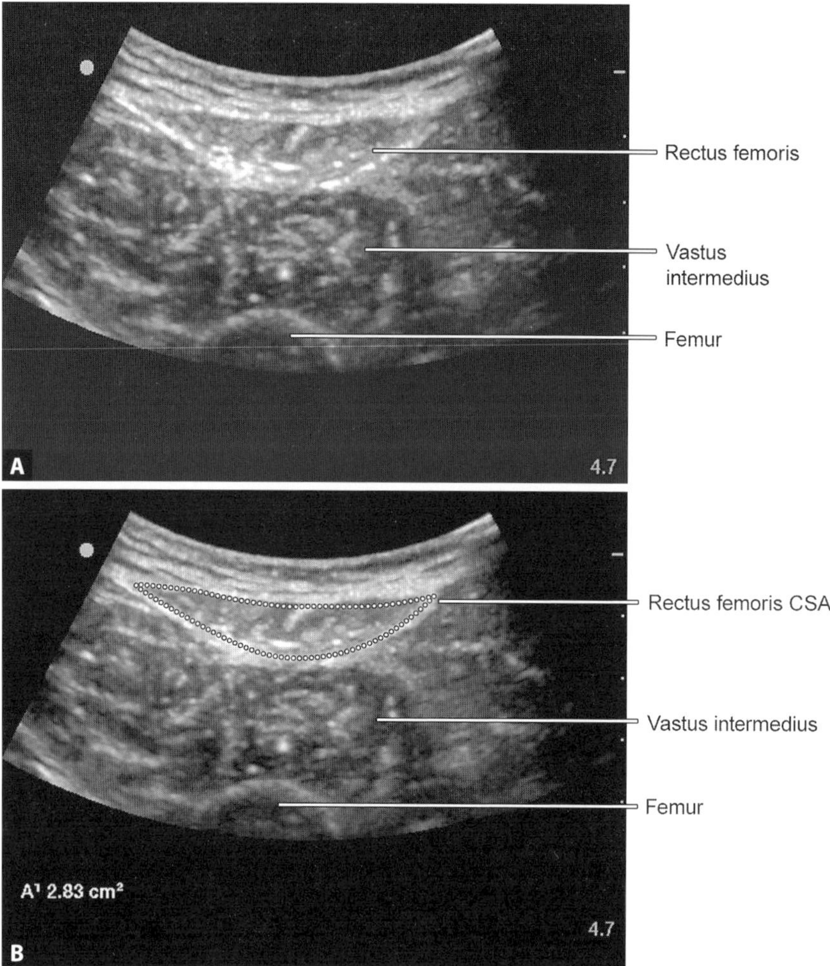

Figs. 4A and B: (A) Sonoanatomy of the rectus femoris muscle using a curvilinear probe, acquired at the level of 3/5 of the distance between the anterior superior iliac spine (ASIS) and the superior patellar border (SPB), with minimal transducer compression; (B) Manual tracing of the rectus femoris muscle to calculate its cross-sectional area (RF CSA).

architectural arrangement of sarcomeres inserting into the aponeurosis, with a larger angle indicating greater sarcomere density and, consequently, higher force-generating capacity. A progressive decline in PA over time has been associated with reduced muscle strength.

Measurement of the PA is typically performed on the RF muscle, using the same anatomical landmarks as those employed for MT and CSA. The ultrasound probe must be aligned longitudinally, parallel to the muscle fibers, to accurately visualize the fascicle trajectory and aponeurotic interface **(Figs. 5A and B)**.[10,12]

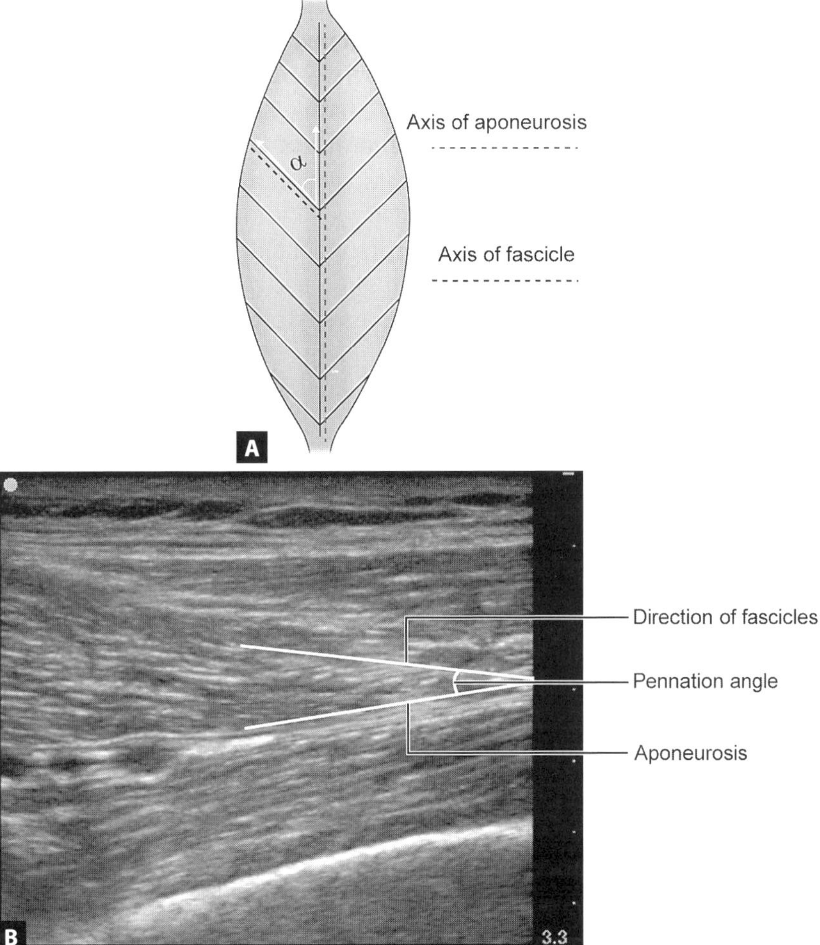

Figs. 5A and B: (A) Schematic illustration of the pennation angle (α) in a pennate muscle. The angle is formed between the axis of the muscle fascicles and the aponeurosis into which they insert; (B) Ultrasound image showing measurement of the pennation angle of the rectus femoris muscle, with the transducer aligned parallel to the longitudinal axis of the muscle.

Fascicle length can be estimated using the following formula:[19]

Fascicle length = Muscle thickness/sin (pennation angle)

While architectural parameters such as PA and FL offer valuable insights into muscle function and strength, their incorporation into nutritional assessment protocols remains limited. Until robust data are available, these parameters should be interpreted cautiously and considered adjunctive to established quantitative measures.

Muscle Echogenicity

Muscle echogenicity has emerged as a qualitative marker of muscle integrity and composition. Increased echogenicity from baseline is hypothesized to reflect pathological infiltration by adipose tissue, fibrous connective tissue, or myonecrosis.[10,20] These structural alterations are believed to precede measurable reductions in muscle mass, positioning echogenicity as a potential early marker of muscle degradation or dysfunction.

The anatomical landmark and probe placement for assessing echogenicity of the RF and VI muscles are identical to those used for CSA measurements. Echogenicity is quantified using computer-assisted grayscale analysis, employing either the trace method or the square method. Among these, the square method demonstrates superior interrater reliability. A standardized 2 × 2 cm square is placed over the ROI within each muscle, and grayscale values are extracted using the histogram function of the ultrasound software. These values range from 0 (black/dark) to 255 (white), expressed in arbitrary units (AU).[21,22]

CLINICAL APPLICATIONS AND CORRELATION WITH PATIENT-CENTERED OUTCOMES

Skeletal muscle ultrasound has demonstrated significant utility in the care of critically ill patients, particularly in nutritional assessment and prognostication. Its applications include:[10,14,15,18,23,24]

- *Identification of patients at high risk for malnutrition*, based on reduced muscle mass and quality
- *Recognition of individuals likely to benefit from nutritional and rehabilitative interventions*
- *Guidance of nutritional therapy*, including individualized calorie and protein targets
- *Serial monitoring to evaluate the efficacy of therapeutic interventions*
- *Prediction of short- and long-term complications*, such as ICU-acquired weakness (ICU-AW), prolonged mechanical ventilation, and increased mortality risk.

A five-site musculoskeletal ultrasound protocol—targeting proximal upper- and lower-limb muscles—has shown reasonable correlation with LBM as assessed by dual-energy X-ray absorptiometry (DEXA).[25] In a landmark study, Puthucheary et al. reported a 12.5% reduction in RF CSA within the first 7 days of ICU admission.[26] Multiple studies have since validated the role of lower-limb ultrasound measurements as surrogate markers of LBM, highlighting their potential to:

- Stratify patients by nutritional risk
- Guide targeted interventions to mitigate muscle loss.
- Inform individualized protein and energy supplementation strategies based on estimated muscle stores.[23,27-29]

Emerging data underscore the clinical relevance of skeletal muscle ultrasound in critically ill patients, particularly in identifying nutritional risk and predicting outcomes. A meta-analysis by Venco et al. revealed that older age and higher BMI were paradoxically associated with lower baseline muscle mass, challenging traditional assumptions that lower BMI correlates with sarcopenia.[14] This finding highlights the phenomenon of *sarcopenic obesity*, wherein excess adiposity masks underlying muscle depletion, and underscores the value of ultrasound in detecting high-risk phenotypes.

Several prospective studies have documented a rapid decline in RF CSA and QMLT within the first 7 days of ICU admission.[23] Baseline reductions in QMLT, RF CSA, and PA have been associated with elevated nutritional risk (mNUTRIC ≥5) and increased 60-day mortality.[24] Furthermore, decreased MLT and RF CSA correlate with fewer ICU-free and ventilator-free days, as well as higher ICU mortality.[10]

Interventional studies have demonstrated the utility of muscle ultrasound in guiding and evaluating therapeutic strategies. A high-protein nutritional protocol was shown to attenuate QMLT loss and reduce malnutrition rates in critically ill patients.[30] Other trials have employed ultrasound to assess the impact of intermittent feeding, supplemental parenteral nutrition, and in-bed cycling on muscle preservation.[23,29]

Importantly, changes in RF echo-intensity between day 1 and day 7 of ICU admission have emerged as strong predictors of ICU-AW at hospital discharge.[23] These findings support the integration of muscle ultrasound into routine ICU care, not only for nutritional assessment but also for prognostication and individualized therapy.

TECHNICAL LIMITATIONS AND PRACTICAL ISSUES IN IMPLEMENTATION

A major barrier to widespread clinical adoption of skeletal muscle ultrasound in critically ill patients is the lack of standardized image acquisition protocols and preconditions. Numerous factors influence image quality and reliability—including ultrasound machine settings (e.g., gain, depth, examination mode, focus), patient positioning, timing relative to prior physical activity, degree of probe compression, anatomical landmark selection, and image capture methodology. Without uniformity across these parameters, comparability between studies and populations remains limited.

This methodological heterogeneity has also hindered the establishment of clinically meaningful cutoff values for changes in muscle CSA or thickness. Although multiple meta-analyses have demonstrated acceptable inter- and intraoperator reproducibility for parameters, such as QMLT, RFMT, and RF CSA, the variability in acquisition techniques significantly compromises external validity and generalizability.[14,15]

ASSESSMENT STANDARDIZATION: A GUIDE TO AVOIDING COMMON PITFALLS

Standardization of skeletal muscle ultrasound is essential to ensure reproducibility, comparability across studies, and clinical applicability. The following factors should be considered when designing or implementing a standardized protocol.[10,12,14,15]

- *Transducer type and frequency:* A high-frequency linear probe is most commonly used. Although some studies have employed curvilinear probes, uniformity in probe type is critical to maintain consistency across measurements.
- *Technical settings:* Ultrasound machine parameters—including gain, depth, focus, and examination mode—must be kept consistent and explicitly reported to ensure image comparability.
- *Number of sonographers:* When multiple operators are involved in serial assessments, interobserver variability should be accounted for. Operator consistency or appropriate training can help mitigate this issue.
- *Operator training:* Adequate training in musculoskeletal ultrasound is essential to minimize measurement error and improve reliability.
- *Transducer pressure:* Probe compression can significantly affect measurements, reducing MLT by up to 50%. RF CSA is less sensitive to pressure variations. While some authors advocate maximal compression to enhance image resolution—especially in edematous patients—there is no consensus on the optimal pressure. Maximal compression has been described as the highest pressure tolerable by the patient without discomfort. In the absence of standardization, it may be prudent to record MLT under both minimal and maximal compression during longitudinal assessments.
- *Patient positioning:* Variations in bed elevation, hip flexion, or standing posture can influence CSA measurements. Most studies employ the supine position, which should be consistently used and documented.
- *Landmarking consistency:* Measurements of MLT and CSA are typically performed at the site of maximal muscle bulk—commonly at the midpoint or at the junction of the upper two-thirds and lower one-third of the line connecting the ASIS and SPB. Consistent landmarking is essential for serial assessments and should be clearly specified.
- *Fluid status:* Severe peripheral edema may render ultrasound images nondiagnostic. While edema may influence echogenicity, further evidence is needed to clarify this relationship.
- *Exercise or limb movement prior to scanning:* Maximal contractions or recent limb activity can alter MLT and CSA measurements. It is recommended to avoid exercise for at least 30 minutes prior to scanning.

CURRENT EVIDENCE AND ADOPTION IN GUIDELINES

The integration of skeletal muscle ultrasound into clinical nutrition and sarcopenia assessment is gaining momentum, supported by evolving consensus and guideline documents:

- *ESPEN guidelines (2019):* The European Society for Clinical Nutrition and Metabolism (ESPEN) included ultrasound among the modalities that *may* be used to assess LBM but emphasized further validation before routine clinical adoption.[31]
- *GLIM framework (2019 and 2025):* The Global Leadership Initiative on Malnutrition (GLIM)—a collaborative effort by ASPEN, ESPEN, and other international societies—proposed a diagnostic framework for malnutrition requiring at least one phenotypic and one etiologic criterion. Low muscle mass is recognized as a phenotypic criterion. The 2025 GLIM consensus update explicitly acknowledges ultrasound as a viable method for assessing muscle mass, contingent upon the availability of reference values and adequate operator expertise.[32]
- *SARCUS Working Group (European Geriatric Medicine Society):* The SARCUS group has published a systematic review summarizing the evidence for peripheral muscle ultrasound in sarcopenia assessment. Their recommendations include protocol standardization for geriatric populations, which may be adapted for use in critically ill patients.

These developments reflect growing recognition of ultrasound as a practical, bedside tool for assessing muscle quantity and quality. However, widespread adoption will depend on further validation, standardization of acquisition protocols, and training across clinical settings.[12]

OTHER MODALITIES IN NUTRITIONAL ASSESSMENT—BODY COMPOSITION ASSESSMENT TOOLS

Body composition assessment involves quantifying the relative proportions of LBM, adipose tissue, and bone mass. Several modalities are employed for this purpose, including bioimpedance analysis (BIA), computed tomography (CT), and dual-energy X-ray absorptiometry (DEXA). These techniques offer objective insights into body composition and are increasingly used to complement clinical nutritional evaluations.

Bioimpedance Analysis

Bioimpedance analysis estimates body composition by passing low-amplitude electrical currents through the body and measuring impedance, which comprises both resistance and reactance. Using predictive equations, BIA can derive parameters such as extracellular water (ECW), total body water (TBW), and fat-free mass (FFM). A key output is the *phase angle,* considered a surrogate marker for cellular integrity and LBM. However, BIA relies on assumptions—such as a stable intracellular-to-extracellular water (ICW:ECW) ratio—that may not hold true in critically ill patients. Fluid shifts, edema, and altered hydration status can compromise accuracy in this population.[1,27]

Computed Tomography

Computed tomography assesses body composition by exploiting the differential radiodensity of tissues such as fat, muscle, and bone. Using specialized software, the CSA of each tissue type is quantified by summing the pixels corresponding to that tissue in a given axial image. Muscle CSA at the L3 vertebral level and total psoas CSA are commonly used as surrogate markers of whole-body muscle mass and sarcopenia. Despite its precision, CT imaging is generally unsuitable for routine LBM assessment in critically ill patients. Limitations include high radiation exposure, inability to perform serial evaluations, and the logistical challenges of transporting hemodynamically unstable patients to radiology suites.[1,23,27]

Dual-energy X-ray Absorptiometry

Dual-energy X-ray absorptiometry provides whole-body estimates of bone mineral density, fat mass, and LBM. While both CT and DEXA offer high accuracy, their use in critically ill patients is limited by logistical constraints, radiation exposure (CT), and the need for patient transport.

AREAS FOR FUTURE RESEARCH

Key areas for investigation include:

- *Optimal anatomical landmarks* for each sonographic parameter to improve reproducibility and anatomical fidelity
- *Comparative studies on probe compression techniques*, evaluating the impact of minimal versus maximal pressure on measurement accuracy and clinical relevance
- *Development of standardized acquisition and reporting protocols*, encompassing machine settings, patient positioning, and operator training
- *Establishment of normative reference ranges and diagnostic cutoffs* for critically ill populations, stratified by age, sex, and clinical condition
- *Determination of minimal clinically important differences (MCID)* in ultrasound parameters that correlate with meaningful changes in patient-centered outcomes such as mortality, ICU-AW, and duration of mechanical ventilation.

Such research will be instrumental in validating skeletal muscle ultrasound as a robust tool for nutritional and functional assessment in critical care.

CONCLUSION

Skeletal muscle ultrasound is emerging as a pivotal modality in the nutritional assessment and management of critically ill patients. Its utility spans three key domains: (1) *diagnosis of malnutrition,* (2) *guidance of nutritional interventions,* and (3) *monitoring of therapeutic efficacy.* It has the potential to become an integral component of malnutrition diagnosis, enabling identification of patients who may benefit from targeted nutritional strategies and facilitating longitudinal tracking of muscle changes in response to illness and intervention. Its accessibility, bedside applicability, and noninvasive nature make it particularly suited for the ICU setting. However, the accurate and meaningful application of this modality hinges on *standardization of technique, rigorous operator training,* and *continued research* to refine its clinical utility. With these foundations, skeletal muscle ultrasound holds promise as a transformative tool in critical care nutrition and rehabilitation.

REFERENCES

1. Mundi MS, Patel JJ, Martindale R. Body composition technology: Implications for the ICU. Nutr Clin Pract. 2019;34(1):48-58.
2. Looijaard WGPM, Dekker IM, Stapel SN, Girbes ARJ, Twisk JWR, Oudemans-van Straaten HM, et al. Skeletal muscle quality as assessed by CT-derived skeletal muscle density is associated with 6-month mortality in mechanically ventilated critically ill patients. Crit Care. 2016;20(1):386.
3. Mueller C, Compher C, Ellen DM; American Society for Parenteral and Enteral Nutrition (A.S.P.E.N.) Board of Directors. A.S.P.E.N. Clinical Guidelines: Nutrition screening, assessment, and intervention in adults. JPEN J Parenter Enteral Nutr. 2011;35(1):16-24.
4. Lee Z, Heyland DK. Determination of nutrition risk and status in critically ill patients: what are our considerations? Nutr Clin Pract. 2019;34(1):96-111.
5. Rahman A, Hasan RM, Agarwala R, Martin C, Day AG, Heyland DK. Identifying critically-ill patients who will benefit most from nutritional therapy: further validation of the “modified NUTRIC” nutritional risk assessment tool. Clin Nutr. 2016;35(1):158-62.
6. Price KL, Earthman CP. Update on body composition tools in clinical settings: computed tomography, ultrasound, and bioimpedance applications for assessment and monitoring. Eur J Clin Nutr. 2019;73(2):187-93.
7. Compher CW, Fukushima R, Correia MITD, Gonzalez MC, McKeever L, Nakamura K, et al. Recognizing malnutrition in adults with critical illness: guidance statements from the Global Leadership Initiative on Malnutrition. JPEN J Parenter Enteral Nutr. 2025;49(4):405-13.
8. Powles AEJ, Martin DJ, Wells ITP, Goodwin CR. Physics of ultrasound. Anaesth Intensive Care Med. 2018;19(4):202-5.
9. Ralston MR, McCreath G, Lees ZJ, Salt IP, Sim MAB, Watson MJ, et al. Beyond body mass index: exploring the role of visceral adipose tissue in intensive care unit outcomes. BJA Open. 2025;14:100391.

10. Mourtzakis M, Parry S, Connolly B, Puthucheary Z. Skeletal Muscle Ultrasound in Critical Care: A Tool in Need of Translation. Ann Am Thorac Soc. 2017; 14(10):1495-503.
11. Formenti P, Umbrello M, Coppola S, Froio S, Chiumello D. Clinical review: peripheral muscular ultrasound in the ICU. Ann Intensive Care. 2019;9:57.
12. Perkisas S, Baudry S, Bauer J, Beckwée D, De Cock AM, Hobbelen H, et al. Application of ultrasound for muscle assessment in sarcopenia: towards standardized measurements. Eur Geriatr Med. 2018;9(6):739-57.
13. Casey P, Alasmar M, McLaughlin J, Ang Y, McPhee J, Heire P, et al. The current use of ultrasound to measure skeletal muscle and its ability to predict clinical outcomes: a systematic review. J Cachexia Sarcopenia Muscle. 2022;13(5):2298-309.
14. Venco R, Artale A, Formenti P, Deana C, Mistraletti G, Umbrello M. Methodologies and clinical applications of lower limb muscle ultrasound in critically ill patients: a systematic review and meta-analysis. Ann Intensive Care. 2024;14(1):163.
15. Weinel LM, Summers MJ, Chapple LA. Ultrasonography to measure quadriceps muscle in critically ill patients: a literature review of reported methodologies. Anaesth Intensive Care. 2019;47(5):423-34.
16. Paris MT, Mourtzakis M, Day A, Leung R, Watharkar S, Kozar R, et al. Validation of bedside ultrasound of muscle layer thickness of the quadriceps in the critically ill patient (VALIDUM Study): a prospective multicenter study. JPEN J Parenter Enteral Nutr. 2017;41(2):171-80.
17. Seymour JM, Ward K, Sidhu PS, Puthucheary Z, Steier J, Jolley CJ, et al. Ultrasound measurement of rectus femoris cross-sectional area and the relationship with quadriceps strength in COPD. Thorax. 2009;64(5):418-23.
18. Umbrello M, Formenti P, Artale A, Assandri M, Palandri C, Ponti S, et al. Association between the ultrasound evaluation of muscle mass and adverse outcomes in critically ill patients: a prospective cohort study. Anesth Analg. 2025;140(2):427.
19. Korhonen MT, Mero AA, Alén M, Sipilä S, Häkkinen K, Liikavainio T, et al. Biomechanical and skeletal muscle determinants of maximum running speed with aging. Med Sci Sports Exerc. 2009;41(4):844.
20. Puthucheary ZA, Phadke R, Rawal J, McPhail MJW, Sidhu PS, Rowlerson A, et al. Qualitative ultrasound in acute critical illness muscle wasting. Crit Care Med. 2015;43(8):1603-11.
21. Parry SM, El-Ansary D, Cartwright MS, Sarwal A, Berney S, Koopman R, et al. Ultrasonography in the intensive care setting can be used to detect changes in the quality and quantity of muscle and is related to muscle strength and function. J Crit Care. 2015;30(5):1151.e9-14.
22. Vieira L, Rocha LPB, Mathur S, Santana L, de Melo PF, da Silva VZM, et al. Reliability of skeletal muscle ultrasound in critically ill trauma patients. Rev Bras Ter Intensiva. 2019;31(4):464-73.
23. Van Ruijven IM, Stapel SN, Molinger J, Weijs PJM. Monitoring muscle mass using ultrasound: a key role in critical care. Curr Opin Crit Care. 2021;27(4): 354-60.
24. Lee ZY, Ong SP, Ng CC, Yap CSL, Engkasan JP, Barakatun-Nisak MY, et al. Association between ultrasound quadriceps muscle status with premorbid functional status and 60-day mortality in mechanically ventilated critically ill

patient: a single-center prospective observational study. Clin Nutr Edinb Scotl. 2021;40(3):1338-47.

25. Paris MT, Lafleur B, Dubin JA, Mourtzakis M. Development of a bedside viable ultrasound protocol to quantify appendicular lean tissue mass. J Cachexia Sarcopenia Muscle. 2017;8(5):713-26.
26. Puthucheary ZA, Rawal J, McPhail M, Connolly B, Ratnayake G, Chan P, et al. Acute skeletal muscle wasting in critical illness. JAMA. 2013;310(15):1591-600.
27. Looijaard WGPM, Molinger J, Weijs PJM. Measuring and monitoring lean body mass in critical illness. Curr Opin Crit Care. 2018;24(4):241.
28. Zaher S. Incorporating ultrasonography to the nutritional assessment process in intensive care settings to improve the prescription of enteral and parenteral nutrition: benefits, practicality, and challenges. Saudi Med J. 2024;45(7):653-7.
29. McNelly AS, Bear DE, Connolly BA, Arbane G, Allum L, Tarbhai A, et al. Effect of Intermittent or Continuous Feed on Muscle Wasting in Critical Illness: A Phase 2 Clinical Trial. Chest. 2020;158(1):183-94.
30. Fetterplace K, Deane AM, Tierney A, Beach LJ, Knight LD, Presneill J, et al. Targeted Full Energy and Protein Delivery in Critically Ill Patients: A Pilot Randomized Controlled Trial (FEED Trial). JPEN J Parenter Enteral Nutr. 2018;42(8):1252-62.
31. Singer P, Blaser AR, Berger MM, Alhazzani W, Calder PC, Casaer MP, et al. ESPEN guideline on clinical nutrition in the intensive care unit. Clin Nutr. 2019;38(1):48-79.
32. Cederholm T, Jensen GL, Correia MITD, Gonzalez MC, Fukushima R, Pisprasert V, et al. The GLIM consensus approach to diagnosis of malnutrition: a 5-year update. Clin Nutr. 2025;49:11-20.

CHAPTER

Gut Failure in Intensive Care Unit: Cause, Consequence, and Outcomes

Santosh Kumar Paiaulla, Palepu B Gopal

"All disease begins in the gut."

—**Hippocrates** (*c. 460–370 BC*)

HISTORY

Ancient insights remain relevant in critical care today. Hippocrates introduced "digestion" ("Pepsis") as central to health, famously stating, "All disease begins in the gut." Claude Bernard highlighted homeostasis and linked barrier breakdown in cholera to systemic toxin entry, establishing the gut's role in overall stability.[1] By the late 20th century, loss of gut absorption and barrier integrity—termed "intestinal failure"—was recognized as a major factor in critical illness, with gut-derived toxins seen as drivers of multiple organ failure (MOF).[2]

INTRODUCTION

Gut failure in the intensive care unit (ICU) is the loss of gastrointestinal (GI) function, impacting digestion, absorption, barrier, and immune roles. Once viewed as secondary in critical illness, the gut is now seen as central to systemic inflammation and organ failure. Critically ill patients are prone to gut failure from factors like decreased blood flow, inflammation, vasopressors, ventilation, and microbiome changes. Consequences include reduced motility, mucosal atrophy, increased permeability, bacterial translocation, and abdominal compartment syndrome (ACS). This chapter covers the causes, mechanisms, clinical impact, and treatments of gut failure in the ICU.

EVOLUTION OF DEFINITION OF GUT FAILURE IN INTENSIVE CARE UNIT

The GI tract was not considered an organ of concern in ICU. Emphasis was on heart, lungs, kidneys, and liver. The gut was thought of more of a "by-stander" of systemic failure.

In the late 1980s and early 1990s, researchers proposed that the gut could drive systemic inflammation. Deitch et al. suggested bacterial translocation from the gut might trigger systemic inflammatory response syndrome (SIRS) and MOF. By the early 2000s, intensivists observed gut dysfunction—such as ileus, feeding intolerance, and GI bleeding—in ICU patients, though definitions remained unclear.[3] As awareness of the gut's impact on clinical outcomes grew, efforts focused on creating a gut dysfunction score. In 2009, Reintam et al. introduced the gastrointestinal failure (GIF) score, incorporating feeding intolerance and intra-abdominal hypertension (IAH).[4] The European Society of Intensive Care Medicine (ESICM) working groups have recognized GIF as a distinct clinical condition and recommended its inclusion in organ failure scoring systems. Recent definitions describe gut failure as a state where the GI tract cannot maintain nutrition, barrier function, or immune homeostasis, thereby contributing to critical illness.[5]

CAUSES OF GUT FAILURE IN INTENSIVE CARE UNIT

In the ICU, the gut is particularly susceptible to fail due to its high metabolic demand, high dependence on perfusion, and its vital role in immune and barrier functions. Due to the absence of definitive clinical indicators for gut failure, early identification often goes unnoticed. Understanding the etiology and often overlapping causes of gut failure is crucial for prevention, identification, prompt intervention, and improved clinical outcomes in the ICU **(Table 1)**.

ETIOLOGY OF GUT FAILURE IN INTENSIVE CARE UNIT

Splanchnic Hypoperfusion and Ischemia

During shock (septic, cardiogenic, or hypovolemic), blood shifts from the splanchnic circulation to support vital organ perfusion. This process can lead to intestinal mucosal ischemia and compromised epithelial junctions, increasing gut permeability and the potential for bacterial translocation.[6]

TABLE 1: Major etiological factors of associated gut failure in ICU.[6-12]

Etiological factor	*Mechanism of failure*
Splanchnic hypoperfusion	Mucosal ischemia, barrier breakdown
Sepsis/systemic inflammation	Epithelial apoptosis and dysbiosis
Mechanical ventilation (PEEP)	Reduced perfusion, ileus
Vasopressors	Mesenteric vasoconstriction
Drugs (opioids and sedatives)	Hypomotility, feeding intolerance
Delayed enteral feeding	Mucosal atrophy, increased permeability
IAH/ACS	Vascular compression, ischemia
Surgical/traumatic injury	Disruption of bowel continuity

(ACS: abdominal compartment syndrome; IAH: intra-abdominal hypertension; ICU: intensive care unit; PEEP: positive end-expiratory pressure)

Sepsis and Systemic Inflammation

Sepsis-induced gut epithelial apoptosis, disruption of tight junctions, causes gut barrier dysfunction. Endotoxemia and inflammatory cytokines amplify mucosal injury and impair regeneration.[7]

Intra-abdominal Hypertension and Abdominal Compartment Syndrome

Elevated intra-abdominal pressure (IAP) (>12 mm Hg) compromises mesenteric perfusion. Severe cases (ACS) cause direct bowel ischemia and organ compression.[8]

Mechanical Ventilation and High Positive End-expiratory Pressure

Increased intrathoracic pressure leads to decreased venous return and splanchnic hypoperfusion. Prolonged ventilation promotes gastric stasis and ileus.[9]

Vasopressor Use

Though necessary for perfusion, vasopressors (especially high-dose norepinephrine) cause vasoconstriction of mesenteric vessels, worsening ischemia.[10]

Pharmacologic Effects

- Opioids and sedatives reduce gut motility leading to delayed gastric emptying and ileus.
- Antibiotics disrupt gut microbiota, causing dysbiosis and *Clostridium difficile* infection.[11]

Nutritional Factors

The hypothesis of prolonged fasting or delayed enteral nutrition (EN) causing mucosal atrophy, decreased secretory IgA, and barrier dysfunction is supported by stronger evidence than ever before.[12] Lack of luminal nutrition impairs gut integrity and alters microbiota.

Surgical and Traumatic Insults

Abdominal surgery, bowel surgery, and trauma can alter gut anatomy and physiology. Postoperative surgical complications can further worsen gut failure **(Table 2)**.

Gut failure in critically ill patients is not a mere GI issue—it is now recognized as a principal contributor to systemic problems and adverse clinical outcomes. It is both an indicator and a motor of systemic deterioration.

TABLE 2: Consequences of gut failure in ICU.[2,11,13-17]

Factor	*Mechanism*	*Effect on GI tract*
Splanchnic hypoperfusion	Reduced blood flow to gut	Ischemia and mucosal injury
Sepsis and inflammation	Cytokine surge → epithelial damage	Barrier dysfunction and immune activation
Intra-abdominal pressure/ACS	Vascular compression → ischemia	Reduced perfusion and edema
Mechanical ventilation (high PEEP)	↑ Thoracic pressure → ↓ gut perfusion	Ischemia and translocation risk
Vasopressors	Mesenteric vasoconstriction	Mucosal ischemia
Opioids/sedatives	↓ Motility → ileus	Bacterial overgrowth and stasis
Nutritional factors	Villous atrophy and barrier dysfunction	Impairs gut immunity and gut microbiota
Surgical and traumatic insults	Altered anatomy and physiology	Loss of gut barrier integrity and ileus

(ACS: abdominal compartment syndrome; GI: gastrointestinal; ICU: intensive care unit; PEEP: positive end-expiratory pressure)

Ileus and Feeding Intolerance

- Gut failure usually presents with delayed gastric emptying, distension, and high gastric residual volumes (GRVs) leading to feeding intolerance, delayed enteral feeding, and malnutrition in ICU.[11]
- Dependency on parenteral nutrition (PN) is associated with risks for infection, liver derangement, and metabolic complications.[13]

Loss of Barrier Function

The intestinal mucosa aids as a critical barrier avoiding gut microbes and toxins from entering systemic circulation. In the context of gut failure:

- Disruption of tight junctions occurs due to ischemia and inflammation
- Increased porousness allows translocation of bacteria, endotoxins (e.g., lipopolysaccharides), and antigens into the bloodstream.

Gut-driven endotoxemia is an identified factor linked with SIRS, sepsis, and MOF.[2]

Contribution to Systemic Inflammation and Multiple Organ Dysfunction Syndrome

Gut-derived mediators such as tumor necrosis factor-α (TNF-α), interleukin-6 (IL-6), and interleukin-1β (IL-1β) promote:

- Endothelial dysfunction

- Leaky capillaries
- Progressive organ dysfunction (lungs, kidneys, and liver).

This "gut-lymph" hypothesis postulates that nonbacterial inflammatory products entering from gut into systemic circulation via the lymphatics, fuel MOF.[14]

Infection and Sepsis Risk

- Bacterial translocation surges bloodstream infections
- Dysbiosis is due to antibiotics and illness, and PN wipes out gut commensals and augments overgrowth of pathogenic bacteria and fungi.
- *Lack of enteral stimulation:* Absence of EN lumen leads to mucosal atrophy and inadequate secretion of protective factors like secretory immunoglobulin A (IgA).
- *Altered microbiome:*
  - ↓ *Firmicutes:* Decline of commensal bacteria
  - ↑ *Proteobacteria:* Overgrowth of pathogenic bacteria and decreased production of short-chain fatty acids leads to increased risk of necrotizing enterocolitis (NEC) and inflammatory bowel disease (IBD).
- *Gut barrier dysfunction:* PN is associated with increased intestinal permeability, "leaky gut", allowing translocation of bacteria and endotoxins into systemic circulation.
- *Immune regulation:* Gut-associated lymphoid tissue (GALT) function is impaired, weakening mucosal immunity.
- Increased incidence of ventilator-associated pneumonia (VAP), intra-abdominal infections, central line-associated bloodstream infections (CLABSI).[15]

Prolonged Intensive Care Unit Stay and Organ Support

Patients with gut failure often require:

- Longer durations of mechanical ventilation
- Increased vasopressor support
- Renal replacement therapy (RRT).

These interventions increase ICU costs, length of stay, and consequent complications.[11]

Long-term Consequences

Even after ICU discharge, patients may suffer from:

- Chronic gut dysfunction (e.g., post-ICU ileus and motility disorders)
- Short bowel syndrome if surgical resection was needed.
- Post-intensive care syndrome (PICS).[16]

Mortality Impact

Gut failure is independently linked with increased ICU and hospital mortality.

- Ischemic bowel disease
- Gut-driven fulminant sepsis
- Unsolved feeding intolerance.[17]

GUT FAILURE SCORING SYSTEMS IN THE INTENSIVE CARE UNIT

Multiple scoring systems have been projected to recognize, quantify, and check GI dysfunction and gut failure in ICU patients. Although there is no universal homogeneity, the following are the most documented tools in research and practice **(Fig. 1)**.

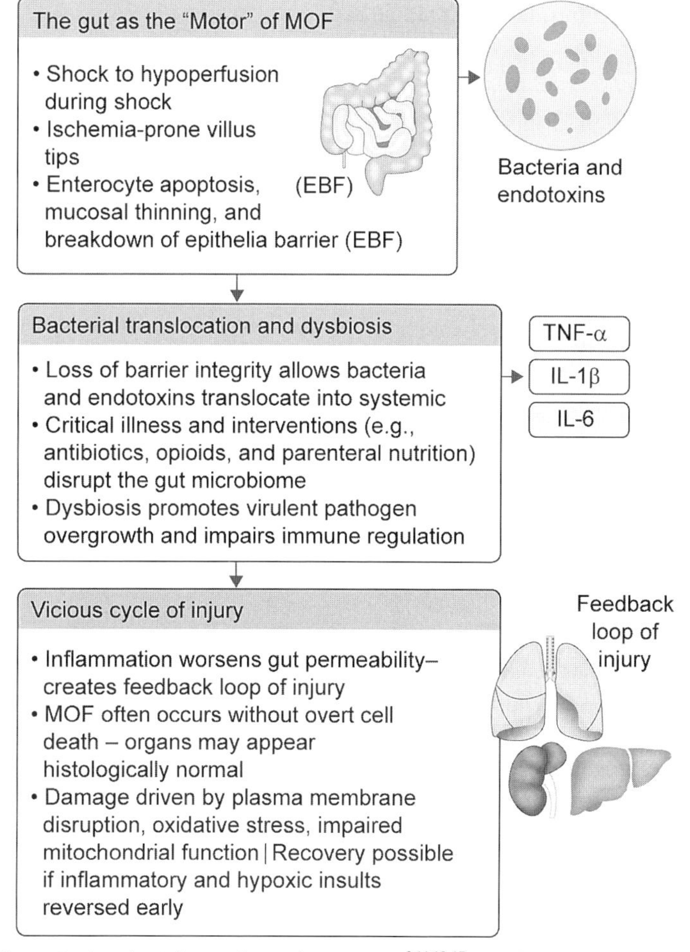

Fig. 1: Pathophysiology of gut-driven MOF.[2,11,13-17] (IL-1β: interleukin-1β; IL-6: interleukin-6; MOF: multiple organ failure; TNF-α: tumor necrosis factor-α)

Gastrointestinal Failure Score[18]

Proposed by: Reintam et al., 2008[18]

Purpose: To quantify GI dysfunction in critically ill patients.

Scoring:

GIF score	Criteria
0	Normal GI function
1	Enteral feeding with <50% of needs, no symptoms
2	Feeding intolerance or intra-abdominal hypertension (IAH)
3	Both feeding intolerance and IAH
4	Abdominal compartment syndrome (ACS)

Gastrointestinal Dysfunction Score[19]

Proposed by: Reintam Blaser et al., 2020[19]

Purpose: A simplified and more structured approach endorsed by ESICM.

Gastrointestinal dysfunction score (GIDS) components (Daily score: 0–4):

GIDS	Definition
0	No GI symptoms
1	Enteral feeding <50% of calculated needs
2	EN stopped due to GI symptoms (vomiting, distension, GRV >500 mL)
3	IAH >12 mm Hg
4	ACS or massive GI bleeding

Acute Gastrointestinal Injury Grading[11]

Proposed by: ESICM Working Group on Abdominal Problems, 2012[11]

Purpose: A clinical framework to classify the severity of GI dysfunction.

Acute gastrointestinal injury (AGI) grades:

Grade	Description
AGI I	At risk of developing GI dysfunction (e.g., postoperative ileus)
AGI II	GI dysfunction (symptomatic, requires interventions but EN possible)
AGI III	GI failure (EN not possible, signs of organ dysfunction, e.g., shock, IAH)
AGI IV	Severe GI failure with life-threatening impact (e.g., ACS and massive bleeding)

DIAGNOSIS OF GUT FAILURE IN INTENSIVE CARE UNIT

Diagnosis of gut failure in ICU is challenging due to the absence of a single biomarker or unanimously accepted criteria. Therefore, diagnosis is clinical, based on a pattern of signs, symptoms, and supportive findings that mirror GI dysfunction or failure.

Symptoms and Signs[20]

- *Feeding intolerance (FI)—a usual clinical feature:*
  - High GRVs (>500 mL)
  - Vomiting or regurgitation
  - Abdominal distension or pain
  - Diarrhea or constipation
  - Absent or hypoactive bowel sounds
  - Ileus
  - Signs of IAH
- *Failure of nutritional delivery:*
  - Failure to start or continue EN due to GI dysfunction
  - <50% of calculated energy needs via EN for ≥3 days
- *Presence of abdominal complications:*
  - Abdominal compartment syndrome
  - Significant GI bleeding
  - Suspected or confirmed mesenteric ischemia

Supportive Diagnostics and Tools[21]

Intra-abdominal Pressure

- Measured via bladder pressure
- *IAH:* IAP ≥12 mm Hg
- *ACS:* IAP >20 mm Hg with new organ dysfunction

Gastric Residual Volume

Gastric residual volume >250–500 mL may show delayed gastric emptying (controversial as a strict threshold).

Bedside Ultrasound

- Assesses bowel distension, peristalsis, and fluid collections
- Noninvasive assessment of ileus or pseudo-obstruction.

Ultrasound (USG) abdomen to assess bowel motility: Real-time imaging can show presence or absence of bowel movements supporting a diagnosis of adynamic ileus.

Ultrasound can reveal free fluid, bowel wall thickening, or air-fluid levels.

Imaging (CT Abdomen)

- For detecting ischemia, bowel wall oedema, or obstruction
- Supports the diagnosis of secondary causes such as ACS and bowel ischemia.

Biomarkers (Experimental)

- *Citrulline:* Low levels may show enterocyte mass.

- *Intestinal fatty acid-binding protein (I-FABP):* Prove enterocyte injury.
- *Diamine oxidase (DAO):* Connected with mucosal barrier damage.

TREATMENT OF GUT FAILURE IN THE INTENSIVE CARE UNIT

Management of gut failure in ICU is complex and needs modification to individual needs. Cornerstones of treatment are as follows:

- Restore gut perfusion and motility
- Preserve mucosal barrier integrity
- Support nutrition
- Prevent complications such as bacterial translocation, sepsis, and MOF.

Hemodynamic Optimization

Goal: Restore Splanchnic Perfusion and Prevent Ischemia[22]

- Maintain mean arterial pressure (MAP ≥65 mm Hg) to ensure gut perfusion.
- Use dynamic fluid responsiveness assessment (e.g., passive leg raise and pulse pressure variation.
- Use vasopressors judiciously; norepinephrine is preferred.

Nutritional Support[23]

Enteral Nutrition First Strategy

Recommend EN within 24–48 hours if possible.

- Start with trophic feeding and advance as tolerated
- Track feed intolerance (e.g., high GRVs, distension, and vomiting).

If EN fails:

- Use postpyloric feeding
- If EN stays intolerable after 5–7 days, consider PN.

Prevention and Management of Intra-abdominal Hypertension[8]

- Monitor IAP in at-risk patients
- Provide adequate sedation
- Decompress with nasogastric or rectal tubes
- Consider surgical decompression if ACS develops (IAP >20 mm Hg + organ dysfunction) **(Fig. 2)**.

Antibiotics and Infection Control[6]

- Empirical antibiotics if bacterial translocation or gut ischemia are suspected.

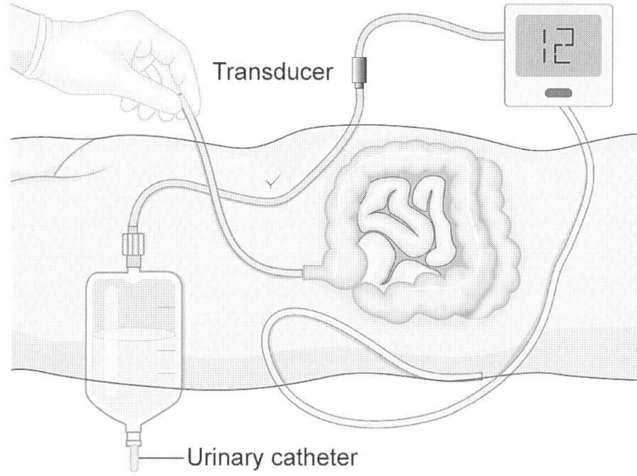

Fig. 2: Intra-abdominal pressure monitoring.[8]

- Modification of therapy based on culture sensitivity profile and source control (e.g., peritonitis and abscess).

Surgical Intervention

Indicated for:
- ACS not responding to medical measures
- Bowel ischemia or infarction
- Perforation or uncontrolled bleeding
- Obstructive pathology.

Scoring and Monitoring

Use tools like:
- Gastrointestinal failure score
- Gastrointestinal dysfunction score
- Acute gastrointestinal injury grading

Monitor progression and response to therapy.

INTENSIVE CARE UNIT GUT PROTECTION BUNDLE

The checklist is provided in **Table 3**.

OUTCOMES OF GUT FAILURE IN THE INTENSIVE VARE UNIT

Increased Mortality[24]

Gut failure is an independent factor associated with higher ICU and hospital mortality. Reported ICU mortality rates as high as 40–60% in patients with documented GI dysfunction or failure.

TABLE 3: Checklist to prevent gut failure in ICU.[8,11,23]

Component	*Action*	*Rationale*
Early hemodynamic optimization	• Target MAP ≥65 mm Hg • Avoid prolonged hypoperfusion • Use dynamic fluid assessments for fluid responsiveness	Keeps splanchnic perfusion to prevent ischemia
Early enteral nutrition (EN)	• Start EN within 24–48 hours unless contraindicated • Use trophic feeds initially	Preserves mucosal barrier and motility
Optimize vasopressor dose	• Titrate to the lowest effective dose • Prefer norepinephrine over others	Decreases mesenteric vasoconstriction and ischemic risk
Monitor bowel function	Daily assessment of bowel sounds, distension, and gastric residual volume	Early detection of ileus or feeding intolerance
Prokinetics	Use metoclopramide or erythromycin for gastric motility delay	Prevents ileus and improves tolerance to EN
Avoid overuse of sedatives and opioids	• Use sedation protocols and pain bundles (e.g., SAT/SBT) • Minimize opioid use	Decreases GI dysmotility and paralytic ileus
Intra-abdominal pressure (IAP)	• Measure IAP in high-risk patients (burns, trauma, and fluid overload) • Act on IAH early	Avoids progression to abdominal compartment syndrome
NG/OG decompression	For vomiting, distension, and high GRVs	Decreases risk of aspiration and feeding intolerance
Electrolyte balance	• Correct Mg^{2+}, K^{+}, and Ca^{2+} levels • Avoid hyperglycemia	Supports smooth GI muscle and neuromuscular function
Infection control and sepsis management	• Prompt source control • Right antibiotics	Avoids sepsis-induced gut barrier dysfunction

(GI: gastrointestinal; GRVs: gastric residual volumes; ICU: intensive care unit; NG: nasogastric; OG: orogastric)

Prolonged Intensive Care Unit and Hospital Stay[25]

Gastrointestinal dysfunction is associated with prolonged duration of mechanical ventilation, delayed weaning, and extended ICU stay. Enteral feeding intolerance leads to insufficient caloric intake, malnutrition, muscle wasting, and immune suppression.

Contribution to Multiorgan Failure

The GI tract is frequently regarded as a key contributor to the development of multiple organ dysfunction syndrome (MODS). Inadequate perfusion and ischemia compromise the integrity of the mucosal barrier, leading to bacterial translocation and systemic inflammation, which may initiate or exacerbate MOF.

Infection and Sepsis[2]

Compromised gut integrity is ideal milieu for bacterial and fungal translocation, increasing the risk of secondary infections. Gut-driven sepsis is a major cause of hospital-acquired infections in ICU patients.

- Pathogen overgrowth and dysbiosis increase susceptibility to multidrug-resistant organism (MDRO) colonization.
- Fungal translocation, chiefly *Candida* species, remains common in immune compromised or long-stay ICU patients.

Nutritional Deficiency and Sarcopenia

Gut failure leads to:

- Feed intolerance and malabsorption
- Protein-energy malnutrition
- Reduced lean body mass and impaired immune function.

Long-term Consequences in Survivors[26]

Patients surviving critical illness with gut failure may experience:

- Chronic GI dysfunction (e.g., malabsorption and chronic diarrhea)
- Short bowel syndrome (after surgical resection)
- Dependence on long-term PN
- Persistent fatigue, weight loss, and suboptimal quality of life.

CONCLUSION

Gastrointestinal failure is the ICU's silent organ dysfunction-common, deadly and usually overlooked. Structured assessment allows early recognition and early recognition of the fatal cascade. Integrating GI failure scores into organ failure scores is vital to improve ICU outcomes.

REFERENCES

1. Sródka A. The short history of gastroenterology. J Physiol Pharmacol. 2003;54 Suppl 3:9-21.
2. Deitch EA. The role of intestinal barrier failure and bacterial translocation in the development of systemic infection and multiple organ failure. Arch Surg. 1990;125(3):403-4.

3. Yannopoulos D, McKnite SH, Metzger A, Lurie KG. Intrathoracic pressure regulation for intracranial pressure management in normovolemic and hypovolemic pigs. Crit Care Med. 2006;34(12 Suppl):S495-500.
4. Reintam A, Parm P, Kitus R, Kern H, Starkopf J. Gastrointestinal failure score in critically ill patients: a prospective observational study. Crit Care. 2008;12(4):R90.
5. Reintam Blaser A, Malbrain MLNG, Starkopf J, et al. Gastrointestinal failure in the ICU: a narrative review. Intensive Care Med. 2020;46:1777-89. doi:10.1007/s00134-020-06184-w
6. Deitch EA. Gut-origin sepsis: evolution of a concept. Surgeon. 2012;10(6):350-6.
7. Clark JA, Coopersmith CM. Intestinal crosstalk: a new paradigm for understanding the gut as the "motor" of critical illness. Shock. 2007;28(4):384-93.
8. Kirkpatrick AW, Roberts DJ, De Waele J, Jaeschke R, Malbrain ML, De Keulenaer B, et al. Intra-abdominal hypertension and the abdominal compartment syndrome: updated consensus definitions and clinical practice guidelines from the World Society of the Abdominal Compartment Syndrome. Intensive Care Med. 2013;39(7):1190-206.
9. an der Voort PHJ, et al. Hemodynamic effects of positive end-expiratory pressure during mechanical ventilation in critically ill patients. Chest. 2004;126(3):820-5.
10. Dünser MW, et al. The effects of vasopressor therapy on intestinal blood flow in critically ill patients: a review. Intensive Care Med. 2006;32(10):1424-31. doi:10.1007/s00134-006-0254-4.
11. Reintam Blaser A, Malbrain ML, Starkopf J, Fruhwald S, Jakob SM, De Waele J, et al. Gastrointestinal function in intensive care patients: terminology, definitions and management. Recommendations of the ESICM Working Group on Abdominal Problems. Intensive Care Med. 2012;38(3):384-94.
12. Alverdy JC, et al. The gut as the motor of multiple organ dysfunction in critical illness. Crit Care Clin. 2009;25(3):649-65. doi: 10.1016/j.ccc.2009.06.001.
13. Wischmeyer PE. Clinical review: the role of the gut in critical illness. Crit Care. 2011.
14. Fink MP. Intestinal epithelial hyperpermeability: update on the pathogenesis of gut mucosal barrier dysfunction in critical illness. Curr Opin Crit Care. 2003;9(2):143-51.
15. Berg RD. Bacterial translocation from the gastrointestinal tract. Trends Microbiol. 1995;3(4):149-54.
16. Doig GS et al. Early enteral nutrition in critically ill patients: a prospective cohort study. Crit Care. 2005.
17. Reintam Blaser A et al. Gastrointestinal failure score and outcome of critically ill patients: a prospective observational multicentre study. Crit Care. 2015.
18. Reintam A, Parm P, Kitus R, Starkopf J, Kern H. Gastrointestinal failure score in critically ill patients: a prospective observational study. Crit Care. 2008;12(4):R90. Erratum in: Crit Care. 2008;12(6):435.
19. Reintam Blaser A, et al. Gastrointestinal dysfunction in the ICU: the status of definitions and scoring systems. Intensive Care Med. 2020;46(10):1777-89. doi: 10.1007/s00134-020-06184-w.
20. Reintam Blaser A, et al. Gastrointestinal dysfunction in critically ill patients: consensus and guidance from the ESICM Working Group on Abdominal Problems. Intensive Care Med. 2012;38(3):384-394. doi: 10.1007/s00134-011-2459-y.

21. Malbrain MLNG, et al. Recommendations for the diagnosis and management of gastrointestinal dysfunction and failure in critical illness: a WINFOCUS consensus statement. World J Crit Care Med. 2014;3(6):47-64. doi: 10.5492/wjccm. v3.i6.47.
22. Dünser MW, et al. The effects of vasopressors on intestinal blood flow in critically ill patients. Intensive Care Med. 2006;32(10):1424-31.
23. McClave SA, Taylor BE, Martindale RG, Warren MM, Johnson DR, Braunschweig C, et al. Guidelines for the Provision and Assessment of Nutrition Support Therapy in the Adult Critically Ill Patient: Society of Critical Care Medicine (SCCM) and American Society for Parenteral and Enteral Nutrition (A.S.P.E.N.). JPEN J Parenter Enteral Nutr. 2016;40(2):159-211. Erratum in: JPEN J Parenter Enteral Nutr. 2016;40(8):1200.
24. In a prospective study by Reintam et al. (2008), patients with gastrointestinal failure had a significantly higher 28-day mortality compared to those without.
25. Montejo JC, Grau T, Acosta J, et al. (2010). Multicenter, prospective, randomized, single-blind study comparing the efficacy and gastrointestinal tolerance of two enteral nutrition formulas in critically ill patients. Critical Care, 14(2), R13. https://doi.org/10.1186/cc8862.
26. Heyland DK, Dhaliwal R, Jiang X, Day AG. Identifying critically ill patients who benefit the most from nutrition therapy: the development and initial validation of a novel risk assessment tool. Crit Care. 2011;15(6):R268.

CHAPTER 4

Organ Crosstalk in the Critically Ill: What is new?

Roshni Sharma, Binila Chacko

INTRODUCTION

"Bad talk" can raise a fire to burn relationships, while "good talk" can build people. Organ crosstalk works in a comparable way inside the human body. Physiological organ crosstalk helps to support homeostasis in the body; pathological organ crosstalk leads to organ dysfunction.

TYPES OF ORGAN CROSSTALK

There are two types of organ crosstalk that have been described in literature:

1. *Physiological organ crosstalk* ***(Fig. 1)****:* Organ crosstalk can be a part of physiological processes, helping to keep homeostasis in the body. Examples of some of these physiological reflexes include:
   - Those occurring between the brain and heart—baroreceptors, chemoreceptors, Cushing reflex, Bainbridge reflex, and Bezold-Jarisch reflex[1]
   - Between the lungs and the brain—the Hering-Breuer inflation reflex[2]
   - Between the gut and the brain—vomiting and vagovagal reflexes

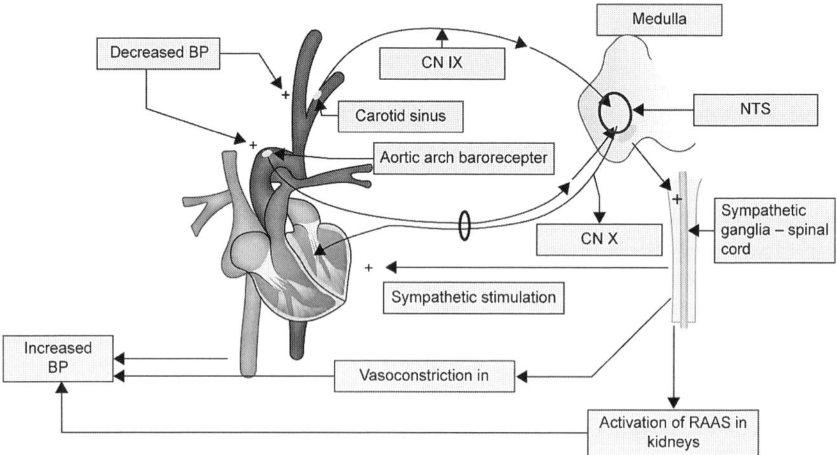

Fig. 1: Example of physiological organ crosstalk—the baroreceptor reflex. (BP: blood pressure; CN: cranial nerve; NTS: nucleus tractus solitarius; RAAS: renin–angiotensin–aldosterone system)

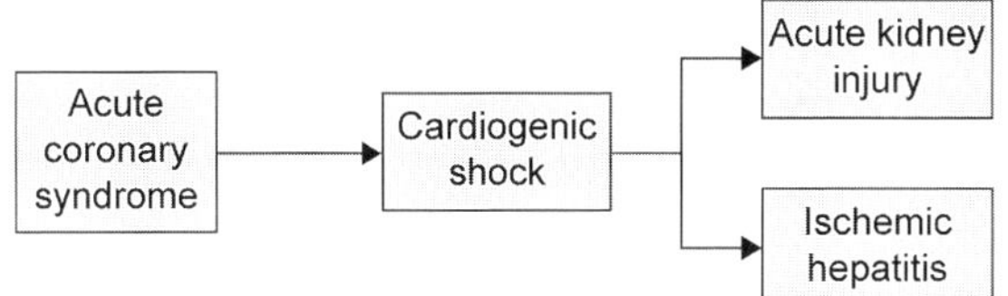

Fig. 2: Pathological organ crosstalk in series.

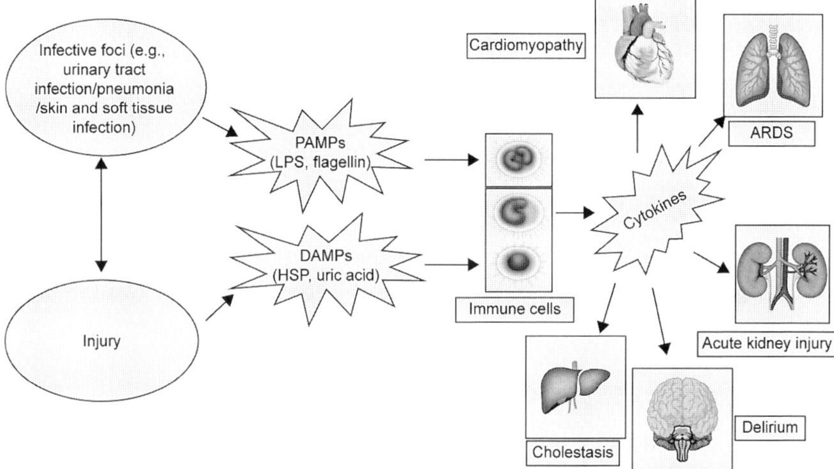

Fig. 3: Pathological organ crosstalk in parallel. (ARDS: acute respiratory distress syndrome; DAMPs: danger-associated molecular patterns; HSP: heat shock protein; LPS: lipopolysaccharide; PAMPs: pathogen-associated molecular patterns)

- Between the brain, the lungs, the systemic vasculature, and the kidneys—the renin-angiotensin-aldosterone system (RAAS)[3]

2. *Pathological organ crosstalk:* Literature describes pathological crosstalk occurring in series or parallel.[4] The end point is a multiorgan dysfunction.
   - *Series **(Fig. 2)**:* Pathological organ crosstalk in series involves one organ dysfunction leading to the dysfunction of other organs one after another. An example of pathological organ crosstalk in series could be that which occurs in cardiogenic shock, wherein acute coronary syndrome results in acute kidney injury (AKI) and ischemic hepatitis.[5,6]
   - *Parallel **(Fig. 3)**:* In parallel organ crosstalk, there is independent but simultaneous failure of multiple organs. An example of this is septic shock, wherein sepsis leads to AKI, acute respiratory distress syndrome (ARDS), sepsis-induced cholestasis, and delirium.[7] It involves the activation of cytokines and interaction between pathogen-associated molecular patterns (PAMPs) and damage-associated molecular patterns (DAMPs) leading to disruption in the homeostatic mechanisms in the human body, amounting to multiorgan dysfunction.[7,8]

MECHANISMS OF ORGAN CROSSTALK

Understanding how organ injury propagates requires examining not only the patterns of interaction (series vs. parallel) but also the underlying biological mechanisms driving this communication. Organ crosstalk occurs when the function or injury of one organ affects other organs. This interaction can happen at two levels:

1. *Cellular level:*[9] At the cellular level, organ crosstalk involves signal interactions between:
    - Inflammatory cells (e.g., macrophages, T-cells, and B-cells)
    - Cytokines and chemokines
    - Intracellular signaling pathways

    These signals can either promote inflammation or contribute to tissue repair.
2. *Interorgan level:* At the organ-to-organ level, circulating molecules carry messages across the body. These signals allow distant organs to "communicate," but in critical illness, they can trigger multiorgan damage.[8]

Key Mechanisms Leading to Organ Injury (Fig. 4)

There are several mechanisms that lead to organ injury following this interaction. While these are diverse, they converge to produce systemic effects. In the critically ill, injury in one organ rarely remains isolated; instead, it sets off a chain reaction leading to dysfunction in multiple organs, as summarized in **Table 1**.

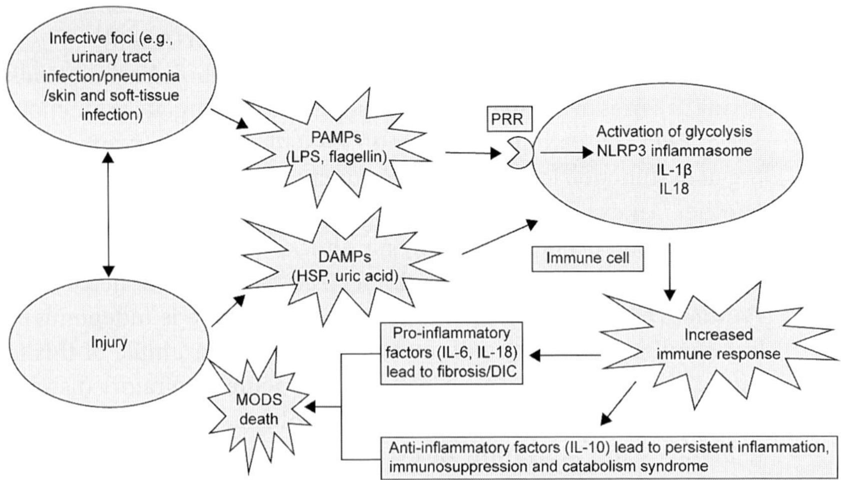

Fig. 4: Pathological organ crosstalk mechanisms. (DIC: disseminated intravascular coagulation; HSP: heat shock protein; LPS: lipopolysaccharide; MODS: multiple organ dysfunction syndrome; PAMPs: pathogen-associated molecular patterns; PRR: pattern recognition receptor)

TABLE 1: Various organ crosstalks.

Organ crosstalk	*Mechanisms*	*Management*
Brain–heart crosstalk	Acute brain injury → catecholamine surge → diastolic/systolic dysfunction, ischemia, arrhythmias, neurogenic stunned myocardium, and Takotsubo cardiomyopathy	Beta-blockers (ultra-short acting, selective), inotropes (levosimendan > dobutamine), avoid vasopressors, if possible, consider IABP or ventricular support if refractory
Brain–lung crosstalk	TBI → catecholamine/ inflammatory surge → ARDS, neurogenic pulmonary edema, VILI, VAP; dysbiosis and lung microbiome alterations increase infection risk	Early lung-protective ventilation, prevent VAP, optimize oxygenation, monitor for dysbiosis; early microbiome modulation may help
Brain–microbiome crosstalk	Brain injury alters gut microbiota within 2 hours → dysbiosis → inflammatory activation (NF-κB and IL-6), gut barrier dysfunction, systemic inflammation; can affect kidney and CNS	Probiotics, microbiota transplantation, early enteral nutrition, minimizing unnecessary antibiotics
Brain–liver crosstalk	TBI activates microglia → systemic cytokine surge → liver releases SAA-1 → worsens neuroinflammation; liver highly sensitive to systemic inflammation	Monitor liver function, research into SAA-1 blockers; supportive management of liver dysfunction
Brain–kidney crosstalk	TBI → sympathetic activation → RAAS stimulation → renal vasoconstriction → ischemia; SIADH/CSW causes hyponatremia; risk of AKI	Ultra-selective β1-blockers (landiolol and esmolol), prefer inotropes (levosimendan), monitor electrolytes; avoid vasopressors if possible
Brain–gut crosstalk	Brain injury → splanchnic hypoperfusion + dysbiosis → barrier disruption, stress ulcers, gastroparesis, ↑ risk of multiorgan failure	Early enteral nutrition, PPI/H2 blockers, manage IAH, explore BPC 157 in trials
Brain–muscle crosstalk	Crosstalk via myokines → prolonged immobility worsens brain recovery; exercise improves hippocampal volume, cognition	Early mobilization, physiotherapy, and ICU rehabilitation

Contd...

Contd...

Organ crosstalk	*Mechanisms*	*Management*
Brain–skin crosstalk	Brain injury alters neuroimmunologic signaling → skin immune dysfunction → infections, dermatitis, and drug eruptions	Skin care, infection prevention, and manage immune dysregulation
Kidney–lung crosstalk	AKI → ↑ pulmonary edema, respiratory failure; ARDS can worsen AKI; mechanical ventilation increases AKI risk	Optimize fluid balance, lung-protective ventilation, early AKI detection, RRT as needed
Kidney–heart crosstalk	AKI → volume overload, metabolic derangements → arrhythmias, acute heart failure (type 3 CRS); conversely, acute cardiac events → AKI (type 1 CRS)	Fluid and electrolyte optimization, early detection of CRS, RRT if severe
Kidney–vascular crosstalk	AKI → ischemia and endothelial dysfunction; sepsis causes interstitial inflammation, thrombosis; tubuloglomerular feedback disrupted	Hemodynamic optimization, avoid prolonged hypotension, early sepsis management
Kidney–liver crosstalk	AKI → toxin accumulation →↑ hepatic load; liver dysfunction (e.g., cirrhosis) → hepatorenal syndrome via RAAS and NO-mediated vasodilation	Treat underlying liver disease, consider vasoconstrictors and albumin in HRS, RRT if needed
Kidney–gut crosstalk	AKI → dysbiosis, uremic toxins, gut barrier dysfunction → multiorgan injury; gut inflammation worsens AKI	Probiotics, prebiotics, gut barrier protection, treat sepsis early
Kidney–brain crosstalk	AKI → uremic toxins, cytokine activation → encephalopathy, seizures, coma; cerebrovascular injury → AKI	RRT for severe AKI, avoid neurotoxic metabolites, antioxidants, RAAS modulation

(AKI: acute kidney injury; ARDS: acute respiratory distress syndrome; CNS: central nervous system; HRS: hepatorenal syndrome; IABP: intra-aortic balloon pump; IAH: intra-abdominal hypertension; ICU: intensive care unit; IL-6: interleukin-6; NF-κB: nuclear factor-kappa B; PPI: proton pump inhibitor; RAAS: renin–angiotensin–aldosterone system; RRT: renal replacement therapy; TBI: traumatic brain injury; CRS: cardiorenal syndrome; VAP: ventilator-associated pneumonia; VILI: ventilator-induced lung injury)

- *Release of cytokines (PAMPs and DAMPs)*:
  - *DAMPs*:[8]
    - Released from injured or stressed cells (mitochondria, nucleus, and cytosol)
    - Include:
      - Protein DAMPs: HMGB1, heat shock proteins, and S100
      - Nonprotein DAMPs: DNA, nucleotides, and uric acid
  - *PAMPs:*[8,10]
    - Released by microorganisms (e.g., LPS from bacterial and viral RNA)
    - Recognized by pattern recognition receptors (PRRs) like toll-like receptors (TLRs) and NOD-like receptors (NLRs)
  - *Effect:* Binding of PAMPs/DAMPs to PRRs triggers cytokine release [tumor necrosis factor-α (TNF-α), interleukin-1 (IL-1), and interleukin-6 (IL-6)], chemokines, and growth factors → inflammation and organ injury.
  - *Examples:*[8]
    - HMGB1: Cardiotoxic, increases endothelial permeability
    - Histones: Toxic to heart and endothelium
    - Extracellular CRP1: Activates NLRP3 inflammasome → cytokine storm → ARDS and endothelial dysfunction
    - RAGE activation: Triggers widespread proinflammatory cytokines → multiorgan dysfunction
- *Immune cell interaction:*[11]
  - Macrophages, T-cells, and B-cells communicate extensively
  - *Example:* Heart–gut axis, where gut immune cells influence heart inflammation via microbiota
- *Metabolic dysregulation:* Adipose tissue secretes proteins, lipids, and microRNAs that link obesity, metabolic syndrome, and cardiovascular disease.[12,13]
- *Neurohumoral mechanisms:* The autonomic nervous system and hypothalamic-pituitary axis mediate brain–organ crosstalk via neurotransmitters and hormones. Example—paroxysmal sympathetic hyperactivity after traumatic brain injury.[14]

From Single Organ Injury to Multiorgan Dysfunction—the Impact Of Organ Crosstalk (Table 1)

Organ crosstalk is bidirectional and involves neural, humoral, immune, and metabolic pathways. While **Table 1** provides detailed descriptions, some important patterns are worth highlighting.

- *Brain–organ crosstalk:* Acute brain injury can precipitate cardiac dysfunction (Takotsubo cardiomyopathy and arrhythmias),[15,16] lung injury (neurogenic pulmonary edema, and ARDS),[17] and systemic dysbiosis[18] that propagates inflammation and organ damage. The brain-gut-microbiome axis is particularly important, with dysbiosis leading to systemic inflammation and immune dysregulation.[18]

- *Kidney-organ crosstalk:* AKI worsens outcomes in the heart, lungs, liver, and brain through toxin accumulation, immune activation, and hemodynamic changes.[19-21] Conversely, cardiac, pulmonary, and hepatic dysfunction frequently trigger secondary AKI (cardiorenal, lung-kidney, and hepatorenal syndromes).[22-25]
- *Gut-liver-microbiome axis:* Gut barrier failure in critical illness permits bacterial translocation, fueling systemic inflammation, hepatic dysfunction, and septic encephalopathy.[26-28] Dysbiosis amplifies injury but also represents a therapeutic target (probiotics and fecal transplantation).
- *Heart-lung-kidney axis:* Myocardial injury, ARDS, and renal dysfunction often coexist in sepsis and shock, each amplifying the other via cytokine release, altered perfusion, and immune-metabolic stress.[29,30]

These interorgan links explain why single-organ injury in critical illness so often evolves into multiorgan dysfunction.[30]

Over the next few sections, we will look at few typical conditions where organ crosstalk is most striking. Sepsis exemplifies pathological crosstalk, where inflammatory, immune, and metabolic pathways amplify injury across multiple organs.[30] Similarly, sepsis-related ARDS highlights how the lungs both influence and are influenced by distant organ dysfunction, making these syndromes key models for understanding maladaptive organ communication.[31]

ORGAN CROSSTALK IN SEPSIS

Sepsis is dysregulated immune response to an infection that leads to organ dysfunction.[32] Septic shock is a severe form of sepsis with significant circulatory, cellular, and metabolic dysfunction. Initially an insult/injury leads to activation of innate immune system, particularly the inflammasomes which in turn causes release of proinflammatory cytokines such as IL-6, TNF-α and interferon-γ (IFN-γ) along with activation of coagulation system.[32] This leads to a shifting of metabolism from oxidative phosphorylation to the glycolytic pathway causing organ dysfunction.[33] To restore organ function, switching back of the metabolism from glycolytic pathway to oxidative phosphorylation is necessary.

Counter-regulatory mechanisms attempt to modulate the inflammatory process. Corticosteroids play a key role, and inadequate activity may cause critical illness-related corticosteroid insufficiency (CIRCI),[34] where supplementation can improve outcomes. Failure to control hyperinflammation leads to refractory shock and multiorgan dysfunction, while survivors may develop persistent inflammation, immunosuppression, and catabolism syndrome (PICS).[35] The balance between hyperinflammation and immune suppression is influenced by organ crosstalk. Extracorporeal therapies such as high-volume hemofiltration and hemadsorption have been explored to reduce inflammatory mediators, but their effects on organ crosstalk remain unclear.[36]

The following types of organ crosstalk may occur in sepsis:

- *Heart-lung-kidney crosstalk:*[29] Sepsis causes release of inflammatory mediators such as IL-6 and TNF-α. These in turn effect the functioning of the heart, lungs, and kidneys creating a vicious cycle:
    - Heart—inflammatory mediators cause myocardial injury and release of cardiokines [e.g., atrial natriuretic factor (ANF), brain natriuretic peptide (BNP), transforming growth factor β-1 (TGFβ1), and angiotensin II] resulting in vasoplegia, oxidative stress and autonomic dysfunction, and heart rate variability → RAAS and β-stimulation → cardiac dysfunction, decreased perfusion, decreased organ function
    - Lung—sepsis often precipitates ARDS → increased production of IL-1, IL-6, and TNF-α → increased capillary permeability, hypoxemia, and hypercarbia → ventilator associated injury
    - Kidney—oxidative stress reduces glomerular function → increased IL-6 and TNF-α → uremia, fluid overload, metabolic acidosis, and electrolyte dysfunction.

  Together, these changes accelerate multiorgan dysfunction. Renal replacement therapy can help by clearing toxins and fluid, but its ability to modify organ crosstalk remains uncertain. The brain also modulates lung inflammation. Proper activation of the cholinergic pathway may reduce inflammatory damage, but overactivation can increase susceptibility to infection and worsen lung injury. Lung-protective ventilation strategies and sedatives such as morphine, dexmedetomidine, and propofol may exert anti-inflammatory benefits, limiting secondary brain injury.
- *Gut-microbiome-liver-brain crosstalk:* The gut microbiota maintains digestion, immunity, and defense against pathogens. In sepsis, barrier disruption leads to bacterial and toxin translocation, resulting in ileus, feeding intolerance, and bleeding. Antibiotics, vasopressors, opioids, and mechanical ventilation further promote dysbiosis. Normally, gut microbiota produce short-chain fatty acids with anti-inflammatory effects, but their loss worsens systemic inflammation.[37]

  Gut dysfunction worsens liver injury.[38] Under septic stress, the liver produces inflammatory cytokines and hepatokines (e.g., adropin, FGF-21, and hepassocin), fueling systemic inflammation, insulin resistance, coagulopathy, and cardiovascular dysfunction. Liver failure synergizes with renal dysfunction to amplify toxin accumulation.

In the brain, as mentioned earlier, there is activation of glial cells and neuroinflammation which leads to secretion of corticotropin-releasing hormone (CRH) and cortisol as well as adrenaline, vasopressin and serotonin. This in turn leads to disruption of microbiota-gut-brain axis homeostasis as well as the blood-brain barrier, hence causing neurological dysfunction (septic encephalopathy) including impaired concentration and apathy. This can progress to delirium, confusion, and coma.

- *Adipose tissue-muscle-bone crosstalk:* Adipose tissue releases adipokines[12] (leptin, adiponectin, resistin, and TNF-α) that regulate systemic inflammation, while brown adipose tissue secretes "batokines"[39] (FGF-21, IL-6, and microRNAs) influencing metabolism and immunity. Their precise role in sepsis is unclear. Leptin is proinflammatory.

  Muscle and bone also contribute. Muscles secrete myokines (IL-6, irisin, myostatin, and FGF-21), while bone produces osteokines (osteocalcin and sclerostin), affecting muscle mass and nutrient metabolism.[40] Muscle wasting in sepsis promotes osteoporosis, while disturbances in vitamin D, calcium, and phosphate metabolism disrupt bone-muscle-kidney-liver communication. Collectively, this axis modulates systemic inflammation and recovery, but current understanding is limited.

  Organ crosstalk in sepsis occurs between native organs, artificial organs, or combinations of both. Current management strategies, based on clinical improvement and biomarkers, have not substantially reduced mortality. A promising avenue is identifying impaired organ crosstalk before overt dysfunction develops.

ORGAN CROSSTALK IN SEPSIS-RELATED ACUTE RESPIRATORY DISTRESS SYNDROME (TABLE 2)

Sepsis-related ARDS can be classified as pulmonary (PSA) or extra-pulmonary (ESA).[31] The underlying mechanisms are multifactorial.

- *Systemic inflammation:* Infection triggers cytokine release, endothelial activation, and coagulation, resulting in microthrombosis, hypoperfusion, and ischemic hypoxia. Organ-specific effects amplify systemic injury—pulmonary edema worsens hypoxia, liver, and kidney dysfunction reduce toxin clearance, and the spleen releases cytokines. Yet, why the lungs remain particularly vulnerable in sepsis remains unclear, raising the question of whether systemic inflammation has organ-specific bias.[41]
- *Microbiome disruption:* In ESA, intestinal barrier dysfunction and dysbiosis enable bacterial translocation, while pulmonary endothelial injury facilitates toxin entry into alveoli.[42] Microbial metabolites such as lipopolysacharides (LPS) mediate organ crosstalk and reshape immune responses. Emerging therapeutic strategies include: (1) Barrier-protective

agents (e.g., terlipressin) to reduce gut translocation, (2) selective digestive decontamination to prevent secondary infections, and (3) microbiota-directed therapies (e.g., fecal microbiota transplantation) to restore microbial balance.

- *Cascade of cell injury and death:* Organ injury releases mediators that propagate local and systemic immune alterations. Macrophages play a central role—during sepsis, they undergo phenotypic changes in the heart, liver, lungs, and kidneys. Pyroptotic macrophages transmit death signals

TABLE 2: Organ crosstalk between lung and extrapulmonary organs in PSA.

Type of organ crosstalk	*Manifestations*	*Mechanisms involved*	*Therapeutic implications*
Lung–brain crosstalk	• Cognitive decline • Neurocognitive deficits • Atrophy • Anxiety and depression	• Barrier disruption and bacterial translocation → microglia activation → inflammation • Direct lung brain neural pathways independent of inflammation	• Therapeutic strategies include targeting inflammation, repairing the barrier, and remodeling microbiota • Modulating CRH responses could alleviate acute symptoms, or disrupting biofilms could combat chronic immune evasion
Lung–kidney crosstalk	Acute kidney injury (AKI)	• Lung injury → platelet-dependent injury to kidneys • Mechanical ventilation → inflammation → AKI	• More research is needed to study platelet-dependent injury and target the same • Balance between lung protective ventilation and minimizing AKI
Lung–gut crosstalk	Intestinal injury → disruption of intestinal barrier → bacterial translocation and problems associated with it	*Bidirectional:* • Lung injury → inflammation → intestinal injury by pathogens and cytokines • Intestinal injury → aggravates lung injury (feed forward loop)	• Interventions like Bcl-2 overexpression or epidermal growth factor halt apoptosis, restore villus architecture, and improve survival • Restoring microbiota homeostasis and blocking intestinal apoptosis may disrupt the lung-gut axis

Contd...

Contd...

Type of organ crosstalk	*Manifestations*	*Mechanisms involved*	*Therapeutic implications*
Lung–liver crosstalk	Hepatic dysfunction	*Bidirectional:* Lung → liver • Direct invasion by organism • Sepsis-driven immune dysregulation • Hepatotoxic agents like drugs Liver → lung • Hepatic NF-κB/ STAT3 signaling • Dysregulated acute-phase reactions	• Hepatic protection and usage of liver safe antimicrobials. Further development of liver safe antimicrobials • Targeting specific acute-phase pathways or transcriptional regulators such as STAT3
Lung–heart crosstalk	• Acute cardiac injury and remodeling • Long term—cardiac scarring	• Systemic inflammation • Direct pathogen-related injury • Necroptosis	Routine cardiac assessment for symptomatic patients

(CRH: corticotropin-releasing hormone; NF-κB: nuclear factor-kappa B)

to neutrophils via mitochondria-containing microvesicles, promoting neutrophil death and neutrophil extracellular trap (NET) formation.[43] This initiates a domino-like cascade of cell death across organs.

Unanswered questions include whether this crosstalk drives long-term dysfunction in distant organs and whether targeting dominant cell-death pathways in sepsis-related ARDS could offer therapeutic benefit.

The various organ crosstalk that occurs in ARDS is described in **Tables 2 and 3**.

Sepsis-related ARDS involves extensive lung–organ crosstalk, which differs in pulmonary (PSA) and extra-pulmonary (ESA) sepsis.

In *PSA*, lung–brain interactions manifest as cognitive decline, depression, and anxiety due to barrier disruption, bacterial translocation, and microglial activation;[44] potential therapies include anti-inflammatory strategies, microbiota modulation, and CRH pathway targeting.

- Lung–kidney crosstalk contributes to AKI through platelet-dependent mechanisms and mechanical ventilation, highlighting the need for balancing lung-protective ventilation with renal safety.[45,46]
- *The lung–gut axis operates bidirectionally:* Lung inflammation worsens intestinal barrier injury and vice versa, forming a feed-forward

TABLE 3: Organ crosstalk between lung and extrapulmonary in ESA.

Type of organ crosstalk	*Manifestations*	*Mechanisms involved*	*Therapeutic implications*
Brain–lung crosstalk	• Encephalopathy • Ventilator-associated pneumonia • Post-stroke pneumonia	• "Blast injury" hypothesis • Two-hit theory • Brain–gut–lung triple blow hypothesis	• Maintenance of stable blood pressure • Prevention of pulmonary infections • Preservation of gut microbiota (all above require further clinical validation)
Kidney–lung crosstalk	Kidney injury → lung injury	• Ligand-receptor interaction [osteopontin (OPN) is the prime mediator in AKI-induced lung injury. AKI → upregulation of OPN → CD44 receptors in lungs → lung injury] • Metabolic reprogramming (shift from oxidative phosphorylation to aerobic glycolysis in renal tubular cells) • Neuro-immunomodulation (renal afferent vagus nerve → activate brain C1 neurons → splenic anti-inflammatory IL-10 production → may protect from lung injury)	• Targeting OPN may have a therapeutic potential • Targeting mitochondrial dysfunction may be of therapeutic benefit • Clinical trials using the cholinergic anti-inflammatory pathway (leading to increased splenic IL-10 production) show favorable outcomes for lung injury
Gut–lung crosstalk	Gut injury → lung injury	• Gut microbial translocation • Metabolite-mediated gut–lung axis • Direct migration of gut immune cells to the lungs (γδ T17 cells migration to lungs → IL-17A → lung injury)	Further studies to find out the role of other immune cell types in extrapulmonary sepsis are needed

Contd...

Contd...

Type of organ crosstalk	*Manifestations*	*Mechanisms involved*	*Therapeutic implications*
Liver–lung crosstalk	Hepatic dysfunction → lung injury	• Systemic accumulation of toxins and impaired pathogen clearance • Hypercoagulability → pulmonary microthrombosis and platelet activation → worsening of lung injury • Detachment of NETs from hepatic vasculature → pulmonary vascular embolization • Increased bile acids → decreased surfactant • Indirectly through liver–gut–lung axis	Hepatic protection and usage of liver safe antimicrobials. Further development of liver safe antimicrobials
Heart–lung crosstalk	Heart injury → lung injury	• Systemic inflammation • Circulatory abnormalities • Metabolic abnormalities	Crosstalk between hearts and lungs needs further studies

(IL-10: interleukin-10)

loop. Strategies include microbiota restoration and antiapoptotic interventions.[31]

- Lung–liver crosstalk involves bidirectional injury via immune dysregulation, direct invasion, hepatotoxic drugs, and NF-κB/STAT3 signaling, suggesting benefit from liver-safe antimicrobials and targeted pathway modulation.[31]
- Lung–heart crosstalk contributes to acute cardiac injury, remodeling, and necroptosis, warranting routine cardiac monitoring.[47]

In *ESA:*

- Brain–lung interactions underlie encephalopathy and pneumonia through mechanisms such as the "two-hit" and "brain–gut–lung" hypotheses.[31]
- Kidney–lung crosstalk is mediated by osteopontin (OPN)–CD44 signaling, metabolic reprogramming, and vagus-mediated neuroimmune modulation;[48-50] therapeutic targets include OPN, mitochondrial protection, and IL-10-based anti-inflammatory pathways.

- Gut-lung interactions involve microbial translocation, metabolites, and immune cell migration (e.g., γδ T17 cells).[51]
- Liver-lung crosstalk causes pulmonary microthrombosis, neuroendocrine tumor (NET) embolization, and surfactant dysfunction.[52]
- Heart-lung crosstalk reflects systemic inflammation, circulatory, and metabolic abnormalities but requires further study.[31]

ROLE OF EXTRACELLULAR VESICLES IN SEPSIS AND ARDS-RELATED ORGAN CROSSTALK

One emerging concept linking sepsis and ARDS-related crosstalk is the role of extracellular vesicles (EVs).[53,54] These vesicles act as messengers, amplifying inflammation and injury across organs. EVs are related to sepsis severity. The role of EVs (exosomes, microvesicles, microsomes, and apoptotic bodies) in organ crosstalk in sepsis-related ARDS is as follows:

- Domino like cascade of cell injury and death as described above
- Modulate immunity—by delivery of LPS/also modulate immune cell functions by influencing neutrophil migration, macrophage functioning, and T and B-cell maturation, improving antigen presentation
- Impair endothelial barrier function
- Alter metabolism—shift from oxidative phosphorylation to aerobic glycolysis
- Promote thrombosis
- Facilitate both short-range and long-range communication, indicating that possible transport pathways for EV-mediated organ crosstalk exist.

Extracellular vesicles may be the potential mechanisms and therapeutic targets for crosstalk between lung and extrapulmonary organs in sepsis-related ARDS. Further research is needed in this area.

ROLE OF ARTIFICIAL INTELLIGENCE IN ORGAN CROSSTALK

Given the complexity of these networks—from cytokines to vesicles—traditional research approaches may be insufficient. Artificial intelligence (AI) offers new ways to map and predict patterns of organ crosstalk.

Artificial intelligence offers a powerful tool to study organ crosstalk, which cannot be fully understood through isolated experiments or limited datasets. By applying machine learning algorithms and computational models, AI enables the integration and analysis of large-scale data, helping to map connections between multiple organs. For example, construction of a pan-organ gerontological geography (GG) map has revealed shared features of multiorgan aging, including tissue disorganization, cellular identity loss, and immunoglobulin accumulation.[55] Wen et al. demonstrated, using support vector machines and multiorgan causal networks, a relationship between Alzheimer's disease and biological age gaps in the brain, liver, musculoskeletal system, and kidneys.[56]

Areas in which AI can be useful in organ crosstalk are as follows:

- *Central and peripheral organ interactions:*[57] Interactions between the central nervous system and peripheral organs have organ-specific regulatory mechanisms mediated through distinct pathways:
    - Neural connections among brain-heart/lung/kidney—autonomic nervous system, respiratory control via brainstem nuclei, bidirectional lung–brain axis, renal via RAAS, and hypothalamic-paraventricular neural circuits.
    - Endocrine and metabolic connections between brain and liver through hypothalamic-pituitary-adrenal (HPA) axis, hepatokines, and hormones.
    - Immune connections in brain-spleen through the cholinergic anti-inflammatory pathway.

  These complex and multilevel connections highlight the difficulty of studying crosstalk, but AI can integrate diverse datasets to uncover insights not visible in single analyses.
- Combination of genomics and proteomics to correlate genetic variations with protein expression and function. Metabolomics plays a crucial role in the integration of omics data. It provides an insight into the metabolic process in cells and organs. Integrating metabolomic data with genomic and proteomic data helps to understand the interaction between these three pathways.[57] Although challenges remain in interpreting molecular roles, this approach may help to create personalized models of sepsis, guiding earlier diagnosis and novel therapeutic strategies.

Despite these advances, challenges remain: The dynamic nature of organ interactions complicates analysis and integrating diverse datasets while establishing standardized methodologies is still a limitation.

CONCLUSION

Organ crosstalk is central to the progression from localized injury to multiorgan dysfunction in critical illness. Physiological crosstalk maintains homeostasis, whereas pathological crosstalk amplifies inflammation, ischemia, and metabolic stress, driving poor outcomes. Mechanistic insights—from cytokine cascades and DAMP/PAMP signaling to microbiome disruption and EV trafficking—have broadened our understanding, but therapeutic translation remains limited.

Sepsis and sepsis-related ARDS exemplify the complexity of organ interactions, with cascading heart–lung–kidney and gut–liver–brain loops accelerating dysfunction. AI and multiomics approaches offer promising tools to map these networks more precisely, while targeted therapies such as immune modulation, microbiome restoration, and extracorporeal interventions are under exploration.

Future research must focus on early detection of maladaptive crosstalk, identification of predictive biomarkers, and development of interventions that restore physiological interorgan communication. A deeper understanding of these interactions may have the potential not only to improve survival but also to reduce long-term sequelae in survivors of critical illness.

REFERENCES

1. Campagna JA, Carter C. Clinical relevance of the Bezold-Jarisch reflex. Anesthesiology. 2003;98(5):1250-60.
2. Dutschmann M, Bautista TG, Mörschel M, Dick TE. Learning to breathe: Habituation of Hering–Breuer inflation reflex emerges with postnatal brainstem maturation. Respir Physiol Neurobiol. 2014;195:44-9.
3. Sparks MA, Crowley SD, Gurley SB, Mirotsou M, Coffman TM. Classical Renin-Angiotensin system in kidney physiology. Compr Physiol. 2014;4(3):1201-28.
4. Saran S, Gurjar M. Brain Crosstalk with Other Organs in ICU Patient. J Neuroanaesth Crit Care. 2019;06(3):299-304.
5. Cruz DN. Cardiorenal Syndrome in Critical Care: The Acute Cardiorenal and Renocardiac Syndromes. Advances in Chronic Kidney Disease. 2013;20(1):56-66.
6. Ciobanu AO, Gherasim L. Ischemic Hepatitis - Intercorrelated Pathology. Maedica (Bucur). 2018;13(1):5-11.
7. Bauer M, Coldewey SM, Leitner M, Löffler B, Weis S, Wetzker R. Deterioration of Organ Function As a Hallmark in Sepsis: The Cellular Perspective. Front Immunol. 2018;9:1460.
8. Cicchinelli S, Pignataro G, Gemma S, Piccioni A, Picozzi D, Ojetti V, et al. PAMPs and DAMPs in Sepsis: A Review of Their Molecular Features and Potential Clinical Implications. Int J Mol Sci. 2024;25(2):962.
9. Armutcu F. Organ crosstalk: the potent roles of inflammation and fibrotic changes in the course of organ interactions. Inflamm Res. 2019;68(10):825-39.
10. Rai V, Mathews G, Agrawal DK. Translational and Clinical Significance of DAMPs, PAMPs, and PRRs in Trauma-induced Inflammation. Archives of Clinical and Biomedical Research. 2022;6(5):673-85.
11. Ren H, Zhu B, An Y, Xie F, Wang Y, Tan Y. Immune communication between the intestinal microbiota and the cardiovascular system. Immunology Letters. 2023;254:13-20.
12. Tilg H, Ianiro G, Gasbarrini A, Adolph TE. Adipokines: masterminds of metabolic inflammation. Nat Rev Immunol. 2025;25(4):250-65.
13. Guay C, Regazzi R. Exosomes as new players in metabolic organ cross-talk. Diabetes Obes Metab. 2017;19 Suppl 1:137-46.
14. Meyfroidt G, Baguley IJ, Menon DK. Paroxysmal sympathetic hyperactivity: the storm after acute brain injury. Lancet Neurol. 2017;16(9):721-9.
15. Krishnamoorthy V, Mackensen GB, Gibbons EF, Vavilala MS. Cardiac Dysfunction After Neurologic Injury: What Do We Know and Where Are We Going? Chest. 2016;149(5):1325-31.
16. Lenstra JJ, Kuznecova-Keppel Hesselink L, la Bastide-van Gemert S, Jacobs B, Nijsten MWN, van der Horst ICC, et al. The Association of Early

Electrocardiographic Abnormalities With Brain Injury Severity and Outcome in Severe Traumatic Brain Injury. Front Neurol. 2020;11:597737.
17. Picetti E, Pelosi P, Taccone FS, Citerio G, Mancebo J, Robba C, et al. VENTILatOry strategies in patients with severe traumatic brain injury: the VENTILO Survey of the European Society of Intensive Care Medicine (ESICM). Crit Care. 2020;24(1):158.
18. Kotfis K, Siwicka-Gieroba D, Dąbrowski W. Brain–Multiorgan Cross-Talk in Critically Ill Patients with Acute Brain Injury. In: Vincent JL (Ed). Annual Update in Intensive Care and Emergency Medicine 2022. Cham: Springer International Publishing; 2022. pp. 317-31.
19. Vieira JM, Castro I, Curvello-Neto A, Demarzo S, Caruso P, Pastore L, et al. Effect of acute kidney injury on weaning from mechanical ventilation in critically ill patients. Crit Care Med. 2007;35(1):184-91.
20. Di Lullo L, Reeves PB, Bellasi A, Ronco C. Cardiorenal Syndrome in Acute Kidney Injury. Semin Nephrol. 2019;39(1):31-40.
21. Li X, Yuan F, Zhou L. Organ Crosstalk in Acute Kidney Injury: Evidence and Mechanisms. J Clin Med. 2022;11(22):6637.
22. Darmon M, Clec'h C, Adrie C, Argaud L, Allaouchiche B, Azoulay E, et al. Acute Respiratory Distress Syndrome and Risk of AKI among Critically Ill Patients. Clin J Am Soc Nephrol. 2014;9(8):1347-53.
23. Palazzuoli A, Ruocco G. Heart-Kidney Interactions in Cardiorenal Syndrome Type 1. Adv Chronic Kidney Dis. 2018;25(5):408-17.
24. Simonetto DA, Gines P, Kamath PS. Hepatorenal syndrome: pathophysiology, diagnosis, and management. BMJ. 2020;370:m2687.
25. Zorrilla-Vaca A, Ziai W, Connolly Jr. ES, Geocadin R, Thompson R, Rivera-Lara L. Acute Kidney Injury Following Acute Ischemic Stroke and Intracerebral Hemorrhage: A Meta-Analysis of Prevalence Rate and Mortality Risk. Cerebrovasc Dis. 2017;45(1-2):1-9.
26. Giridharan VV, Generoso JS, Lence L, Candiotto G, Streck E, Petronilho F, et al. A crosstalk between gut and brain in sepsis-induced cognitive decline. J Neuroinflammation. 2022;19(1):114.
27. Pan S, Lv Z, Wang R, Shu H, Yuan S, Yu Y, et al. Sepsis-Induced Brain Dysfunction: Pathogenesis, Diagnosis, and Treatment. Oxid Med Cell Longev. 2022;2022:1328729.
28. Kim TH, Hong DG, Yang YM. Hepatokines and Non-Alcoholic Fatty Liver Disease: Linking Liver Pathophysiology to Metabolism. Biomedicines. 2021;9(12):1903.
29. Husain-Syed F, McCullough PA, Birk HW, Renker M, Brocca A, Seeger W, et al. Cardio-Pulmonary-Renal Interactions: A Multidisciplinary Approach. J Am Coll Cardiol. 2015;65(22):2433-48.
30. Borges A, Bento L. Organ crosstalk and dysfunction in sepsis. Ann Intensive Care. 2024;14(1):147.
31. Li B, Lin W, Hu R, Bai S, Ruan Y, Fan Y, et al. Crosstalk between lung and extrapulmonary organs in sepsis-related acute lung injury/acute respiratory distress syndrome. Ann Intensive Care. 2025;15(1):97.
32. Singer M, Deutschman CS, Seymour CW, Shankar-Hari M, Annane D, Bauer M, et al. The Third International Consensus Definitions for Sepsis and Septic Shock (Sepsis-3). JAMA. 2016;315(8):801-10.

33. Liu J, Zhou G, Wang X, Liu D. Metabolic reprogramming consequences of sepsis: adaptations and contradictions. Cell Mol Life Sci. 2022;79(8):456.
34. Annane D, Pastores SM, Arlt W, Balk RA, Beishuizen A, Briegel J, et al. Critical illness-related corticosteroid insufficiency (CIRCI): a narrative review from a Multispecialty Task Force of the Society of Critical Care Medicine (SCCM) and the European Society of Intensive Care Medicine (ESICM). Intensive Care Med. 2017;43(12):1781-92.
35. Mira JC, Brakenridge SC, Moldawer LL, Moore FA. Persistent Inflammation, Immunosuppression and Catabolism Syndrome (PICS). Crit Care Clin. 2017;33(2):245-58.
36. Ronco C, Ricci Z, Husain-Syed F. From Multiple Organ Support Therapy to Extracorporeal Organ Support in Critically Ill Patients. Blood Purif. 2019;48(2):99-105.
37. Krautkramer KA, Fan J, Bäckhed F. Gut microbial metabolites as multi-kingdom intermediates. Nat Rev Microbiol. 2021;19(2):77-94.
38. Di Ciaula A, Baj J, Garruti G, Celano G, De Angelis M, Wang HH, et al. Liver Steatosis, Gut-Liver Axis, Microbiome and Environmental Factors. A Never-Ending Bidirectional Cross-Talk. J Clin Med. 2020;9(8):2648.
39. Till A, Fries C, Fenske WK. Brain-to-BAT - and Back?: Crosstalk between the Central Nervous System and Thermogenic Adipose Tissue in Development and Therapy of Obesity. Brain Sci. 2022;12(12):1646.
40. Severinsen MCK, Pedersen BK. Muscle-Organ Crosstalk: The Emerging Roles of Myokines. Endocr Rev. 2020;41(4):594-609.
41. Zi SF, Wu XJ, Tang Y, Liang YP, Liu X, Wang L, et al. Endothelial Cell-Derived Extracellular Vesicles Promote Aberrant Neutrophil Trafficking and Subsequent Remote Lung Injury. Adv Sci (Weinh). 2024;11(38):e2400647.
42. Tang J, Xu L, Zeng Y, Gong F. Effect of gut microbiota on LPS-induced acute lung injury by regulating the TLR4/NF-kB signaling pathway. Int Immunopharmacol. 2021;91:107272.
43. Kuang L, Wu Y, Shu J, Yang J, Zhou H, Huang X. Pyroptotic Macrophage-Derived Microvesicles Accelerate Formation of Neutrophil Extracellular Traps via GSDMD-N-expressing Mitochondrial Transfer during Sepsis. Int J Biol Sci. 2024;20(2):733-50.
44. Hopkins RO, Weaver LK, Collingridge D, Parkinson RB, Chan KJ, Orme JF. Two-year cognitive, emotional, and quality-of-life outcomes in acute respiratory distress syndrome. Am J Respir Crit Care Med. 2005;171(4):340-7.
45. Singbartl K, Bishop JV, Wen X, Murugan R, Chandra S, Filippi MD, et al. Differential effects of kidney-lung cross-talk during acute kidney injury and bacterial pneumonia. Kidney Int. 2011;80(6):633-44.
46. van den Akker JPC, Egal M, Groeneveld ABJ. Invasive mechanical ventilation as a risk factor for acute kidney injury in the critically ill: a systematic review and meta-analysis. Crit Care. 2013;17(3):R98.
47. Reyes LF, Restrepo MI, Hinojosa CA, Soni NJ, Anzueto A, Babu BL, et al. Severe Pneumococcal Pneumonia Causes Acute Cardiac Toxicity and Subsequent Cardiac Remodeling. Am J Respir Crit Care Med. 2017;196(5):609-20.
48. Khamissi FZ, Ning L, Kefaloyianni E, Dun H, Arthanarisami A, Keller A, et al. Identification of kidney injury released circulating osteopontin as causal agent of respiratory failure. Sci Adv. 2022;8(8):eabm5900.

49. Liu C, Wei W, Huang Y, Fu P, Zhang L, Zhao Y. Metabolic reprogramming in septic acute kidney injury: pathogenesis and therapeutic implications. Metabolism. 2024;158:155974.
50. Tanaka S, Abe C, Abbott SBG, Zheng S, Yamaoka Y, Lipsey JE, et al. Vagus nerve stimulation activates two distinct neuroimmune circuits converging in the spleen to protect mice from kidney injury. Proc Natl Acad Sci U S A. 2021;118(12):e2021758118.
51. Xie B, Wang M, Zhang X, Zhang Y, Qi H, Liu H, et al. Gut-derived memory γδ T17 cells exacerbate sepsis-induced acute lung injury in mice. Nat Commun. 2024;15(1):6737.
52. Maiwall R, Kulkarni AV, Arab JP, Piano S. Acute liver failure. Lancet. 2024;404(10454):789-802.
53. Welsh JA, Goberdhan DCI, O'Driscoll L, Buzas EI, Blenkiron C, Bussolati B, et al. Minimal information for studies of extracellular vesicles (MISEV2023): From basic to advanced approaches. J Extracell Vesicles. 2024;13(2):e12404.
54. Lehner GF, Harler U, Haller VM, Feistritzer C, Hasslacher J, Dunzendorfer S, et al. Characterization of Microvesicles in Septic Shock Using High-Sensitivity Flow Cytometry. Shock. 2016;46(4):373-81.
55. Ma S, Ji Z, Zhang B, Geng L, Cai Y, Nie C, et al. Spatial transcriptomic landscape unveils immunoglobin-associated senescence as a hallmark of aging. Cell. 2024;187(24):7025-7044.e34.
56. Wen J, Tian YE, Skampardoni I, Yang Z, Cui Y, Anagnostakis F, et al. The genetic architecture of biological age in nine human organ systems. Nat Aging. 2024;4(9):1290-307.
57. Chen Y, Yang M, Hua Q. Artificial intelligence in central-peripheral interaction organ crosstalk: the future of drug discovery and clinical trials. Pharmacol Res. 2025;215:107734.

CHAPTER 5

Extracorporeal Therapies in Toxicology

Kushal R Kalvit

INTRODUCTION

Extracorporeal therapy (ECTR) in the context of toxicology is an umbrella term that comprises multiple modalities which serve the primary purpose of removal of a toxic substance from the blood. At the same time, it also provides temporary support to one or more failing organs. Although the use of ECTR in poisoning cases is scarce, it remains a lifesaving intervention in selected cases.[1] The use of ECTR as a rescue measure in poisoning dates to >100 years old when it was demonstrated to be useful for the removal of salicylates from animal blood.[2] Unlike the technological advancements and their expanded indications in other domains of the medical world, the evidence-based use of ECTR in toxicology remains elusive. In order to mitigate this issue, a multinational and multidisciplinary group called EXTRIP (extracorporeal treatments in poisoning) was formed to study and formulate evidence as well as expert opinion-based guidelines for the use of ECTR in toxicological cases.[3]

MODALITIES IN EXTRACORPOREAL THERAPY

The various modalities available for the removal of toxic substances from blood are listed below. Each of the therapies have their own pros and cons and would be selected based on the toxic agent in question and the clinical picture.[4]

- *Hemodialysis:* This method filters the blood using a dialysis machine and a semipermeable membrane. It works on the principle of diffusion where the solutes move from a high concentration to lower concentration compartment across a semipermeable membrane. This is the ECTR modality of choice for almost all poisons. It is particularly effective for toxins that are water-soluble, have low molecular weight, and low protein binding.
- *Hemoperfusion:* In this technique, blood is passed through a cartridge containing adsorbent materials like activated charcoal or resins. It is useful for removing substances that are highly protein-bound or lipid-soluble.
- *Continuous renal replacement therapy (CRRT):* Typically used in critically ill patients, CRRT gradually removes toxins and fluids over an extended period. It is suitable for hemodynamically unstable patients who cannot

tolerate standard hemodialysis. It is also a suitable option for the treatment of toxins that warrant repeated ECTR due to the rebound phenomenon. The rebound phenomenon occurs when a toxic agent initially is redistributed into all compartments, removed from the blood by ECTR and then gradually diffuses back into the intravascular compartment from the extravascular/interstitial space. Lithium, dabigatran, vancomycin, and methotrexate often demonstrate a rebound phenomenon.

- *Plasmapheresis (therapeutic plasma exchange):* This procedure works on the principle of centrifugation and removes plasma containing harmful substances and replaces it with donor plasma or a substitute.
- *Exchange transfusion:* This involves replacing the patient's blood with donor blood to reduce toxin levels. It is used rarely but may be effective in severe poisoning cases, especially in neonates.
- *Peritoneal dialysis:* A less commonly used method today, this involves the exchange of fluids through the peritoneal cavity. It is generally reserved for patients in settings where hemodialysis is not available.
- *Extracorporeal membrane oxygenation (ECMO):* ECMO does not remove toxic agent from the body, but it is a vital modality to support the circulation as well as oxygenation in a severely poisoned patient in case of hemodynamic collapse or severe respiratory failure. It basically buys time for other therapies to act and organ function to improve.

DOES IT WORK FOR ALL POISONS?

The removal of a poison with the help of ECTR relies on multiple factors related to the poison itself as well as the clinical condition. The most important physicochemical properties of the toxic agent that determine its removal are volume of distribution, protein binding, and its endogenous clearance.

The volume of distribution (Vd) of a substance is the theoretical volume that would be required to contain the substance at the same concentration it has in the blood or plasma. A toxic agent with low volume of distribution would be restricted largely to the intravascular compartment and, hence, would be easily cleared by an extracorporeal method. On the contrary, agents with a high Vd are distributed widely in the extravascular space and are difficult to remove with ECTR. In general, lipophilic drugs have a higher Vd while hydrophilic drugs have a relatively low Vd. An agent with a volume of distribution >1–1.5 L/kg is poorly dialyzable.[5]

All toxic agents are bound to plasma proteins to some extent. However, owing to the large size and molecular weight of plasma proteins, the protein-bound fraction of poisons cannot be removed by dialysis filters. Substances with a protein binding of >80% are difficult to remove with conventional dialysis filters as they can remove molecules below 15,000 Daltons. However, high cutoff hemofilters can remove molecules with weight up to

50,000 Daltons. Plasmapheresis, on the other hand, can remove molecules of any size.[6,7] The endogenous clearance of a poison plays an important role in the utility of ECTR for treatment of any toxicity. If the endogenous route (hepatic, renal, or otherwise) is highly efficient in clearing the substance and is not dysfunctional, then ECTR would not add any benefit. The endogenous clearance via renal route for metformin is more efficient than extracorporeal removal. Hence, ECTR is not recommended in metformin toxicity unless renal impairment is also present.[8]

SELECTING A POISON FOR EXTRACORPOREAL THERAPY

While choosing ECTR for the management of poisoning, the following points need to be considered and ECTR employed only if the characteristics of that toxic agent fall into one or more of these criteria:[9]

- Exposure to the poison can cause serious mortality or morbidity.
- No antidote is present or antidote is unavailable due to logistical issues.
- Other techniques such as absorption inhibitors or enhanced elimination are of little benefit.
- Poison's endogenous clearance <4 mL/kg/min.
- Volume of distribution of the poison <1–1.5 L/kg and protein binding <80%.

EXTRIP GUIDELINES

The EXTRIP group has formulated guidelines for the international community regarding the indications, type of modality, and duration of ECTR in various poisoning cases. The guidelines are regularly updated and recommendations for newer poisons are added. A quick glance at the guidelines points out two important points that are common to almost all poisons. Firstly, ECTR should be continued till there is sustained and significant clinical improvement irrespective of the serum concentration of the toxic agent. Secondly, even if the choice of ECTR modality in all cases is intermittent hemodialysis (IHD), there would be many situations where IHD would not be tolerated by the patient due to hemodynamic instability or would have to be employed repeatedly due to the rebound phenomenon. In such cases, CRRT or even prolonged intermittent renal replacement therapy (PIRRT) [sustained low-efficiency dialysis (SLED)] is an effective alternative modality. Following is the list of poisons for which the EXTRIP group recommends ECTR therapy.

- *Acetaminophen (APAP) (paracetamol):*[10]
    - *Indications:*
        - APAP level >900 mg/L along with the presence of altered mental state, elevated lactate and metabolic acidosis even if N-acetylcysteine (NAC) is administered.
        - APAP level >1,000 mg/L, and NAC is not administered.

    - APAP level >700 mg/L along with the presence of altered mental state, elevated lactate, and metabolic acidosis, and NAC is not administered.
  - *Contraindications:* ECTR should not be started solely on the basis of APAP level if NAC has been administered.
  - *Modality:* IHD
  - *Duration:* To be continued till sustained clinical improvement seen.
- *Baclofen:*[11]
  - *Indications:* Toxicity from therapeutic baclofen in patients with renal impairment only in the presence of associated coma requiring ventilatory support.
  - *Contraindications:* Severe acute baclofen poisoning in the presence of normal renal function.
  - *Modality:* IHD
  - *Duration:* To be continued till sustained clinical improvement seen (watch for withdrawal symptoms).
- *Barbiturates:*[12]
  - *Indications:*
    - Presence of prolonged coma, refractory shock or toxic signs despite multiple-dose activated charcoal (MDAC) therapy
    - Respiratory depression necessitating mechanical ventilation
    - Rising barbiturate concentration despite MDAC therapy
  - *Modality:* IHD
  - *Duration:* Till clinical improvement observed
- *Beta-blockers:*[13]
  - *Indications:*
    - Atenolol toxicity in patients with renal impairment
    - Sotalol toxicity in patients with renal impairment
    - No recommendation made for or against in patients with β-blocker toxicity and normal renal function
  - *Modality:* IHD
  - *Duration:* Till sustained clinical improvement
- *Carbamazepine:*[14]
  - *Indications:*
    - Refractory seizures
    - Life-threatening arrhythmias
    - Prolonged coma or respiratory depression with ventilatory support
    - Rising carbamazepine concentrations despite MDAC therapy
  - *Modality:* IHD
  - *Duration:* Sustained clinical improvement and carbamazepine concentration below 10 mg/L.

- *Ethylene glycol (EG):*[15]
  - *Indications:*
    - EG concentration >310 mg/dL if fomepizole or ethanol is used.
    - EG concentration >62 mg/dL if no antidote is used.
    - If EG concentration is unavailable, ECTR is recommended if osmol gap is >50 or anion gap >27 mmol/L.
    - Coma, seizures, and in patients with acute kidney injury (AKI)
  - *Modality:* IHD
  - *Duration:* Anion gap is <18 mmol/L and EG concentration is <25 mg/dL.
- *Gabapentin/pregabalin:*[16]
  - *Indications:* Gabapentinoid toxicity in the presence of renal impairment
  - *Modality:* IHD
  - *Duration:* Sustained clinical improvement (monitor for withdrawal symptoms)
- *Lithium:*[17]
  - *Indications:*
    - Coma, seizures, or life-threatening arrhythmias
    - Renal impairment and lithium level >4.0 mEq/L
    - Lithium level >5.0 mEq/L and altered mental state
  - *Modality:* IHD
  - *Duration:* Lithium level <1.0 mEq/L and clinical improvement (serial measurements of lithium needed after cessation of ECTR)
- *Metformin:*[8]
  - *Indications:*
    - Lactate concentration >15–20 mmol/L
    - pH <7.1
    - Failure of standard supportive measures
    - Comorbid conditions such as shock, AKI, liver failure, and coma
  - *Modality:* IHD
  - *Duration:* Lactate <3 mmol/L and pH >7.35
- *Methanol:*[18]
  - *Indications:*
    - Coma, seizures, and new vision deficits (any of these)
    - Persistent metabolic acidosis (pH <7.15) or a serum anion gap >24 mmol/L
    - Renal dysfunction
    - Methanol concentration >700 mg/L (with fomepizole) or >500 mg/L (without fomepizole)
  - *Modality:* IHD
  - *Duration:* Clinical improvement and methanol concentration <200 mg/L

- *Phenytoin:*[19]
  - *Indications:* Prolonged coma and prolonged incapacitating ataxia (do not rely solely on phenytoin concentration)
  - *Modality:* IHD
  - *Duration:* Clinical improvement
- *Salicylates:*[20]
  - *Indications:*
    - Salicylate concentration >100 mg/dL or >90 mg/dL in presence of renal impairment
    - Altered mental status or new-onset hypoxemia
  - *Modality:* IHD
  - *Duration:* Clinical improvement and salicylate concentration <19 mg/dL
- *Thallium:*[21]
  - *Indications:*
    - Any suspicion of thallium poisoning based on history and clinical features
    - Thallium concentration >1 mg/L
  - *Modality:* IHD
  - *Duration:* Continue until thallium concentration is 0.1 mg/L for at least 72 hours.
- *Theophylline:*[22]
  - *Indications:*
    - Theophylline concentration >100 mg/L
    - Seizures, shock, or life-threatening dysrhythmias
  - *Modality:* IHD
  - *Duration:* Clinical improvement or theophylline concentration <15 mg/L
- *Valproic acid:*[23]
  - *Indications:*
    - Valproate concentration >1,300 mg/L
    - Shock or cerebral edema
    - Coma or respiratory depression with ventilatory support
    - Acute hyperammonemia or pH <7.1
  - *Modality:* IHD
  - *Duration:* Clinical improvement or valproate levels between 50 and 100 mg/L.

CONCLUSION

Extracorporeal therapies are indeed a lifesaving intervention in the management of severely poisoned patients. However, the employment of such modalities requires a thorough understanding of the pharmacokinetics of the toxic agent. More importantly, the initiation and cessation of ECTR should largely depend on the clinical picture rather than the laboratory values.

REFERENCES

1. Mowry JB, Spyker DA, Cantilena LR Jr, Bailey JE, Ford M. 2012 Annual Report of the American Association of Poison Control Centers' National Poison Data System (NPDS): 30th Annual Report. Clin Toxicol (Phila). 2013;51(10):949-1229.
2. Abel JJ, Rowntree LG, Turner BB. On the removal of diffusable substances from the circulating blood by means of dialysis. Transactions of the Association of American Physicians, 1913. Transfus Sci. 1990;11(2):164-5.
3. Lavergne V, Nolin TD, Hoffman RS, Roberts D, Gosselin S, Goldfarb DS, et al. The EXTRIP (EXtracorporeal TReatments In Poisoning) workgroup: guideline methodology. Clin Toxicol (Phila). 2012;50(5):403-13.
4. King JD, Kern MH, Jaar BG. Extracorporeal Removal of Poisons and Toxins. Clin J Am Soc Nephrol. 2019;14(9):1408-15.
5. Roberts DM, Buckley NA. Pharmacokinetic considerations in clinical toxicology: clinical applications. Clin Pharmacokinet. 2007;46(11):897-939.
6. Eloot S, Schneditz D, Cornelis T, Van Biesen W, Glorieux G, Dhondt A, et al. Protein-Bound Uremic Toxin Profiling as a Tool to Optimize Hemodialysis. PLoS One. 2016;11(1):e0147159.
7. Gondouin B, Hutchison CA. High cut-off dialysis membranes: current uses and future potential. Adv Chronic Kidney Dis. 2011;18(3):180-7.
8. Calello DP, Liu KD, Wiegand TJ, Roberts DM, Lavergne V, Gosselin S, et al. Extracorporeal treatment for metformin poisoning: systematic review and recommendations from the extracorporeal treatments in poisoning workgroup. Crit Care Med. 2015;43(8):1716-30.
9. Jha VK, Padmaprakash KV. Extracorporeal Treatment in the Management of acute poisoning: what an intensivist should know? Indian J Crit Care Med. 2018;22(12):862-9.
10. Gosselin S, Juurlink DN, Kielstein JT, Ghannoum M, Lavergne V, Nolin TD, et al. Extracorporeal treatment for acetaminophen poisoning: recommendations from the EXTRIP workgroup. Clin Toxicol (Phila). 2014;52(8):856-67.
11. Ghannoum M, Berling I, Lavergne V, Roberts DM, Galvao T, Hoffman RS, et al. Recommendations from the EXTRIP workgroup on extracorporeal treatment for baclofen poisoning. Kidney Int. 2021;100(4):720-36.
12. Mactier R, Laliberté M, Mardini J, Ghannoum M, Lavergne V, Gosselin S, et al. Extracorporeal treatment for barbiturate poisoning: recommendations from the EXTRIP Workgroup. Am J Kidney Dis. 2014;64(3):347-58.
13. Bouchard J, Shepherd G, Hoffman RS, Gosselin S, Roberts DM, Li Y, et al. Extracorporeal treatment for poisoning to beta-adrenergic antagonists: systematic review and recommendations from the EXTRIP workgroup. Crit Care. 2021;25(1):201.
14. Ghannoum M, Yates C, Galvao TF, Sowinski KM, Vo TH, Coogan A, et al. Extracorporeal treatment for carbamazepine poisoning: systematic review and recommendations from the EXTRIP workgroup. Clin Toxicol (Phila). 2014;52(10):993-1004.

15. Ghannoum M, Gosselin S, Hoffman RS, Lavergne V, Mégarbane B, Hassanian-Moghaddam H, et al. Extracorporeal treatment for ethylene glycol poisoning: systematic review and recommendations from the EXTRIP workgroup. Crit Care. 2023;27(1):56.
16. Bouchard J, Yates C, Calello DP, Gosselin S, Roberts DM, Lavergne V, et al. Extracorporeal treatment for gabapentin and pregabalin poisoning: systematic review and recommendations from the EXTRIP workgroup. Am J Kidney Dis. 2022;79(1):88-104.
17. Decker BS, Goldfarb DS, Dargan PI, Friesen M, Gosselin S, Hoffman RS, et al. Extracorporeal Treatment for Lithium Poisoning: Systematic Review and Recommendations from the EXTRIP Workgroup. Clin J Am Soc Nephrol. 2015;10(5):875-87.
18. Roberts DM, Yates C, Megarbane B, Winchester JF, Maclaren R, Gosselin S, et al. Recommendations for the role of extracorporeal treatments in the management of acute methanol poisoning: a systematic review and consensus statement. Crit Care Med. 2015;43(2):461-72.
19. Anseeuw K, Mowry JB, Burdmann EA, Ghannoum M, Hoffman RS, Gosselin S, et al. Extracorporeal treatment in phenytoin poisoning: systematic review and recommendations from the EXTRIP (Extracorporeal Treatments in Poisoning) Workgroup. Am J Kidney Dis. 2016;67(2):187-97.
20. Juurlink DN, Gosselin S, Kielstein JT, Ghannoum M, Lavergne V, Nolin TD, et al. Extracorporeal treatment for salicylate poisoning: systematic review and recommendations from the EXTRIP workgroup. Ann Emerg Med. 2015;66(2):165-81.
21. Ghannoum M, Nolin TD, Goldfarb DS, Roberts DM, Mactier R, Mowry JB, et al. Extracorporeal treatment for thallium poisoning: recommendations from the EXTRIP workgroup. Clin J Am Soc Nephrol. 2012;7(10):1682-90.
22. Ghannoum M, Wiegand TJ, Liu KD, Calello DP, Godin M, Lavergne V, et al. Extracorporeal treatment for theophylline poisoning: systematic review and recommendations from the EXTRIP workgroup. Clin Toxicol (Phila). 2015;53(4):215-29.
23. Ghannoum M, Laliberté M, Nolin TD, MacTier R, Lavergne V, Hoffman RS, et al. Extracorporeal treatment for valproic acid poisoning: systematic review and recommendations from the EXTRIP workgroup. Clin Toxicol (Phila). 2015;53(5):454-65.

CHAPTER 6

Respiratory Drive During Mechanical Ventilation: Monitoring and Modulation

Jacob George Pulinilkunnathil

INTRODUCTION

Respiratory drive is the overall measure of the intensity of the brain's respiratory center output that initiates and regulates every breath. Abnormalities of respiratory drive are common in the intensive care unit (ICU) and are clinically significant, particularly in those requiring mechanical ventilation.[1,2] Both excessive and insufficient respiratory drive can lead to lung and diaphragmatic injury—patient self-inflicted lung injury (P-SILI), ventilator-induced lung injury (VILI), and ventilator-induced diaphragmatic dysfunction (VIDD).[1,2] Recognition of these adverse effects has shifted the focus from gas exchange alone to modulation of respiratory drive to optimize lung and diaphragmatic function.

PHYSIOLOGY OF RESPIRATORY DRIVE

Neural Control of Breathing

Spontaneous breathing is controlled by a central control system comprising neurons in the brain stem and cerebral cortex. The cerebral cortex primarily mediates voluntary (behavioral) control of breathing, while involuntary control is predominantly brainstem-mediated.[3] In the medulla, the dorsal and ventral respiratory groups maintain the basic pattern of respiration. The pneumotaxic and apneustic areas in the pons fine-tune medullary discharges and regulate the depth and rate of respiration.[3] Mechanoreceptors (stretch receptors) located in the bronchial smooth muscle are responsible for the Hering-Breuer reflex. Neural signals descend via phrenic and intercostal neurons to activate the diaphragm and accessory muscles **(Fig. 1)**.[3]

Determinants of Drive

Respiratory drive is influenced by three principal feedback systems: (1) Chemical, (2) metabolic, and (3) cortical.

$PaCO_2$ as the Primary Stimulus

The central chemoreceptors are located on the ventrolateral surface of the medulla. They sense changes in the pH of cerebrospinal fluid (CSF), which reflects arterial CO_2 content. A rise in $PaCO_2$ causes acidic CSF pH, stimulating

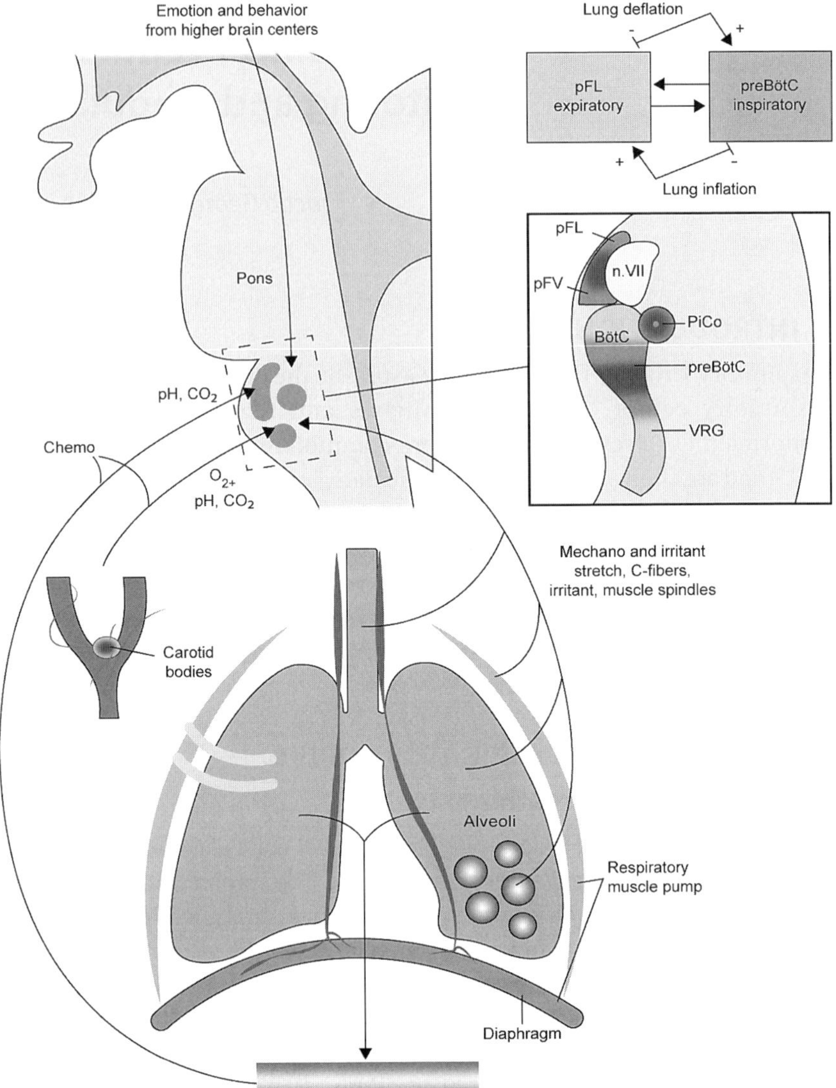

Fig. 1: Control of respiration. The respiratory centers are located in the brain stem and receive information from various sources. Central chemoreceptors are located near the ventral parafacial nucleus (pFV) and peripheral chemoreceptors are located in the carotid bodies. Mechanoreceptors and the irritant receptors are located in the chest wall, airway, lungs, and respiratory muscles. Emotional and behavioral feedback originate in the cerebral cortex and hypothalamus. The pre-Bötzinger complex (preBötC) is located between the ventral respiratory group (VRG) and the Bötzinger complex (BötC). The post-inspiratory complex (PiCo) is located near the Bötzinger complex. The lateral parafacial nucleus (pFL) controls expiratory activity.

Source: Adapted from Jonkman AH, de Vries HJ, Heunks LMA. Physiology of the Respiratory Drive in ICU Patients: Implications for Diagnosis and Treatment. Crit Care. 2020;24:104.[3]

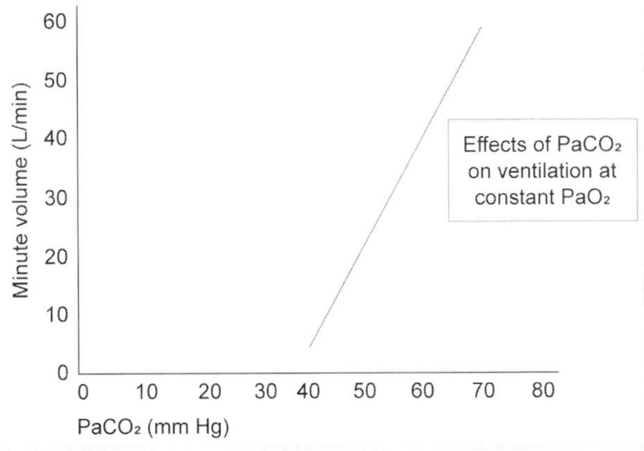

Fig. 2: Relation of $PaCO_2$ and minute ventilation at constant PaO_2.

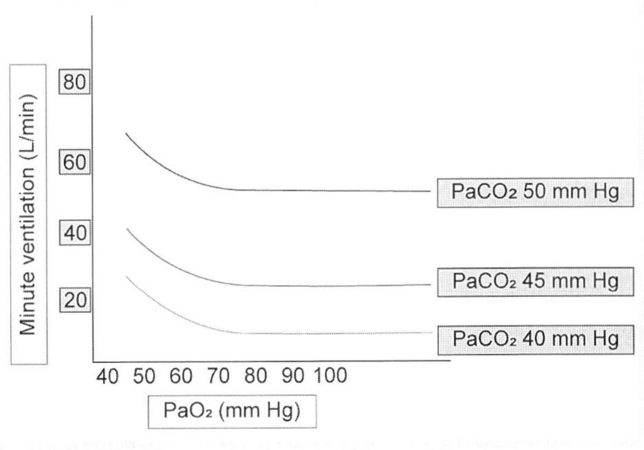

Fig. 3: Effects of hypoxia and ventilation at various levels of $PaCO_2$.

the medullary center to increase minute ventilation. The ventilatory response to $PaCO_2$ is often depicted as a CO_2 response curve under normal conditions, the curve is linear between ~40–80 mm Hg $PaCO_2$, and minute ventilation increases by about 2–3 L/min for every 1 mm Hg increase in $PaCO_2$ as shown in **Figure 2**.[3] Sleep, narcotics, or anesthetics shift the curve rightward and flatten the slope (reduced drive), while hypoxemia or metabolic acidosis shift it leftward and steepen the slope (enhanced drive).

Oxygen (PaO_2) Influence

Peripheral chemoreceptors in the carotid and aortic bodies respond to hypoxemia and modulate the respiratory drive. Their activity remains modest until PaO_2 falls below ~60 mm Hg, after which the ventilatory response increases sharply.[3] Hypoxemia potentiates the CO_2 response and the ventilation increases during hypoxemia, as illustrated in **Figure 3**.

TABLE 1: Summary of various stimulus for respiratory drive and the effect on ventilation.

Stimulus	*Primary sensors*	*Ventilatory effect*	*Curve effect*
↑$PaCO_2$	Central chemoreceptors	Strong ↑ ventilation	Linear ↑ slope
↓PaO_2 (<60 mm Hg)	Peripheral chemoreceptors	Augments CO_2 drive	Leftward/steeper
↓pH (metabolic acidosis)	Peripheral and central	Augments drive	Leftward/steeper
Sleep and narcotics	Central	Depress drive	Rightward/flatter

pH (Metabolic) Effects

Metabolic acidosis augments the minute-ventilation response to CO_2, further steepening the slope of the CO_2 response curve, while alkalosis blunts it.[3]

The stimulus, sensors, and effects on ventilation are summarized in **Table 1**.

Brain–Ventilation Curve, Metabolic Hyperbola, and the "Dogleg" Phenomenon

A comprehensive understanding of respiratory drive requires integrating two fundamental relationships:

- Metabolic hyperbola—plots $PaCO_2$ against minute ventilation ($\dot{V}E$). $PaCO_2$ varies inversely with $\dot{V}E$, producing a hyperbolic curve.
- Brain (ventilation-$PaCO_2$) curve—describes the ventilatory response to $PaCO_2$. Above the eupneic $PaCO_2$ it rises nearly linearly, reflecting chemosensitivity.

Their intersection sets the operating $PaCO_2$ and $\dot{V}E$. During wakefulness, a minimum ventilatory plateau persists even as $PaCO_2$ falls, creating the characteristic "dogleg" inflection—evidence of a wakefulness drive independent of chemical stimulation (marked as 4 in **Figure 4**).[3,4] During sleep or heavy sedation, this plateau disappears, and ventilation ceases once $PaCO_2$ reaches the apneic threshold. Critical illness can steepen, flatten, or shift these curves, explaining the clinical scenarios of varied respiratory drive in the ICU **(Fig. 4)**.[4]

PATHOPHYSIOLOGY OF ABNORMAL RESPIRATORY DRIVE IN CRITICAL ILLNESS

High Respiratory Drive

Excessive drive may be due to increased stimulation of chemoreceptors from hypercapnia, metabolic acidosis, or hypoxemia; mechanical factors

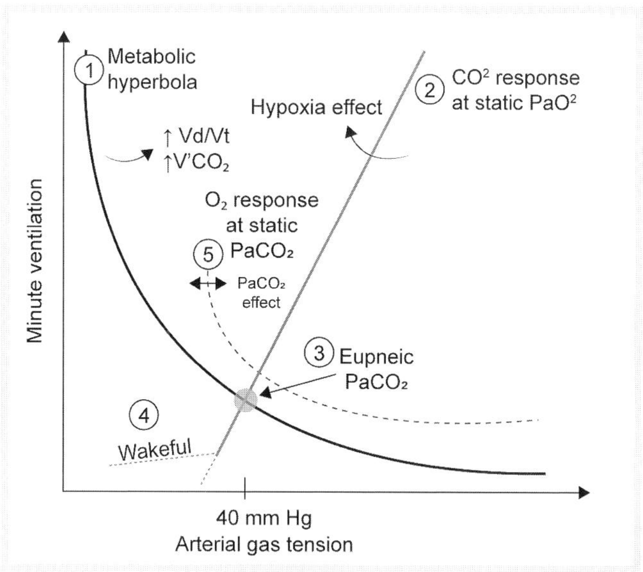

Fig. 4: Control of breathing. (1) The metabolic hyperbola plots changes in minute ventilation and $PaCO_2$; (2) The ventilatory response to $PaCO_2$ at fixed oxygen saturation; (3) The eupneic $PaCO_2$ is the intercept between the CO_2 response curve and the metabolic hyperbola; (4) In a wakeful state apnea does not normally occur (dogleg phenomenon) while during sleep or sedation apnea occurs when the actual $PaCO_2$ drops below eupneic CO_2; (5) The ventilatory response to PaO_2 is minimal, >60 mm Hg, below which it increases exponentially.

such as atelectasis or increased dead space; or cortical stimulation from pain, anxiety, or patient-ventilator dyssynchrony. This results in large transpulmonary pressures, diaphragmatic myotrauma, and hemodynamic compromise.[5-7]

Low Respiratory Drive

Low drive often reflects overassistance, deep sedation, or brain stem depression, which are associated with adverse outcomes including VIDD and asynchrony. Observational data show that an intermediate range of inspiratory effort during the first 72 hours of mechanical ventilation is associated with better outcomes.[5,7]

MONITORING RESPIRATORY DRIVE

Because the neuronal activity of the brain stem cannot be measured directly, respiratory drive in critically ill patients is inferred from physiologic surrogates. The current methods for monitoring respiratory drive can be classified into direct measures, semidirect measures, and clinical surrogates as below.[1,2,5]

Direct Measures of Respiratory Drive

Electrical Activity of the Diaphragm

The electrical activity of the diaphragm (EAdi) and the average rate of increase of EAdi (EAdi/dt), serve as the closest measure for respiratory drive in patients with intact phrenic nerves and neuromuscular junctions. EADi is measured using a specialized type of nasogastric catheter with integrated electrodes, thus measuring the diaphragmatic electromyography (EMG) activity. The normal value for EAdi range from 10 to 20 μV in nonintubated patients and 5 to 20 μV in patients on ventilatory support. Neuromuscular efficiency (NME) index—the ratio of the maximal negative airway pressure deflection to the corresponding EAdi amplitude during the occlusion (in $cmH_2O/\mu V$) is also used as a marker of respiratory drive.[1,2]

Diaphragmatic Electromyography

Electromyography can capture the electrical signals from the diaphragm and assess the contraction. It is more of a research tool due to technical challenges and not performed routinely in ICU.[1]

Surrogate Measures of Respiratory Drive

Airway Occlusion Pressure at 100 ms (P0.1)

This is the measure of the maximum negative airway pressure generated during the first 100 ms of a breath with the airway occluded. This value is independent of lung mechanics; readily displayed on most modern ventilator and remains valid even in mild-moderate respiratory muscle weakness. This requires averaging ≥3 readings and awareness of ventilator-specific measurement techniques. Clinical target: 1–4 cmH_2O in most patients; 2.5–5 cmH_2O in COPD; 3–6 cmH_2O in acute respiratory distress syndrome (ARDS).[1,2]

Esophageal Pressure (P_{es}) and Pressure–time Product

An esophageal balloon catheter provides a gold standard measure of inspiratory effort and can be used to calculate the pressure–time product (PTP) and transdiaphragmatic pressure (Pdi). These metrics closely reflect the energy cost of breathing and help to detect patient–ventilator dyssynchrony.[1,2]

Inspiratory swings in central venous pressure (CVP) may reflect inspiratory effort (tidal swing) and can be readily measured in patients with central lines. However, this is not widely validated.[1]

Indirect Measures

Respiratory rate, tidal volume, accessory muscle activity, dyspnea, and visible asynchrony provide rough estimates of the respiratory drive. These are confounded by sedation, ventilator settings, and muscle weakness, and cannot differentiate between central and peripheral causes of an altered drive.[1]

Diaphragm Ultrasound

Diaphragm thickening fraction (TFdi): Diaphragmatic thickening fraction and excursion measured by ultrasound may provide indirect insight into inspiratory effort. A low TFdi suggests diaphragm dysfunction. Measuring requires training and consistency and might be difficult in the obese ICU patient or in those with dressings.[1,2]

MODULATION OF RESPIRATORY DRIVE

The goal of respiratory-drive modulation is to achieve a "safe zone"—a neural output strong enough to maintain adequate ventilation and prevent atelectasis, but not so strong that it causes P-SILI, hemodynamic compromise, or exhaustion.[2,5,6] Because drive arises from a complex interplay of chemoreceptor input, cortical influences, and mechanical feedback, a stepwise and individualized strategy is essential.

Correcting Underlying Physiologic Drivers

Hypoxemia

Most individuals increase their ventilation to approximately 3–6 times baseline when PaO_2 falls to around 40 mm Hg (corresponding to an SpO_2 of approximately 75%). Supplemental oxygen, appropriate positive end-expiratory pressure (PEEP), and recruitment maneuvers help to correct the hypoxia and reduce peripheral chemoreceptor stimulation. Care must be taken to avoid hyperoxia, which can be deleterious in patients with chronic hypercapnia [e.g., chronic obstructive pulmonary disease (COPD)].[2,5]

Metabolic and respiratory acidosis increases the ventilation by stimulating the chemoreceptors. This is counteracted by an increase in ventilation, to lower $PaCO_2$ by increasing alveolar minute ventilation or correcting increased dead space. Other causes of metabolic acidosis (e.g., sepsis, diabetic ketoacidosis, and lactic acidosis) need to be addressed by treating the cause such as adequate fluid resuscitation, insulin therapy, infection control, or renal replacement therapy.

Ventilator Adjustments

Optimizing mechanical ventilation is often the most effective and instant tool. Care should be taken to titrate the ventilator settings as underassistance leads to excessive effort, while overassistance suppresses respiratory drive and promotes diaphragm disuse.[1,2] Pressure support can be titrated to achieve a target P0.1 of roughly 1–4 cmH_2O or an esophageal pressure swing of 5–10 cmH_2O. Selecting the optimal PEEP prevents derecruitment and hypoxemia, thereby reducing the peripheral chemoreceptor stimulation.

However, an overly high PEEP may impede the venous return causing significant hemodynamic compromise and also worsen ventilation by an increase in dead space.

Mode Selection

Newer ventilatory modes with closed loop technology such as neurally adjusted ventilatory assistance (NAVA), adaptive support ventilation (ASV), or proportional assist ventilation (PAV) adjust assist in real time to the patient's own effort, preserving physiologic variability while preventing over- or underassistance. The commonly used modes such as volume- or pressure-controlled modes may be preferred in conditions like severe ARDS where tight control over tidal-volume and plateau pressures are required. However, they require constant monitoring of respiratory drive and ventilator asynchrony. Flow starvation or early cycling can trigger double-triggering and breath stacking, which in turn increases VIDD.[2]

Pharmacologic Modulation

Sedation or analgesia may be needed when nonpharmacologic measures are insufficient.

Opioids blunt the respiratory centers and provide analgesia. These can be particularly helpful when metabolic acidosis or pain is the primary driver. Careful titration is required to avoid apnea in patients who are not on controlled modes of ventilation.

Propofol provides both sedation and some reduction in drive. It has a rapid onset of action, allows tight control but carries risk of hypotension and propofol infusion syndrome at high doses.

Dexmedetomidine, a newer agent, offers conscious sedation with relatively mild respiratory depression, mild analgesia making it attractive for patients in ICU. Bradycardia and hypotension need to be watched for.

Benzodiazepines are generally avoided because of an increased risk of delirium, hypotension, and unpredictable suppression of respiratory drive.

Neuromuscular blockade is reserved for severe ARDS for the initial 48 hours, or in patients with refractory dyssynchrony or life-threatening P-SILI. Whenever used, they should be used for the shortest possible duration and paired with strategies to prevent diaphragmatic atrophy.[2,5]

Extracorporeal Support

Extracorporeal membrane oxygenation or extracorporeal CO_2 removal ($ECCO_2R$) can be considered when hypoxic or hypercapnic stimuli remain uncontrolled despite optimizing the ventilator settings and correction of reversible causes. These extracorporeal techniques provide adequate provide systemic oxygenation and facilitate CO_2 removal, permitting rest to the lungs, and avoiding further VILI. Venovenous ECMO supports oxygenation and

CO_2 clearance in severe ARDS cases with refractory hypoxia, despite proning and neuromuscular blockade, while $ECCO_2R$ is aimed at CO_2 clearance, to control respiratory acidosis and thereby reduce ventilatory drive. Once extracorporeal support is initiated, clinicians should titrate ventilator settings to "lung-rest" parameters with continuous reassessment by P0.1, esophageal pressure, or EAdi.[1,2,5] This is to ensure that neural drive is appropriately reduced without causing oversuppression leading to diaphragmatic atrophy. Regular monitoring also helps to guide the timing of weaning from extracorporeal support as the native lung function recovers.[1,2,5]

PRACTICAL BEDSIDE APPROACH

A systematic bedside framework helps clinicians to translate physiologic principles into daily practice.

Quantitative Assessment

- *Airway occlusion pressure (P0.1):* P0.1 offers a quick estimate of drive. Target range is 1–4 cmH_2O in most adults.
- *Esophageal pressure (P_{es}):* Provides direct measurement of inspiratory effort and allows calculation of the PTP.
- *Electrical activity of the diaphragm (EAdi):* Real-time index of neural drive, useful in proportional ventilation modes.
- *Blood gases and capnography:* Complement monitoring by confirming adequacy of ventilation and acid–base status.

Identify the Cause

Evaluate metabolic status (pH, lactate, and bicarbonate), review analgesia and sedation levels, examine ventilator settings for mismatch or patient discomfort and investigate for the underlying pathology such as pneumonia, sepsis, pulmonary embolism, or neurologic injury.

Intervention

Treat the precipitant: correct hypoxemia, acidosis, or sepsis; optimize the ventilator: titrate assist, adjust flow, and cycling; titrate sedation/analgesia: prefer short-acting agents; avoid over suppression of the respiratory drive.

Reassess

After each change, repeat measurements (P0.1, P_{es}, or EAdi) and clinical observation. The patient should remain comfortable, with stable gas exchange and an intermediate level of inspiratory effort. Multidisciplinary communication with nursing staff and respiratory therapists should be undertaken to guide titration throughout the day.

Troubleshooting Scenarios

High P0.1 (>5 cmH_2O): Check for pain, acidosis, or flow starvation; increase support or treat cause.

Low P0.1 (<1 cmH_2O): Lighten sedation, reduce support, or assess for neuromuscular weakness.[1,2]

RESEARCH GAPS AND FUTURE DIRECTIONS

Although physiological rationale is strong, high-quality randomized trials defining ideal targets for P0.1 or EAdi and demonstrating improved patient-centered outcomes remain scarce. Future research should explore individualized thresholds, integration of automated drive monitoring into closed-loop ventilation, and long-term outcomes of drive-guided strategies.[2,5]

CONCLUSION

Monitor: Quantifying respiratory drive is feasible at the bedside using P0.1, esophageal pressure, or EAdi.[1,2]

Modulate: Correct underlying causes, adjust ventilator settings, and titrate sedatives to keep drive in an intermediate range.[1,2,5]

Protect: Maintaining balanced drive helps to avoid P-SILI, VILI, and VIDD, and facilitates timely liberation from mechanical ventilation.[2,5-7]

REFERENCES

1. Telias I, Abbott M, Brochard L. Monitoring respiratory drive and effort during mechanical ventilation. J Transl Crit Care Med. 2021;3:13.
2. Consalvo S, Accoce M, Telias I. Monitoring and modulating respiratory drive in mechanically ventilated patients. Curr Opin Crit Care. 2025;31:30-7.
3. Jonkman AH, de Vries HJ, Heunks LMA. Physiology of the respiratory drive in ICU patients: implications for diagnosis and treatment. Crit Care. 2020;24:104.
4. Giosa L, Collins PD, Shetty S, Lubian M, Del Signore R, Chioccola M, et al. Bedside Assessment of the Respiratory System During Invasive Mechanical Ventilation. J Clin Med. 2024;13(23):7456.
5. Vaporidi K, Akoumianaki E, Telias I, Goligher EC, Brochard L, Georgopoulos D. Respiratory drive in critically ill patients: pathophysiology and clinical implications. Am J Respir Crit Care Med. 2020;201:20-32.
6. Balzani, Eleonoraa; Alcala, Glasiele CB; Bellani, Giacomoa C; Pesenti, Antoniod. Patient self-inflicted lung injury an important phenomenon. Current Opinion in Critical Care 32(1):p 9-16, February 2026.
7. Goligher EC, Dres M, Fan E, Rubenfeld GD, Scales DC, et al. Mechanical Ventilation-induced Diaphragm Atrophy Strongly Impacts Clinical Outcomes. Am J Respir Crit Care Med. 2018;197(2):204-13.

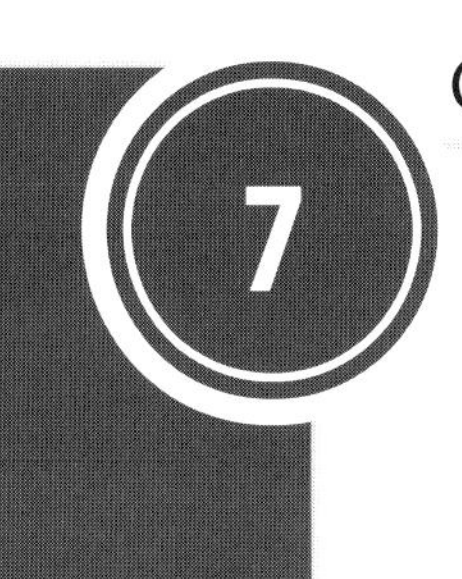

CHAPTER

Cerebral Autoregulation and Monitoring: Recent Advances in Neurocritical Care

Balkrishna Nimavat, Kapil Gangadhar Zirpe

INTRODUCTION

Blood pressure is not a constant figure in human physiology; it varies with diurnal pattern, physical activities, and posture. Constant change in arterial blood pressure is threat to tissue/organ perfusion irrespective to their basal functional/metabolic need. To overcome this problem of human biology, adapt system called autoregulation where they maintain constant perfusion of blood flow despite variation in arterial blood pressure. Cerebral autoregulation (CA) defined as homeostatic ability of brain and cerebral vasculature to adjust global and regional blood flow to meet metabolic demands in range of physiological/pathological conditions.[1,2] In this chapter, we have discussed about different mechanisms responsible for CA, types of CA, what are the methods to assess it, and how this understanding translated into meaningful neurocritical care practice.

Concept of autoregulation is not restricted to brain; it is seen in many other organs too **(Table 1)**.[3]

CEREBRAL AUTOREGULATION

Cerebral oxygen delivery (oxygen flux of brain) depends on cerebral blood flow (CBF) + blood oxygen content. CBF while depends on cerebral perfusion pressure (CPP) and inversely related to cerebral vascular resistance (CVR). CBF = CPP/CVR = [mean arterial pressure (MAP) – intracranial pressure (ICP)]/CVR, if ICP is stable then CPP can be replaced by MAP: Give rise to concept of pressure flow autoregulation.[4]

PHYSIOLOGY OF CEREBRAL AUTOREGULATION

Cerebral autoregulation regulated by four different mechanisms (as shown in **Figure 1**).[4]

TABLE 1: Organs with autoregulation mechanism.

Stronger autoregulation	*Moderate autoregulation*	*Weaker autoregulation*
Brain and spinal cord Heart Kidney	Skeletal muscles	*Splanchnic circulation:* Stomach, intestine, liver, and pancreas

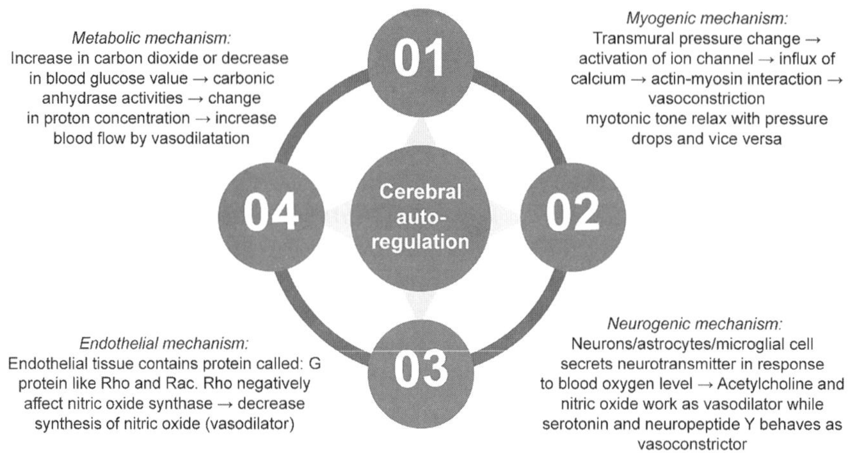

Fig. 1: Factors affecting cerebral autoregulation.

CLASSIC LASSEN AUTOREGULATORY CURVE AND LIMITATION

Original concept of autoregulation in brain was given by Lassen in 1959 (In article, CBF and oxygen consumption in Man), where he shown relationship between change in CBF to CPP. He highlighted that CBF remains constant in relatively wide range of MAP (between 60 and 150 mm Hg) due to phenomenon of cerebral vasculature called CA. Above (upper limit of autoregulation, ULA) and below (lower limit of autoregulation, LLA) the limit of autoregulation curve, CBF becomes pressure dependent. Subsequent data suggest that curve below LLA is even steeper compared to slope of ULA.[5] With advancement in knowledge of neuromonitoring, limitation of classic Lassen's curve get unmasked: (1) Interindividual variability, (2) Mostly represent static autoregulation (in real world CBF and MAP constantly fluctuate), (3) Oversimplification of CA concept, (4) Not fully represent nonlinear nature of CA behavior, and (5) Not considering buffer capacity below lower limit of CA. [6] Joshi et al. demonstrated that limit of CA varies significantly and unpredictably between patients (for some patients, MAP of 40 mm Hg is sufficient for CBF, while in others 90 mm Hg needed to maintain CBF). Regulation of CBF is much more complex than just pressure regulation (as metabolic factors, $PaCO_2$ and neuronal factors also affecting CA). Position and shape of CA curve changes depends on physiological/pathological need and condition (rather than classical Lassen's curve shape).[7]

TYPES OF CEREBRAL AUTOREGULATION

Depends on experimental construct/time scale CA classified as **(Table 2)**.

TABLE 2: Classification of cerebral autoregulation.[8-10]

Static versus (steady-state CA/sCA)	*Dynamic CA (dCA)*
Static CA evaluates overall effect of autoregulatory action, but does not address the time in which this change in CVR achieved (i.e., latency)	Dynamic CA characterized by observing changes in CBF velocity in response to rapid change in MAP/ABP
Derived from: Baseline steady state CBV/CBF and CPP/MAP followed another measurement after manipulating CPP/MAP Static autoregulation can be described by Lassen's curve	*Derived from methods:* • *Utilizing transcranial Doppler (TCD):* Deflation of BP cuff on thigh and observing CBF velocity change • Paced breathing or modulation of PEEP • PRx (concept given by Czosynka et al.)
Static CA reflects ultra-low frequency oscillations.	Dynamic CA reflects very low, low- and high-frequency range oscillations
Static autoregulation looks at long-term change, from minutes to hours	Dynamic autoregulation looks at the immediate change, within seconds to minutes
Give information about CPP range in which CA is active	• Give idea about latency/how quick response of CBF to change in ABP/pressure changes • Dynamic CA methods are helpful in pathological conditions such as IC hypertension, TBI, AIS, ICH. (As it addresses time in which change in CVR achieved)
Difficult to control confounding factors during static measurement (like effect of anesthesia medication or change in CO_2 level)	PRx, ARI, Mx, and TFA are some of the example indices for dynamic CA

(ABP: arterial blood pressure; ARI: autoregulation index; CA: cerebral autoregulation; CBF: cerebral blood flow; CBV: cerebral blood volume; CPP: cerebral perfusion pressure; CVR: cerebral vascular resistance; ICH: intracranial hypertension; PRx: pressure reactivity index; MAP: mean arterial pressure; Mx: mean flow index; TBI: traumatic brain injury; TFA: transfer function analysis)

CLASSIFICATION OF CEREBRAL AUTOREGULATION MONITORING DEVICES

See **Table 3**.

TYPES OF ANALYTIC METHOD ASSESS CEREBRAL AUTOREGULATION

See **Table 4**.

Invasive Method to Monitor Cerebral Autoregulation

Brain tissue oxygen tension ($PbtO_2$): $PbtO_2$ is a surrogate marker of regional/local CBF. It is an invasive (Clark) probe that represents the balance between

TABLE 3: Classification of cerebral autoregulation monitoring devices.[10,11]

Continuous monitoring devices versus	*Intermittent (over finite time period) monitoring devices*	
Example		
	Most of imaging-based techniques	
Spatially resolved/ frequency resolved/time resolved NIRS	Xe-CT	
fNIRS	CTP	
Diffuse correlation spectroscopy (DCS)	PET	
Transcranial Doppler [TCD (semi-intermittent)]	*MRI:* DWI, PWI, DSC, PWI, ASL, and fMRI	
Depends on invasiveness of device:		
Noninvasive	*Minimally invasive*	*Invasive*
Neuroimaging methods	Positron emission tomography along with magnetic resonance imaging (IV contrast)	Brain tissue oxygen tension ($PbtO_2$)
Transcranial Doppler	Xe-CT (inhalational agent)	Microdialysis
Near-infrared spectroscopy (NIRS)		ICP
Laser Doppler flowmetry (LDF) (can be combined/ conjugate with invasive component/methods)		

(ASL: arterial spin labeling; CTP: computed tomography perfusion; DSC: dynamic susceptibility contrast; DWI: diffusion-weighted imaging; fMRI: functional MRI; PET: positron emission tomography; PWI: perfusion-weighted imaging)

oxygen delivery and oxygen consumption at brain-tissue level. Normal value of $PbtO_2$ is 35–50 mm Hg and value <15 mm Hg is the risk of hypoperfusion and poor outcome. Value below 10 mm Hg correlates with irreversible ischemic injury.[13]

Limitations of $PbtO_2$ method: Probe availability and bleeding/infection risk with probe.

Oxygen reactivity index (ORx): ORx is a moving correlation coefficient between $PbtO_2$ and CPP. $PbtO_2$ values are derived every 30s and moving correlation window between 30 minutes and 1 hour. Jaeger et al. study found association between ORx with GOS and independent association of ORx to

TABLE 4: Types of analytic method to assess cerebral autoregulation.[12]

Frequency-based analysis/ algorithm	*Time-based analysis/ algorithm*	*Time-frequency analysis*
Assess the dCA by an analyzing how brain responds to BP fluctuation at different frequencies	Helpful for monitoring dCA and capture even nonlinear relationship between pressure and flow	Analyze how signals related to blood pressure and blood flow change over both time and frequency
Helpful in identifying whether CA is intact or not	Less affected by physiological noise signal	Give better insight about dynamic nature of CA
High coherence and lack of phase in low frequency range suggest impaired CA	Helps in tailored CPP for individual to improve outcome	
Indices		
• TF gain • TF phase • Coherence	Time regression/time correlation analysis	• Wavelet transform • Cross-wavelet spectrum
	Cerebral oximetry index (COx)	
	Total hemoglobin index (THx)	
	Laser Doppler reactivity index (LDx)	
	Pressure reactivity index (PRx)	
	Low-frequency autoregulation index (LAx)	
	Autoregulation index (ARI)	
	Mean flow index (Mx), systolic flow index (Sx), and diastolic flow index (Dx)	
	Oxygen reactivity index (ORx) or tissue oxygenation index (TOI)	

(dCA: dynamic cerebral autoregulation)

delayed cerebral ischemia (DCI) in subarachnoid hemorrhage (SAH) group of patients [13] **(Table 5)**.

Pulse amplitude index (PAx): It correlates the pulse amplitude (AMP) change of ICP waveform with change in MAP. Noninvasive PAx (nPAx) is a novel device for monitoring ICP and PAx.[14] PAx is a new modified index of

TABLE 5: Comparison of different invasive and noninvasive methods.[18]

Method	*Principle*	*CBF area covered*	*Continuous or intermittent*	*Advantage*	*Limitation*
TCD	Doppler principle	Vascular territory	Semi-intermittent	• High-frequency signal and noninvasive • Bedside tool	• Operator dependent • Cumbersome • Difficult to get signal window • Limited to anterior circulation • Limited validity over temporal course
NIRS	Absorbance difference between oxy- and de-oxy Hb	Global	Continuous	• Noninvasive • Bedside tool	
$PbtO_2$	Invasive Clark electrode to detect difference between oxygen supply and consumption	Local	Continuous	Invasive	• Local brain tissue perfusion • Depends on probe position
$AVDO_2$	Oxygen difference between jugular vein and arterial blood	Global	Intermittent	Invasive (need arterial line and jugular bulb catheter)	• Repeated ABP challenge can give secondary brain injury • Low sensitive to focal insult
LDF	Works on doppler shift principle	Local	Continuous	Assessment of microcirculation	Probe placement can affect value
Microdialysis		Local	Continuous		Probe-related complication

Contd...

Contd…

Method	*Principle*	*CBF area covered*	*Continuous or intermittent*	*Advantage*	*Limitation*
CTP	Time dependent decay in IV contrast	Global	Intermittent	High accuracy	• Radiation exposure • All intermittent methods have limited validity over temporal course
Xe-enhanced CT	Special tracer distribution used to detect CBF	Global	Intermittent	High accuracy	All augmented ABP method associated with secondary insult to brain
PET	Augmentation of MAP/CPP ≥20 mm Hg manipulation used to see change in CBF	Global	Intermittent	High accuracy	• IV contrast exposure • Limited validity over temporal course
MRI	Acetazolamide injection used for ABP manipulation and observed CBF	Global	Intermittent	• ASL technique required IV access • Suitable in steno-occlusive disease	• Time-consuming and difficult to conduct in critically ill patient • Limited validity over temporal course

(ABP: arterial blood pressure; ASL: arterial spin labeling; $AVDO_2$: arteriovenous jugular oxygen difference; CBF: cerebral blood flow; CPP: cerebral perfusion pressure; CTP: computed tomography perfusion; LDF: laser Doppler flowmetry; MAP: mean arterial pressure; NIRS: near-infrared spectroscopy; $PbtO_2$: brain tissue oxygen tension; PET: positron emission tomography; TCD: transcranial Doppler) cerebrovascular reactivity. PAx performs as good as established index like PRx in group of traumatic brain injury (TBI) patients and have more promising association even at lower values of ICP.[15]

Microdialysis: Intracranial microdialysis is a surrogate marker of regional CBF. Glutamate (an excitatory neurotransmitter) is released during cerebral ischemia. The concentration is inversely proportional to cerebral perfusion and can be regarded as a surrogate marker of CBF. Limitation of microdialysis method is unable to detect global change in metabolism/flow (as restricted to focal area) and probe-related complications.[16]

Laser doppler flowmetry (LDF): LDF is excellent tool to monitor continuous real time local CBF. It works on principle of Doppler shift, i.e., the frequency change (wavelength) that light waves undergo when they are reflected by moving objects such as red blood cells. LDF can be noninvasive (if probe applied to forehead) or invasive (in brain tissue) depends on probe placement. To get idea about CA LDF combined with invasive (ABP or ICP) or minimally invasive tool (TCD). Limitation of LDF are: (1) Give idea about regional CBF (as small area of brain CBF covered) and (2) probe placement may affect value.[17]

Arteriovenous jugular oxygen difference ($AVDO_2$): $AVDO_2$ can be used as surrogate of CBF. As name suggests, $AVDO_2$ assessed the difference in oxygenation between jugular vein and arterial blood. Autoregulation considers intact if there is no change in CBF after an ABF challenge.[18]

Noninvasive Methods to Monitor Cerebral Autoregulation

Near-infrared spectroscopy (NIRS): NIRS is not a novel method; it was introduced in 1970s with purpose of monitoring tissue oxygen level (while pulse oximetry used to monitor arterial oxygen saturation of Hb). It transmits and absorbs the near infrared length light (700–1,000 nm) and detects the difference between oxygenated to deoxygenated Hb. Ratio of oxygenated Hb to total Hb known as "tissue oxygenation index (TOI)". SPO_2, ScO_2, rSO_2, and other such indices are examples of TOI. Transcranial Doppler (TCD) and NIRS are noninvasive methods to monitor CA, but NIRS seems less cumbersome, not required frequent calibration and continuous monitoring are easier.

NIRS limitation: There is lack of standardization. The variety of commercially available monitors measure different parameters and proprietary algorithms. Preprocessing techniques such as signal acquisition frequency, data filtering, and artifact removal are varying among investigators. Index-specific cutoffs and methods for identifying curve features (upper and lower limits or optimal blood pressure) are not yet validated.[19]

Transcranial Doppler: TCD-based tests are feasible at bedside and does not require ABP challenge (if compared to radiological imaging where ABP manipulation needed to see change in CBF). TCD findings are operator dependent and need good acoustic window. Due to anatomical reasoning, TCD-based indices are more helpful in anterior circulation pathology and had limited validity over temporal course. Transient hyperemic response test (THRT), autoregulatory index (ARI), flow index (Mx and Sx), and transfer functional analysis are the indices derived from TCD tool[18] **(Table 5)**.

Minimally Invasive/Radiological/Imaging Based

^{133}Xenon (Xe) washout technique: Consider as gold standard method to monitor CBF.

Method: Scintillation counter monitor regional decay in radioactivity of ^{133}Xe observed after intracarotid or intraaortic injection.

Interpretation: The slope of the washout curve is proportional to regional CBF. The curve is biexponential, the fast and slow components representing blood flow in gray and white matter.[17]

Computed tomography perfusion (CTP): Perfusion of CT scan compared to other methods is more readily available and quantification of perfusion is easier than MRI. Disadvantage of CTP is doubling irradiation exposure (one before vasomotor stimulus and other after). Choice of vasomotor stimulus in radio-imaging are: (1) Controlling CO_2 level by either hyperventilating or apnea, or by (2) Injection of acetazolamide: Carbonic anhydrase inhibitor converts CO_2 into bicarbonates and provokes hypercapnia and acidosis, which leads to vasodilatation and increased CBF by 20–30%.[20]

Positron emission tomography (ET) Use ^{15}O labeled H_2O (special tracer) distribution to detect CBF. Consider multiple metabolic factors but required IV cannula and radiation exposure. Various indices can be derived from PET scans such as oxygen extraction fraction (OEF) and cerebral metabolic rate of oxygen ($CMRO_2$) are helpful in assessment of neurovascular coupling and understanding ischemic penumbra in stroke patients.[21]

MRI: Compared to other radioimaging method MRI gives infracentimetric spatial resolution + temporal resolution of about 1 second. Many MRI methods proposed for assessment of CA like BOLD contrast, arterial spin labeling (ASL), MR angiography, and susceptibility contrast by gadolinium injection. Out of all methods ASL is the best one due to its capability of quantifying CBF. ASL is one of the methods selected for studying healthy subject physiology and in cognitive neuroscience field, i.e., neurodegenerative disorders. fMRI widely used for estimating vascular reserve and risk of stroke in steno-occlusive disease in order to improve treatment choice.[20]

CEREBRAL AUTOREGULATION IN PATHOLOGICAL CONDITIONS

Traumatic Brain Injury

Despite advancement in modern medicine, morbidity and mortality in TBI is still significantly high. Brain trauma foundation guidelines (and most of neurocritical care literature) suggest CPP target of 60–70 mm Hg. Such cutoff does not consider CA concept that is even more complex than perceived. TBI disrupts the CA mechanism and, thus, predicting CPP for that particular individual became extremely difficult. This gives rise to concept of optimal cerebral perfusion pressure (CPPopt) and pressure reactivity index (PRx). Early observational data suggest that targeting CPP near to CPPopt (personalized for that individual) improves neurological outcome.[2]

Cerebrovascular reactivity [pressure reactivity index (PRx)]: Concept was given by Czosnyka et al. in 1997. It defined as Pearson correlation coefficient between MAP and ICP. (30 consecutive monitoring values of MAP and ICP, each of 10s, i.e., 30 multiplies 10s: 300 seconds, i.e., 5 minutes data). It creates linear association between slow waves component of MAP and ICP. Positive PRx (positive correlation coefficient between MAP and ICP) suggests rise in ICP with rise in MAP, i.e., indicates impaired CA. Negative PRx indicates intact CA, i.e., lower ICP in response to increased MAP.

Autoregulation curve (CPPopt): Collecting PRx and CPP values over time and plotting them give rise to U-shaped curve. CPPopt is the value of CPP when PRx is minimal (nadir PRx in U-shaped curve correlates to CPPopt).

Evidence for CPPopt-guided therapy: COGiTATE study (multicenter RCT pilot study) compared standard CPP target (according to BTF: 60–70 mm Hg) versus CPPopt-guided therapy, shown some signal of favorable neurological outcome and less mortality in CPPopt group[2] **(Table 6)**.

Mean flow index (Mx) is a time-domain method based on strength of correlation between spontaneous slow fluctuations in mean CPP and FV.

Interpretation: Lack or negative correlation between CPP and FV represents functional autoregulation (higher index represents impaired autoregulation). Mx > 0.3 indicates disturbed autoregulation and lower than 0.05 good autoregulation. Values between 0.05 and 0.3 are window of uncertainty.[22]

Frequency-based mathematical methods:

TF gain: TF gain describes how much of input signal variation transmitted to output signal. It is the ratio of FV (amplitude of output) to ABP (amplitude of input).

Interpretation: With intact autoregulation, the low frequency (LF) fluctuations in FV related to fluctuations in ABP are largely suppressed, resulting in low TF gain, whereas a high gain represents impaired CA.

TABLE 6: Summary of autoregulatory indices.[18,24]

Index	*Input signal*		*Interpretation*	*Data/evidence*
ARI	ABP (arterial BP) and Fv (flow velocity)	*Parametric model with 10 strengths of autoregulation:* Observing CBF response to change in ABP	ARI 0: No CA ARI 9: Perfect CA	Low ARI correlates with unfavorable clinical outcome and severity of angiographic vasospasm. ARI might help in stratifying therapy in SAH management and can be used as early warning tool in SAH
Flow index: Mx, Sx, and Dx	ABP (CPP) and Fv	• Pearson correlation between CPP and mean Fv • Sx and Dx calculated from systolic and diastolic flow velocity respectively	Higher value suggestive of impaired autoregulation	Fair correlation with high Mx value to higher NIHSS and infarct size in ischemic stroke
PRx	ABP and ICP	Correlation between 30 consecutive 10s means of ABP and ICP	Higher value impaired autoregulation	MAP below PRx-derived MAPopt-5 was associated with mortality after cardiac arrest and nonsurvivors had a narrower range of intact CAR than survivors
PAx/nPAx	ABP and amplitude of ICP	Correlation between 30 consecutive 10s means of ABP and amplitude of ICP	Higher value impaired autoregulation	PAx performs as good as PRx in group of traumatic brain injury (TBI) patients and have more promising association even at lower values of ICP

Contd...

Contd...

Index	*Input signal*		*Interpretation*	*Data/evidence*
TOx, COx, and THx/HVx	ABP (CPP) and NIRS oxygenation	Correlation between 30 consecutive 10s means of HR and NIRS oxygenation	Higher value impaired autoregulation	A COx value of <0.3 indicates intact autoregulation and the MAP with the lowest COx is considered the MAP_{opt}. Helps in personalized MAP target
Transfer function analysis	ABP and Fv ABP and NIRS oxygenation	Derived from the transfer function of fast Fourier transform of ABP and Fv signals	Low phase, high gain, and high coherence suggestive of impaired autoregulation	TFA data shows association of low phase with worse outcome and larger ICH volume. Hematoma volume was independently associated with ipsilateral phase
ORx	ABP (CPP) and $PbtO_2$	Correlation between 30 consecutive 10s means of ABP and $PbtO_2$	Higher value impaired autoregulation	ORx (more precisely TOxa) can predict DCI and unfavorable Glassgow Outcome Score (GOCs) in SAH

(ABP: arterial blood pressure; CBF: cerebral blood flow; COx: cerebral oximetry index; CPP: cerebral perfusion pressure; Dx: diastolic flow velocity index; HVx: hemoglobin volume index; MAP: mean arterial pressure; Mx: mean flow velocity index; NIRS: near-infrared spectroscopy; $PbtO_2$: brain tissue oxygen tension; Sx: systolic flow velocity index; THx: total hemoglobin reactivity index; TOx: tissue oxygenation index)

TF phase: Represents autoregulation filter inertia. Normally, there is a degree of shift (delay) between sinusoidal (Fourier) components of input signal (ABP) and output signal (FV).

Intact autoregulation is associated with highly positive phase values (90° and more) for LF decreasing down to 0 for high frequencies (of heart rate and above). Impaired autoregulation shows no active response (no "inertia" effects), manifested as 0 phase shift at all frequencies.

Coherence: Coherence reflects the degree of linear correlation between the input and output amplitudes of the Fourier components at each frequency point. Linear systems with high signal-to-noise ratios (SNR), and a univariate input–output relationship, coherence will approach one. On the other hand, coherence will approach 0 if SNR is low, systems are highly nonlinear or if there are other variables influencing the output.[23]

Interpretation:
In TFA analysis: Impaired autoregulation characterized by low phase, high gain, and high coherence.[24]

Ischemic Stroke

Transcranial Doppler TFA studies (Reinhard et al., Guo et al., Peterson et al., Castro et al., and Xiong et al.) observed low phase in affected hemisphere. They also got some signal of: (1) Low phase and higher infarct size at 24 hours, (2) Higher mRS/NIHSS score correlation with low phase, (3) CA impairment in bilateral lacunar infarct/large infarct, and (4) CA impairment resolved at 3 months. TCD-Mx (Reinhard et al.) shows fair correlation with high Mx value to higher NIHSS and infarct size. TCD-ARI (Saeed et al., Guo et al., and Xiong et al.) findings show that cortical infarct had lower ARI compared to subcortical. Small vessel disease worsens CA impairment. In acute phase, ARI similar to control group reduces over 2 weeks and recovered over 1–3 months.[25]

Intracerebral Bleed

Earlier data on perfusion CT (Gould et al., 2013) has shown that static CA is not altered much in intracerebral hemorrhage. TCD-TFA data shows association of low phase with worse outcome and larger ICH volume (Oeinck et al.). Hematoma volume was independently associated with ipsilateral phase (Ma et al.). ICP PRx (Diedler et al.) observed that mortality was lower when CPP was close to their CPPopt.[25]

Subarachnoid Hemorrhage

Subarachnoid hemorrhage (SAH) is a stroke subtype associated with high mortality and morbidity. This poor outcome is related to biphasic insult/nature of primary disease process, i.e., primary bleeding related injury and later secondary to DCI (impaired micro- and macrocirculation due to vasospasm).

CONSCIOUS clinical trial, use of clazosentan: Endothelin-1 receptor antagonist shows to reduce macrocirculation angiospasm but failed to improve clinical outcome (that shift focus to radiologically invisible cerebral microcirculation/autoregulation).

Transient hyperemic response test (THRT):
Concept: Dynamic assessment method for autoregulation. Compression of carotid artery ipsilateral to insonified MCA leads to change in CPP and

activate myogenic component of autoregulation. If microcirculation dilates in response to reduction in pressure, suggest intact CA.

Method: TCD used to measure middle cerebral artery blood flow velocity (MCA-BFV). Compression of carotid artery done to decrease CPP for 3–5 seconds and then released. It gives rise to brief hyperemic response when pressure/flow restored.

Interpretation: THRT scored as intact or perturbed depends on whether transient hyperemic BFV is 10% higher than the precompression BFV.

Alternative approach/Thigh cuff approach: Where thigh cuff inflated to 200 mm Hg for 2 minutes and then released. BFV response mapped and autoregulatory index (ARI) derived from it. 0 indicates no autoregulation and 9 indicates intact autoregulation.

Evidence: Fontana et al.[26] observed in their study that early deterioration of CA (based on ARI) correlates with unfavorable clinical outcome and severity of angiographic vasospasm. Dynamic autoregulation index (ARI) might help in stratifying therapy in SAH management and can be used as early warning tool in SAH.[27]

Oxygen reactivity index:

Oxygen reactivity index (ORx) can be measured by invasive or noninvasive method. ORx represents slow wave correlation between oxygen saturation and blood pressure. Budohoski et al.[28] in their prospective study shown that ORx (more precisely TOxa) can predict DCI and unfavorable Glassgow Outcome Score (GOCs) in SAH.

Cardiac Arrest

Hypoxic ischemic brain injury (HIBI) is associated with increasingly high morbidity and mortality. HIBI is a part of post ROSC syndrome/postcardiac arrest consequences. Two pathological processes associated with such devastated outcome: (1) Primary insult due to stoppage of heart activity/blood flow, and (2) Reperfusion injury once ROSC achieved. Study shows that majority of patients in the acute phase after cardiac arrest, CA is either absent or right-shifted.[29]

PRx and MAPopt: PRx can be used as surrogate marker for CA. Relationship between PRx and MAP gives idea about the MAP at which cerebral autoregulation (CAR) is most intact known as MAP_{opt}. Kirschen et al. have shown in their study that MAP below PRx-derived MAP_{opt}-5 was associated with mortality after cardiac arrest and nonsurvivors had a narrower range of intact CAR than survivors.[30]

SURGICAL PATIENTS (CARDIAC AND NONCARDIAC SURGERY

- *Evidence in cardiac surgery:* Cardiopulmonary bypass surgeries are associated with high incidence of neurological complications, i.e., stroke,

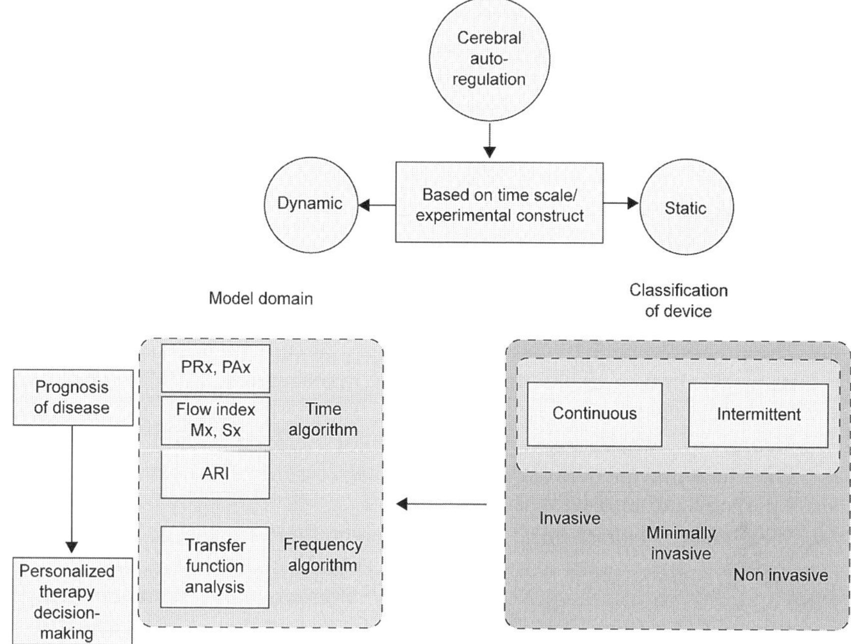

Fig. 2: Chapter infographic.

delirium, and cognitive impairment. Exact pathophysiology is not well understood but cerebral dysregulation is one of the possible factors for such neurological insult. In one systemic review 17 out of 20 studies reported impaired CA with CPB.[31] Another prospective observational study data in postoperative cardiac surgery patients show that impaired CA was associated with high postoperative delirium. They used tissue oximetry index (NIFS oxygenation and MAP to derive TOx) to monitor CA[32] **(Fig. 2)**.

- *Evidence in noncardiac surgery:*
  - *Liver failure and transplant subgroup:* Acute/fulminant liver failure associated with hepatic encephalopathy and cerebral edema. TCD assessment in pretransplant acute liver failure patient shows impaired CA. This impaired CA re-establish to normal after 48–72 hours of posttransplantation.[33] They used static CA as index to monitor CA, i.e., MAP was increased by 20–30 mm Hg [with norad (norepinephrine)] and observing CBv change (ABP manipulation).
  - *Endarterectomy:* Studies have shown that dynamic CA impaired in patient of severe carotid artery stenosis. dCA improved after 1 month of postoperative surgery period (did not improve immediately).[34]

CONCLUSION

There is a paradigm shift in understanding of CA from classic Lassen's curve to dynamic CA. With help of TCD and NIRS devices, monitoring cerebral parameters become real time and noninvasive by nature. Evolution in deep learning artificial intelligence and data science industry gave birth to lots of time/frequency-based algorithm to assess CA in quantified way. Still CA indices are in their infantile phase and need more validation with feasible bedside tool to get more insights.

REFERENCES

1. Holstein-Rathlou NH, Marsh DJ. From blood flow to organ function: The physiology of autoregulatory dynamics. Exp Physiol. 2026;111(1):21-5.
2. Tsigaras ZA, Weeden M, McNamara R, Jeffcote T, Udy AA, Anstey J, et al. The pressure reactivity index as a measure of cerebral autoregulation and its application in traumatic brain injury management. Crit Care Resuscit. 2023;25(4):229-36.
3. Meng L, Wang Y, Zhang L, McDonagh DL. Heterogeneity and Variability in Pressure Autoregulation of Organ Blood Flow: Lessons Learned over 100+ Years. Crit Care Med. 2019;47(3):436-48.
4. Silverman A, Petersen NH. Physiology, Cerebral Autoregulation. In: StatPearls [Internet]. Treasure Island (FL): StatPearls Publishing; 2025.
5. Vu EL, Brown CH, Brady KM, Hogue CW. Monitoring of cerebral blood flow autoregulation: physiologic basis, measurement, and clinical implications. Br J Anaesth. 2025;132(6):1260-73.
6. Tan CO, Taylor JA. On the Judicious Use of Metrics for Cerebral Autoregulation. Eur J Appl Physiol. 2013;113(11):10.1007/s00421-013-2718-4.
7. Moerman A, De Hert S. Why and how to assess cerebral autoregulation? Best Pract Res Clin Anaesthesiol [Internet]. 2019;33(2):211-20.
8. Tiecks FP, Lam AM, Aaslid R, Newell DW. Comparison of static and dynamic cerebral autoregulation measurements. Stroke [Internet]. 1995;26(6):1014-9.
9. Pham T, Fernandez C, Blaney G, Tgavalekos K, Sassaroli A, Cai X, et al. Noninvasive Optical Measurements of Dynamic Cerebral Autoregulation by Inducing Oscillatory Cerebral Hemodynamics. Front Neurol. 2021;12:745987.
10. Sainbhi AS, Gomez A, Froese L, Slack T, Batson C, Stein KY, et al. Non-Invasive and Minimally-Invasive Cerebral Autoregulation Assessment: A Narrative Review of Techniques and Implications for Clinical Research. Front Neurol [Internet]. 2022;13:872731.
11. Klein SP, Depreitere B, Meyfroidt G. How I monitor cerebral autoregulation. Crit Care. 2019;23(1):1-3.
12. Kostoglou K, Bello-Robles F, Brassard P, Chacon M, Claassen JAHR, Czosnyka M, et al. Time-domain methods for quantifying dynamic cerebral blood flow autoregulation: Review and recommendations. A white paper from the Cerebrovascular Research Network (CARNet). J Cereb Blood Flow Metabol. 2024;44(9):1480-514.
13. Zweifel C, Dias C, Smielewski P, Czosnyka M. Continuous time-domain monitoring of cerebral autoregulation in neurocritical care. Med Eng Phys. 2014;36(5):638-45.
14. Hassett CE, Uysal SP, Butler R, Moore NZ, Cardim D, Gomes JA. Assessment of Cerebral Autoregulation Using Invasive and Noninvasive Methods of Intracranial Pressure Monitoring. Neurocrit Care. 2023;38(3):591-9.

15. Aries MJH, Czosnyka M, Budohoski KP, Kolias AG, Radolovich DK, Lavinio A, et al. Continuous monitoring of cerebrovascular reactivity using pulse waveform of intracranial pressure. Neurocrit Care. 2012;17(1):67-76.
16. Chan MTV, Ng SCP, Lam JMK, Poon WS, Gin T. Monitoring of autoregulation using intracerebral microdialysis in patients with severe head injury. Acta Neurochir Suppl (Wien). 2005;(95):113-6.
17. Sturgess J, Matta B. Chapter 46: Transcranial Doppler Ultrasonography and Other Measures of Cerebral Blood Flow. Essentials of Neuroanesthesia and Neurointensive Care: A Volume in Essentials of Anesthesia and Critical Care. Amsterdam, Netherlands: Elsevier; 2008. pp. 296-300.
18. Svedung Wettervik T, Fahlström M, Enblad P, Lewén A. Cerebral Pressure Autoregulation in Brain Injury and Disorders–A Review on Monitoring, Management, and Future Directions. World Neurosurg. 2022;158:118-31.
19. Bush B, Sam K, Rosenblatt K. The role of near-infrared spectroscopy in cerebral autoregulation monitoring. J Neurosurg Anesthesiol [Internet]. 2019;31(3):269.
20. Krainik A, Villien M, Troprès I, Attyé A, Lamalle L, Bouvier J, et al. Functional imaging of cerebral perfusion. Diagn Interv Imaging. 2013;94(12):1259-78.
21. Wang Z, Mascarenhas C, Jia X. Positron Emission Tomography after Ischemic Brain Injury: Current Challenges and Future Developments. Transl Stroke Res. 2020;11(4):628.
22. Sorrentino E, Budohoski KP, Kasprowicz M, Smielewski P, Matta B, Pickard JD, et al. Critical thresholds for transcranial Doppler indices of cerebral autoregulation in traumatic brain injury. Neurocrit Care. 2011;14(2):188-93.
23. Liu X, Czosnyka M, Donnelly J, Budohoski KP, Varsos GV, Nasr N, et al. Comparison of frequency and time domain methods of assessment of cerebral autoregulation in traumatic brain injury. J Cereb Blood Flow Metabol. 2014;35(2):248.
24. Donnelly J, Budohoski KP, Smielewski P, Czosnyka M. Regulation of the cerebral circulation: bedside assessment and clinical implications. Crit Care. 2025;;20(1):1-17.
25. Castro P, Azevedo E, Sorond F. Cerebral Autoregulation in Stroke. Curr Atheroscler Rep. Curr Atheroscler Rep. 2018;20(8):37.
26. Fontana J, Moratin J, Ehrlich G, Scharf J, Weiß C, Schmieder K, et al. Dynamic Autoregulatory Response After Aneurysmal Subarachnoid Hemorrhage and Its Relation to Angiographic Vasospasm and Clinical Outcome. Neurocrit Care. 2015;23(3):355-63.
27. Fontana J, Wenz H, Schmieder K, Barth M. Impairment of Dynamic Pressure Autoregulation Precedes Clinical Deterioration after Aneurysmal Subarachnoid Hemorrhage. J Neuroimag. 2016;26(3):339-45.
28. Budohoski KP, Czosnyka M, Smielewski P, Kasprowicz M, Helmy A, Bulters D, et al. Impairment of cerebral autoregulation predicts delayed cerebral ischemia after subarachnoid hemorrhage: A prospective observational study. Stroke. 2012;43(12):3230-7.
29. Sundgreen C, Larsen FS, Herzog TM, Knudsen GM, Boesgaard S, Aldershvile J. Autoregulation of cerebral blood flow in patients resuscitated from cardiac arrest. Stroke. 2001;32(1):128-32.
30. Kirschen MP, Majmudar T, Diaz-Arrastia R, Berg R, Abella BS, Topjian A, et al. Deviations from PRx-derived optimal blood pressure are associated with mortality after cardiac arrest. Resuscitation [Internet]. 2022;175:81-7.

31. Caldas JR, Haunton VJ, Panerai RB, Hajjar LA, Robinson TG. Cerebral autoregulation in cardiopulmonary bypass surgery: a systematic review. Interact Cardiovasc Thorac Surg. 2018;26(3):494-503.
32. Chan B, Aneman A. A prospective, observational study of cerebrovascular autoregulation and its association with delirium following cardiac surgery. Anaesthesia. 2019;74(1):33-44.
33. Paschoal-Jr FM, Nogueira RC, Ronconi K de AL, de Lima Oliveira M, Almeida KJ, Rocha IS, et al. TCD assessment in fulminant hepatic failure: Improvements in cerebral autoregulation after liver transplantation. Ann Hepatol. 2024;29(2):101167.
34. Shen ZD, Qu Y, Zhang P, Wang G, Wang Y, Yang Y, et al. Dynamic Cerebral Autoregulation After Carotid Endarterectomy. J Endovas Ther. 2025;32(5):1267-74.

CHAPTER 8

Continuous Intra-abdominal Pressure Monitoring: Is it Worth it?

Suhail Sarwar Siddiqui, Ambuj Yadav

INTRODUCTION

Elevated intra-abdominal pressure (IAP) is recognized as a significant contributor to morbidity and mortality among critically ill patients.[1] Approximately 25% of intensive care patients have intra-abdominal hypertension (IAH), and >50% develop IAH within the first week of intensive care unit (ICU) admission.[2,3] The IAH and abdominal compartment syndrome (ACS) are same spectrum of conditions related to elevated IAP. IAH is the sustained elevation of IAP above 12 mm Hg, while ACS occurs when IAP is significantly higher (>20 mm Hg) associated with new onset organ dysfunction. Even mild but persistent elevations in IAP can compromise blood flow and cause multiple organ dysfunction, e.g., cardiac, respiratory, renal, gastrointestinal (GI), central nervous system, etc. Continuous intra-abdominal pressure (CIAP) monitoring has emerged as a promising alternative to conventional intermittent IAP monitoring, offering real-time data, early detection, and tracking trends in response to interventions. Furthermore, CIAP has shown potential to improve patient outcomes by enabling early diagnosis and timely management of IAH and ACS. Essentially, IAH can progress to ACS if not addressed on time. Despite its frequency and clinical importance, IAH often remains undetected and thus underreported, as IAP monitoring is not a routine practice in most ICUs. A systematic and structured management strategy can significantly improve outcomes. Since clinical examination alone is often unreliable for detecting raised IAP, serial or continuous measurements are essential for diagnosing and managing IAH and ACS. Although various techniques have been developed to measure IAP, transbladder measurement remains one of the most commonly used methods. This technique is favored for its simplicity, cost-effectiveness, and minimal invasiveness, but it is labor-intensive and intermittent. This chapter highlights recent developments in the measurement of CIAP, which will help in early diagnosis, monitoring, and intervention of this critical condition.

INTRA-ABDOMINAL HYPERTENSION GRADING AND PATHOPHYSIOLOGY OF IAH AND ACS

The IAP monitoring is crucial in critical care due to the potential for complications such as IAH and ACS. The reported prevalence of IAH varies

TABLE 1: IAH grading.

Grade	*IAP (mm Hg)*
I	12–15
II	16–20
III	21–25
IV	>25

(IAH: intra-abdominal hypertension; IAP: intra-abdominal pressure)

widely, ranging from 18 to 81%, depending on the threshold used to define elevated IAP (e.g., 12, 15, 18, 20, or 25 mm Hg), as well as the specific patient population studied: such as trauma, surgical, or medical intensive care patients.[3]

Intra-abdominal pressure measurement is recommended by the World Society of Abdominal Compartment Syndrome (WSACS) every 4–6 hours in critically ill patients when any known risk factor for IAH/ACS is present.[4] The standard technique for intermittent IAP monitoring is via the urinary bladder. It should be measured in a completely supine position, at end-expiration with relaxed abdominal muscles using a pressure transducer zeroed at the midaxillary line, with a maximum of 25 mL of sterile saline for instillation.

Normal and elevated IAP: In critically ill patients, a typical IAP ranges between 5 and 7 mm Hg.[4] IAH is a persistent or repeated increase in IAP ≥12 mm Hg.[5] Grading of IAH is given in **Table 1**.

Abdominal compartment syndrome (ACS): ACS occurs when IAP rises above 20 mm Hg and leads to new organ dysfunction or failure, possibly accompanied by abdominal perfusion pressure (APP) <60 mm Hg (APP is the difference between mean arterial pressure and intra-abdominal pressure).

The impact of raised IAP is not limited to intra-abdominal organs but can also affect organs outside, leading to multiorgan failure **(Table 2)**.[6]

Although measuring IAP intermittently via the bladder remains the current standard, this method has certain limitations, including being labor-intensive and potentially delaying the identification of sudden changes in IAP. As a result, CIAP monitoring has emerged as a promising alternative.[2]

ADVANTAGES OF CONTINUOUS INTRA-ABDOMINAL PRESSURE

- *Early identification and timely intervention:* CIAP facilitates the prompt recognition of IAH and ACS, potentially improving clinical outcomes.
- *Real-time monitoring, trend analysis, and targeting abdominal perfusion pressure:* By continuously observing IAP, clinicians can better understand the relationship between IAP and other vital parameters such as urine

TABLE 2: Impact of raised IAP on various organs.[6]

Kidney	• Decreased renal blood flow • Elevated renal parenchymal and venous pressures causing AKI
Respiratory system	• Decreases chest wall compliance • Increase intrathoracic pressure • Reduced lung volumes • Compression atelectasis • Hypoxia and hypercarbia
Hemodynamics	• Impedes venous return • Increases afterload • Reduced cardiac output • Poor organ perfusion and eventually worsening of IAH
Intracranial pressure	Increase intracranial pressure
Gastrointestinal tract	• Decreased gastrointestinal motility • Gastroparesis • Gastroesophageal reflex • Increase GRV • Reduced splanchnic perfusion
Hepatobiliary	• Decrease portal blood flow • Decreased lactate clearance • Deranged liver function

(AKI: acute kidney injury; GRV: gastric residual volume; IAH: intra-abdominal hypertension)

output (UO). Simultaneous CIAP and UO monitoring may enable early diagnosis and treatment of both ACS and AKI, leading to improved kidney function and hemodynamic stability. This can assist in targeting abdominal perfusion pressure (APP), assessing therapeutic responses and adjusting treatment strategies effectively.

- *Decreased manual workload:* CIAP reduces the need for repeated manual IAP checks, potentially alleviating the burden on healthcare staff. CIAP monitoring aims to provide a more dynamic and timely assessment of IAP compared to traditional intermittent techniques. Here are some established and emerging methods for CIAP monitoring **(Table 3)**.[2]

METHODS OF INVASIVE CONTINUOUS INTRA-ABDOMINAL PRESSURE

- *Direct intraperitoneal pressure measurement:* This technique involves placing a catheter directly into the peritoneal cavity to assess IAP. Although it provides a direct and potentially more precise measurement, it is considered more invasive than indirect approaches and carries a greater risk of infection and other complications. Despite these drawbacks, it may

TABLE 3: Methods of continuous intra-abdominal pressure monitoring.[2]

Invasive	*Less/noninvasive*
• Direct intraperitoneal pressure measurement via intraperitoneal catheter • Intravesical pressure monitoring • Intragastric pressure monitoring	• Strain gauge • Respiratory inductance plethysmography (RIP) • Abdominal tensiometry • Ultrasound-based techniques – Ultrasound tonometry – Measurement of abdominal wall thickness (AWT) – Doppler assessments – Laser ultrasound • Bioelectrical impedance • Microwave reflectometry • Digital capsules (ingestible)

be appropriate in specific situations, such as during surgical interventions or in patients with an open abdomen, where continuous and accurate monitoring is essential.

- *Intravesical pressure monitoring (via bladder):* This approach involves using a three-way Foley catheter equipped for continuous irrigation, where the irrigation port serves to measure IAP in real time. This eliminates the need for intermittent clamping, which is traditionally required in standard methods. Clinical studies have demonstrated that this technique closely correlates with conventional intermittent measurements, suggesting it as a reliable alternative. Potential risks such as backflow of fluids and catheter-associated infections should be considered. Another advanced system, the *Accuryn Monitoring System* by Potrero Medical, employs a specially designed urinary catheter featuring an additional air-filled balloon at its tip. This setup allows for continuous and accurate measurement of IAP, UO, and core body temperature, offering high-resolution and near-continuous monitoring capabilities.[7]
- *Intragastric pressure monitoring (via stomach):* This method involves using a balloon-tipped nasogastric tube (e.g., Spiegelberg) to estimate CIAP. When properly positioned, these techniques can be fully automated and provide continuous IAP trends.

LESS/NONINVASIVE TECHNIQUES OF CONTINUOUS INTRA-ABDOMINAL PRESSURE

- *Strain gauges:* Strain gauges can be incorporated into systems for noninvasive IAP monitoring. Strain gauges offer a low-cost and simple method to detect changes in abdominal wall tension (AWT), which can indirectly correlate with IAP. Strain gauges operate on the principle that their electrical resistance changes proportionally to the force or pressure applied to them, and by extension, to the deformation (strain) they experience. In the context of IAP monitoring, a strain gauge can be attached to the abdominal wall to detect subtle changes in tension caused by fluctuations in IAP. These changes in tension lead to variations in the indentation force on strain gauges alone, which may not provide sufficiently accurate IAP measurements due to potential motion artifacts and other distortions. To improve accuracy and enhance the value of IAP monitoring, strain gauges are often used with other less invasive techniques such as respiratory inductance plethysmography (RIP) or abdominal tensiometry.[2,8]

- *Respiratory inductance plethysmography:* RIP measures respiratory rates and lung volumes by detecting changes in the cross-sectional area of the chest and abdomen during breathing. RIP uses two elastic bands with embedded coils of wire, one around the chest and the other around the abdomen. An alternating current is passed through the coils, generating a magnetic field. As the chest and abdomen expand and contract with respiration, the area of the coil changes, which alters the magnetic field and the inductance. The changes in inductance are converted into digital waveforms, reflecting breathing patterns and lung volumes. While not a primary method for IAP monitoring, changes in breathing patterns measured by RIP can indirectly relate to IAP, especially in conditions where the abdominal wall compliance is altered. Furthermore, IAP measurement by RIP has not yet been validated.[2]
- *Abdominal tensiometry:* Abdominal tensiometry, also known as AWT measurement, is a noninvasive method. The principle relies on the assumption that, similar to pressurized cylinders, there is a direct relationship between the tension of the abdominal wall and the internal pressure within the abdominal cavity. Tensiometry involves applying a punctual force to the abdominal wall and measuring the resulting displacement (indentation) or the force required to produce a specific displacement. AWT is then calculated as the ratio of thrust to displacement. Studies have explored the correlation between AWT and IAP, particularly using urinary bladder pressure as a surrogate for IAP.[9] Abdominal tensiometry is noninvasive, simple, and fast, but these devices need to be standardized to achieve more reliable and repeatable evaluations.
- *Ultrasound-based techniques:* Various ultrasound-based methods—such as ultrasound tonometry, measurement of abdominal wall thickness, Doppler assessments, and laser ultrasound—offer noninvasive and safe options for evaluating IAP.[2] These approaches are appealing due to their bedside applicability and minimal risk. However, their reliability and effectiveness for continuous pressure monitoring across diverse clinical settings need more research.

- *Bioelectrical impedance:* This method estimates IAP by detecting fluctuations in the electrical impedance of the abdominal wall. As a noninvasive technique, it holds potential for bedside monitoring. When properly optimized, abdominal wall bioimpedance can serve as a sensitive and accurate surrogate for continuous IAP monitoring in experimental models—paving the way for potential human application. However, further clinical validation is needed to determine its accuracy in detecting elevated IAP values.[10]
- *Microwave reflectometry:* A microwave system sends electromagnetic waves toward the abdominal wall and analyzes the reflected signals. Fluctuations in the reflected signal's properties are correlated with changes in IAP, allowing for estimation of pressure levels. This innovative and noninvasive technique shows potential as a reliable IAP monitoring tool, though it is still in the experimental stage and requires additional research to confirm its clinical utility.[11]
- *Digital capsules (ingestible):* Ingestible devices are equipped with miniaturized pressure sensors that transmit real-time pressure data wirelessly from inside the GI tract. This innovative, noninvasive method enables continuous IAP monitoring without limiting patient mobility or requiring invasive procedures. While promising in terms of patient comfort and convenience, potential challenges—such as delayed capsule transit or retention—must be considered. A human pilot trial demonstrates that the digital ingestible capsule is a safe and feasible tool for continuously monitoring IAP, with measurements closely matching those from the conventional bladder (intravesical) method during pneumoperitoneum.[12]

LIMITATIONS OF CONTINUOUS INTRA-ABDOMINAL PRESSURE

Continuous intra-abdominal pressure does have some challenges. Accurate and consistent readings depend on patient positioning, bladder volume, and the specific method used. Moreover, patient-specific variables such as body mass index, type of surgery, or underlying conditions like pancreatitis can influence pressure readings, requiring individualized interpretation. Some studies, including those involving three-way Foley catheters, have shown CIAP to be comparable with intermittent techniques, supporting its clinical viability. Technical complexity, lack of validation and the need for specialized training may limit the use of specific CIAP systems.

Furthermore, these systems may not be reliable or accurate enough to be used in clinical practice. Choosing the most suitable approach for CIAP monitoring involves evaluating several factors, such as the patient's clinical status, the level of invasiveness acceptable, the precision needed, and the accessibility of available technologies. Ongoing studies and clinical trials aim to enhance current methods and develop innovative, more accurate and user-friendly solutions for effective CIAP monitoring.

COMPARISON OF INTERMITTENT VERSUS CONTINUOUS IAP MONITORING IN GAUGING THERAPEUTIC INTERVENTION AND ITS CORRELATION TO OUTCOMES

Traditionally, intermittent IAP measurement using the intravesical method has been the gold standard; however, it may miss transient spikes in pressure that can have clinical significance. Malbrain et al. highlighted that continuous IAP monitoring provides superior temporal resolution, allowing for early detection of pathological pressure changes and timely therapeutic responses, possibly reducing the progression to ACS.[6] Liao et al. observed the feasibility and accuracy of a novel swallowable capsular device for continuous IAP monitoring, with excellent correlation to standard bladder pressure measurements and potential for real-time and noninvasive monitoring in surgical patients.[12] Similarly, David et al. validated the use of abdominal wall bioimpedance in a porcine model, showing promise for continuous and noninvasive monitoring.[9] Continuous monitoring enhances the detection of critical pressure changes and correlates with improved hemodynamic management and outcomes in critically ill patients, making it a valuable tool for early intervention in high-risk scenarios where IAP fluctuations are common.

FUTURE DIRECTIONS

- *Noninvasive monitoring techniques:* Emerging technologies such as microwave reflectometry, ultrasound-based evaluation, and swallowable sensor capsules are being investigated to enable real-time, accurate IAP monitoring without invasive procedures.
- *Intelligent systems and automation:* The incorporation of CIAP monitoring with machine learning algorithms and advanced data analytics can automate the recognition of critical pressure elevations, enabling early intervention through timely alerts.
- *Customized patient care:* Future strategies may increasingly focus on individualized IAP monitoring and treatment plans, taking into account each patient's unique clinical status and risk profile to optimize outcomes.

CONCLUSION

Continuous intra-abdominal pressure monitoring can enhance patient care in critical care settings by facilitating early identification, real-time evaluation, and more precise monitoring and management of IAH and ACS.

However, its validation and high-level evidence that it improves outcomes are yet to be proven in large-scale studies. Further research is needed to address challenges in standardization and technological refinement, to enhance the accuracy, ease of use, and seamless integration of CIAP monitoring into everyday clinical practice.

REFERENCES

1. Malbrain ML, Chiumello D, Pelosi P, Bihari D, Innes R, Ranieri VM, et al. Incidence and prognosis of intraabdominal hypertension in a mixed population of critically ill patients: a multiple-center epidemiological study. Crit Care Med. 2005;33(2):315-22.
2. Tayebi S, Gutierrez A, Mohout I, Smets E, Wise R, Stiens J, et al. A concise overview of non-invasive intra-abdominal pressure measurement techniques: from bench to bedside. J Clin Monit Comput. 2021;35(1):51-70.
3. Malbrain ML, Chiumello D, Cesana BM, Reintam Blaser A, Starkopf J, Sugrue M, et al. A systematic review and individual patient data meta-analysis on intra-abdominal hypertension in critically ill patients: the wake-up project. World initiative on Abdominal Hypertension Epidemiology, a Unifying Project (WAKE-Up!). Minerva Anestesiol. 2014;80(3):293-306.
4. Sosa G, Gandham N, Landeras V, et al. Abdominal compartment syndrome. Dis Mon. 2019;65(1):5-19.
5. Kirkpatrick AW, Roberts DJ, De Waele J, Jaeschke R, Malbrain ML, De Keulenaer B, et al. Intra-abdominal hypertension and the abdominal compartment syndrome: updated consensus definitions and clinical practice guidelines from the World Society of the Abdominal Compartment Syndrome. Intensive Care Med. 2013;39(7):1190-206.
6. Malbrain MLNG, De Keulenaer BL, Khanna AK. Continuous intra-abdominal pressure: is it ready for prime time? Intensive Care Med. 2022;48(10):1501-4.
7. Khanna AK, Minear S, Kurz A, Moll V, Stanton K, Essakalli L, et al. Intra-abdominal hypertension in cardiac surgery patients: a multicenter observational sub-study of the Accuryn registry. J Clin Monit Comput. 2023;37(1):189-99.
8. Tang H, Liu D, Guo Y, Zhang H, Li Y, Peng X, et al. A New Device for Measuring Abdominal Wall Tension and Its Value in Screening Abdominal Infection. Med Devices (Auckl). 2021;14:119-31.
9. Chen YZ, Yan SY, Chen YQ, Zhuang YG, Wei Z, Zhou SQ, et al. Noninvasive monitoring of intra-abdominal pressure by measuring abdominal wall tension. World J Emerg Med. 2015;6(2):137-41.
10. David M, Amran O, Peretz A, et al. Optimized electrical bioimpedance measurements of abdominal wall on a porcine model for the continuous non-invasive assessment of intra-abdominal pressure. J Clin Monit Comput. 2020;34(6):1209-14.
11. David M, Raviv A, Guttel A, García Reyes V, Simini F, Pracca F. Non-invasive indirect monitoring of intra-abdominal pressure using microwave reflectometry: system design and proof-of-concept clinical trial. J Clin Monit Comput. 2021;35(6):1437-43.
12. Liao CH, Spain DA, Chen CC, Cheng CT, Lin WC, Ho DR, et al. Feasibility and accuracy of continuous intraabdominal pressure monitoring with a capsular device in human pilot trial. World J Emerg Surg. 2025;20(1):7.

CHAPTER 9

Precision Medicine: Sub-phenotyping in Critical Care

Shaveta Devesar, Prashant Nasa

INTRODUCTION

The evolving landscape in healthcare is precision-based medicine and patient-centered care with an individualized treatment approach. Historically, critical care has relied on broad syndromic definitions for treatment and research purposes. Constructs or syndromes such as sepsis, acute respiratory distress syndrome (ARDS), acute kidney injury (AKI), traumatic brain injury (TBI), and delirium were developed using a combination of clinical, physiological, and biochemical patterns for the identification and grouping of critically ill patients. Although these syndromes help in early diagnosis through easily accessible clinical and physiological variables, the fundamental heterogeneity in underlying etiology and pathophysiological processes challenges their existence. It is further complicated by the inter-individual variation in response to inciting injury and response to interventions. Additionally, these syndromes involve diverse overlapping biological mechanisms, and may present as multiple, yet interconnected critical care syndromes.

The heterogeneity observed in these syndromes is often cited as a significant barrier, both in clinical practice and research. The definition or diagnostic criteria of these syndromes are mainly left broader to improve sensitivity and include the majority of patients, albeit with varied clinical presentations, disease course, and outcomes. Moreover, using these definitions as inclusion criteria for clinical research has its own challenges. The heterogeneity could explain the numerous failed clinical trials on various pharmacological and supportive care interventions that may appear otherwise promising in preclinical models. Furthermore, in some instances, heterogeneity may also account for adverse effects of an intervention observed in certain subgroups of patients while the benefit is observed in others (heterogeneity-of-treatment effect).

A *one-size-fits-all* approach is increasingly viewed as inadequate, prompting a shift toward more personalized interventions that recognize patient and disease heterogeneity.[1,2] Sub-phenotyping these clinical syndromes into distinct subgroups with or without treatable traits offers an opportunity for more targeted, effective interventions in critical care settings. This chapter aims to provide a comprehensive overview of sub-phenotyping in critical care, highlighting the scientific rationale, methodologies employed, evidence, clinical applications, challenges for sub-phenotyping, and future directions for precision-based medicine.

RATIONALE FOR SUB-PHENOTYPING

Delineate Heterogeneity

Sub-phenotyping involves using various measurable traits such as physiological characteristics, imaging and biomarkers to categorize syndromes (phenotype) into distinct and reproducible subgroups **(Table 1)**. Sub-phenotyping is used in critical care to address patient heterogeneity and enable tailored treatment strategies and prognostic enrichment.

Most syndromes in critical care are inherently heterogeneous, featuring patients with overlapping clinical presentations and pathophysiological mechanisms but heterogeneous etiology, molecular, immunological, and physiological characteristics. Sub-phenotyping helps to delineate heterogeneity of syndromes such as sepsis, ARDS, and AKI, and allows

TABLE 1: Definitions of phenotyping terminology used in this chapter.

Terms	*Definition*	*Example*
Phenotype	Clinically observable set of characteristics	ARDS
Subgroup	Categorization of phenotypes using a *cut-off of clinical or physiological* variable	PaO_2/FiO_2 ratio-based classification of ARDS
Sub-phenotype	Clinically *distinct subgroups* of phenotype which can be reliably discriminated, based on a shared set or pattern of measurable or observable characteristics	Biomarkers-based sub-phenotyping into hyper- or hypoinflammatory
Endotype	Sub-phenotype with *distinct underlying functional or biological mechanisms* (e.g., gene expression, protein levels, or biomarkers) that may or may not be associated with a specific treatment response	Specific profile within hyperinflammatory sub-phenotype (e.g., IL-6, complement pathway)
Treatable traits	Set of measurable clinical characteristics and/or biomarkers representing a pathophysiological process and have been linked to outcomes/interventions	Hyperinflammation in ARDS or sepsis

(ARDS: acute respiratory distress syndrome; IL: interleukin; PaO_2/FiO_2: ratio of arterial partial pressure of oxygen to fraction of inspired oxygen)

Source: Adapted from Nasa P, Bos LD, Estenssoro E, van Haren FM, Serpa Neto A, Rocco PR, et al. Consensus statements on the utility of defining ARDS and the utility of past and current definitions of ARDS-protocol for a Delphi study. BMJ Open. 2024;14(4):e082986.

precision-based personalized treatment. For example, sepsis has been redefined by third International Consensus Definitions for Sepsis and Septic Shock (Sepsis 3) as life-threatening organ dysfunction caused by a dysregulated host response to infection. Although the definition shifted its focus on organ dysfunction from nonspecific clinical signs grouped as systemic inflammatory response syndrome (SIRS). However, there is no consideration of the underlying etiology, molecular and immunological pathways leading to organ failure and the presence of pre-existing organ dysfunction.[3] Furthermore, many noninfective conditions present with organ failure and overlap considerably with sepsis. This often accounts for the failure of otherwise promising therapies to demonstrate efficacy in large clinical trials, as differential responses among unrecognized patient subgroups dilute observed treatment effects. Sub-phenotyping aims to resolve these differences, allowing clinicians to—(1) predict which patients will respond to specific therapies; (2) identify mechanisms that drive adverse outcomes; and (3) design targeted clinical trials that enrich for likely responders.

Differential Prognostic and Treatment Implications

Patients categorized into distinct sub-phenotypes may demonstrate unique disease trajectories and varying responses to treatments.[4] The identification of these subgroups facilitates prediction of outcomes (prognostic enrichment) and enables the selection of patients who are most likely to benefit from specific therapeutic interventions (predictive enrichment).[5]

Understanding Pathophysiology

Identifying sub-phenotypes based on biological characteristics provides deeper understanding of the pathophysiological mechanisms underlying the various syndromes and insights into heterogeneity of treatment effect. Besides, these mechanistic studies also explain varied patient trajectories within the same condition and help in prognostication.[6]

METHODOLOGIES FOR SUB-PHENOTYPING

Various approaches are employed to uncover distinct patterns within a broader clinical phenotype, thereby identifying sub-phenotypes. These sub-phenotypes often differ in prognosis, treatment response, or biological pathways. The process typically involves statistical modeling using a combination of clinical and physiological characteristics, biomarkers, and imaging.[3]

Statistical and Clustering Methods

Recent advances in big data analytics and computational biology have facilitated the integration of multidimensional datasets that include multiple variables such as clinical, physiological, imaging, and biological (biomarker) characteristics. The complex statistical tools such as clustering algorithm and latent class analysis (LCA) are used for large scale analyses of clinical, physiological and molecular data to identify critical illness subphenotypes.

Latent Class Analysis

Latent class analysis is a probabilistic method for partitioning patients into latent subgroups within a heterogeneous cohort based on patterns of observed variables (clinical, physiological, or biological).[3]

Clustering Analysis

It is an unsupervised machine learning method that identifies homogenous subgroups based on similar characteristics (clinical, biological, or physiological).[6]

Dynamic Time Warping

Along with hierarchical agglomerative clustering (HAC), dynamic time warping (DTW) identifies sub-phenotypes by analyzing the trajectory of physiological scores, e.g., temporal evolution of Sequential Organ Failure Assessment (SOFA) score over time in sepsis.[7]

Biomarker and Data-driven Approaches

Machine Learning Models

Unsupervised clustering of large datasets including support vector machines, random forests, and deep learning identifies sub-phenotypes with distinct underlying biological mechanisms.[2]

Multiomics

Integrating information genomics, transcriptomics, proteomics, and metabolomics for better characterization of pathophysiology and patient-environment interactions, thereby, identifies exclusive subgroups (sub-phenotypes).

Real-time Sub-phenotyping

Emerging technologies enable point-of-care diagnostic platforms for rapid biomarker measurement (e.g., portable immunodiagnostic assays), which may facilitate real-time clinical decision-making.

Trajectory-based Methods

Using dynamic evolution of various physiological characteristics, distinct subgroups could be identified for patient prognostication and treatment responses (dynamic trajectory of PaO_2 and FiO_2 ratio, organ dysfunction scores).[8]

EVIDENCE FOR SUB-PHENOTYPES IN CRITICAL CARE SYNDROMES

In this section, we will discuss the evidence on three common ICU syndromes—sepsis, ARDS, and AKI. There are other conditions where sub-phenotyping has been described such as TBI and delirium. However, these are beyond the scope of this chapter.

Sepsis

Sub-phenotyping in sepsis has been performed based on the immune response, biomarkers, organ dysfunction, and clinical trajectories. Moreover, the evidence supports sub-phenotyping for mortality prediction, guiding personalized interventions, and/or developing targeted therapies.[2]

Inflammatory (Hyperinflammatory versus Hypoinflammatory) Sub-phenotypes

Previously validated models used for sub-phenotyping ARDS, including clinical data and plasma biomarkers, were used for LCA-based sub-phenotyping in two randomized controlled trials (RCTs) of sepsis—Prospective Recombinant Human Activated Protein C Worldwide Evaluation in Severe Sepsis and Septic Shock (PROWESS-SHOCK) trial and Vasopressin and Septic Shock Trial (VASST) were evaluated. A strong concordance was noted between sepsis and ARDS sub-phenotypes with higher proinflammatory cytokines and lower protein C in the hyperinflammatory sub-phenotype. Moreover, a higher vasopressor requirement and mortality rates were observed in the hyperinflammatory versus hypoinflammatory sub-phenotype ($p < 0.0001$). Notably, significant heterogeneity of treatment effect was found with lower mortality associated with activated protein C in the hyperinflammatory sub-phenotype compared to placebo. However, no treatment interaction was observed in the VASST trial.[9]

Immune Profiling

The immune profiling is based on the host response to the microbial agent. In a large study, four distinct sub-phenotypes were identified across three observational cohorts and three clinical trial populations, and labeled as α, β, γ, and δ. Patients in the α sub-phenotype showed relatively normal laboratory values and minimal organ dysfunction. Those in the β sub-phenotype were typically older, with a greater burden of chronic diseases, and more often presented with AKI. Hypoalbuminemia, higher body temperatures, and elevated markers of systemic inflammation characterized the γ sub-phenotype. In contrast, the δ sub-phenotype was marked by hypotension and elevated serum lactate levels. Importantly, mortality rates were consistently highest among patients in the δ group—up to eight times greater than those in the lowest-risk α group. Additionally, circulating cytokine concentrations were found to be elevated in both the γ and δ phenotypes compared with α and β.[10]

In another study using body temperature, four sub-phenotypes were identified—hyperthermic slow resolvers, hyperthermic fast resolvers, normothermic, and hypothermic. Hyperthermic cohorts had higher levels of both pro- and anti-inflammatory cytokines. However, hypothermic patients had lower levels of inflammatory cytokines, instead higher levels of coagulation biomarkers such as thrombomodulin, Ang-1, and tissue factor as well as higher mortality.[11]

The Molecular Diagnosis and Risk Stratification of Sepsis (MARS) consortium described four sepsis sub-phenotypes, termed Mars1–4.[11] Patients classified as Mars1 had the highest SOFA scores, with a greater incidence of shock and mortality. Their gene-expression profile suggested impaired innate and adaptive immune responses, including downregulation of NFκB1, toll-like receptor signaling, T-cell receptor signaling, and antigen presentation.

Trajectory-based

Sub-phenotyping based on the trajectory of vital signs, laboratory variable, and organ function helps to identify sub-phenotypes. Hao et al. identified three sub-phenotypes using time-series clustering analysis and DTW and labeled as type A to C. Type C with severely impaired organ function noted to have highest inflammatory markers and mortality rate, compared to type A and type B.[12]

Acute Respiratory Distress Syndrome

There is no other syndrome like ARDS in critical care, where considerable heterogeneity exists and with extensive work on sub-phenotyping has been performed. Sub-phenotyping ARDS has been performed based on etiological, physiological, radiological, and biological criteria.

Inflammatory Sub-phenotypes

In ARDS, inflammatory sub-phenotyping divides patients into groups with distinct biological and clinical characteristics, most commonly hyperinflammatory and hypoinflammatory. Patients in the hyperinflammatory subgroup tend to experience poorer outcomes, with higher rates of mortality and multiorgan failure, whereas those in the hypoinflammatory subgroup generally show more favorable prognoses. These categories, defined through a combination of biomarkers and clinical variables, also appear to respond differently to specific therapies such as simvastatin and corticosteroids, highlighting opportunities for a more personalized approach to ARDS management. Post-hoc analysis of large

RCTs indicates that the incidence of hyperinflammatory sub-phenotype is around 30–40%. In a meta-analysis of 12 studies comprising 6,643 patients, based on low certainty of evidence, patients with hyperinflammatory ARDS were found to be associated with a higher risk of death and lower ventilator-free days compared to hypoinflammatory sub-phenotypes.[13]

However, primary challenges with biomarkers are the bedside availability for classification and diagnosis. Besides, most research is retrospective with post-hoc analysis of large RCT. Prospective research and point-of-care biomarker assays are required, before they are adopted in clinical practice.[4]

Radiology-based Sub-phenotyping

Imaging (CT chest)-based categorization of ARDS into focal and nonfocal sub-phenotypes have been studied for personalized ventilation strategies. Patients with focal ARDS received a tidal volume of 8 mL/kg, low positive end-expiratory pressure (PEEP), and early prone positioning. On the other hand, nonfocal ARDS patients received a lower tidal volume (6 mL/kg), higher PEEP, as well as recruitment maneuvers. Although there was no survival benefit between the personalized ventilation compared to control, misclassification of patients into wrong sub-phenotype was associated with higher mortality.[14] This study reflects on the challenges of classification of ARDS at the bedside and potential implications of misclassification.

Lung ultrasound provides a noninvasive alternative to categorize ARDS, but challenges such as interobserver variability, difficulties in image acquisition in patients with obesity or subcutaneous emphysema, and its inability to detect hyperinflation limit its utility. A meta-analysis showed pooled sensitivity of 0.631 [95% confidence interval (CI): 0.45–0.782] and specificity of 0.942 (95% CI: 0.86–0.98) for diagnosis of ARDS. However, the data was inadequate for meta-analysis for sub-phenotyping.[15] An ongoing RCT will provide further evidence in this regard.[16]

Beyond imaging, physiological and radiological data have helped identify ARDS sub-phenotypes such as recruitable and non-recruitable groups, which differ in their responses to therapies and in mortality risk—a trend also observed in COVID-19-related ARDS.

Physiological Variables

Tracking respiratory mechanics like ventilatory ratio and mechanical power over time can identify worsening or stabilizing sub-phenotypes. Using the machine learning with training in the Chinese ARDS Database and further validation in FACTT, SAILS, ALVEOLI, and MIMIC-IV datasets, three longitudinal oxygenation subgroups were identified. The PaO_2/FiO_2 trajectories over time were characterized as persistently low, gradually increasing, and rapidly improving. Mortality varied significantly across these subgroups (62.6% vs. 35.8% vs. 17.4%) and performed better than the Berlin classification of severity. Moreover, treatment heterogeneity with high versus low PEEP was greater in the longitudinal subgroups than the static PaO_2/FiO_2 Berlin-defined groups.[17]

A cluster analysis of 3,875 patients identified three clinical sub-phenotypes of ARDS. Sub-phenotype I (40%) was associated with fewer laboratory abnormalities, less organ failure, lower in-hospital mortality, and the greatest number of ventilator-free and ICU-free days, resembling the hypoinflammatory phenotype. Sub-phenotype II (32%) was characterized by younger age, elevated WBC count, higher temperature, increased heart and respiratory rates, and lower systolic blood pressure—features consistent with the hyperinflammatory phenotype. Sub-phenotype III (28%) included older patients with higher serum creatinine and blood urea nitrogen, lower bicarbonate, fewer ventilator-free and ICU-free days, and the highest mortality, reflecting contributions from organ dysfunction, advanced age, and metabolic acidosis. These findings were validated in three RCTs (ALVEOLI, FACTT, and SAILS), where significant treatment heterogeneity was observed in ALVEOLI and FACTT, though no clear heterogeneity of treatment response was seen in SAILS.[18]

Acute Kidney Injury

Sub-phenotyping AKI has highlighted heterogeneous treatment effects with fluid balance strategies, as well as response to renal replacement therapies.

Creatinine Trajectory

In a cohort of cardiopulmonary bypass, divided into development and validation sets and using LCA, 12 AKI sub-phenotypes were distinguished by different postoperative serum creatinine trajectories over time. The study also incorporated patient demographics, procedural variables, postoperative complications, and long-term outcomes. Importantly, four of these sub-phenotypes were classified as high-risk, demonstrating a substantially greater long-term mortality risk compared with lower-risk groups.[19]

In another cohort of 6,816 ICU patients with any stage of kidney disease: Improving Global Outcomes (KDIGO)-defined AKI, the pattern of kidney function over time was more strongly linked to inpatient mortality than the peak KDIGO stage itself. Patients with a lower maximum KDIGO stage but a gradual decline in renal function (sub-phenotypes C and D) experienced higher ICU mortality than those who presented with a high KDIGO stage but showed rapid recovery within three days (sub-phenotypes A and B).[20] Another recent study on AKI in sepsis patients, using creatinine trajectory, noted a persistent AKI sub-phenotype was more likely associated with worse outcomes and chronic kidney disease.[21]

Biomarker-based Sub-phenotypes

Various biomarkers are used for detection of subclinical AKI, defined as AKI before rise of creatinine. These biomarkers include plasma or urinary neutrophil gelatinase-associated lipocalin (NGAL), urinary kidney injury molecule 1 (KIM-1), urinary tissue inhibitor of metalloproteinase-2 (TIMP-2), and insulin-like growth factor-binding protein 7 (IGFBP7).

In cohorts of septic patients, LCA identified two distinct AKI sub-phenotypes using biomarkers. Patients with elevated biomarker levels [(TIMP–2) · (IGFBP7) > 0.3] following fluid resuscitation were at increased risk of a composite outcome comprising progression to severe AKI (Stage 2/3), need for dialysis, or death. Notably, the incidence of this composite endpoint was comparable among patients with elevated postresuscitation biomarkers, regardless of their preresuscitation biomarker status, and was also similar between those with or without AKI at enrolment as defined by serum creatinine and urine output.[22,23]

Analysis of data from the VASST trial (vasopressin versus norepinephrine in septic shock) further revealed treatment effect heterogeneity, with differing responses to the early initiation of vasopressin between the sub-phenotypes. Patients with less severe septic shock, potentially benefited with early vasopressin initiation, with no survival benefit observed in more severe septic shock.[24]

TABLE 2: Challenges in implementation of current sub-phenotyping of critical care syndromes.

Pitfall	*Description*
Clinical utility	Sub-phenotypes must be prospectively identifiable, measurable, actionable, predictive of treatment response, and reproducible across populations
Generalizability	Models identified and validated in high-resource settings may not translate directly to low-resource environments; global validation is needed
Practicality	Complex sub-phenotypes should be approximated using simple, pragmatic, readily available and point-of-care measurable data for routine implementation
Equity and representation	Underrepresentation of ethnic minorities, children, and pregnant women can limit applicability and exacerbate disparities; patient-centered outcomes are essential
Transparency	Artificial intelligence/machine learning models may be "black boxes," complicating clinician understanding and patient communication
Trial feasibility	Selecting cohort for treatment evaluation increases screening burden, sample size requirements, and raises ethical considerations regarding equipoise

CHALLENGES WITH SUB-PHENOTYPING

The major challenges in data-driven phenotyping are the heterogeneity of current methods, with no standardized or reproducible approaches to identify sub-phenotypes and endotypes across different datasets, and a lack of consolidated strategies to translate these findings into clinical practice. Most models have been developed in specific cohorts and settings, so their generalizability across various health systems and ICUs remains unclear. Prospective validation in diverse populations will, therefore, be essential, before their widespread adoption. Any proposed sub-phenotype should be evaluated for—(1) consistency and reproducibility in independent datasets, (2) biological plausibility, and (3) clinical utility, such as predicting high-risk patients or guiding treatment response **(Table 2)**.

Ultimately, an ideal phenotyping algorithm should inform real-time clinical decision-making and offer added value compared with existing severity scoring systems.

FUTURE DIRECTION

Future direction for sub-phenotyping in critical care includes translating promising research findings into clinically meaningful strategies at bed side that improve patient outcomes. A key priority is the prospective validation of identified sub-phenotypes through large, multicenter international studies. The primary objective is to determine whether sub-phenotypes reliably predict treatment response and improve patient-centered outcomes across diverse populations and healthcare settings. Therefore, the reproducibility and generalizability of the research findings will be critical, particularly as current models have largely been derived from high-resource settings in west (North America and Europe), which may not reflect patient characteristics or critical illness epidemiology in low- and middle-income countries. Adapting and validating sub-phenotyping approaches in these settings will be necessary to ensure global relevance and equity in critical care research.[1]

Another important direction is the development of pragmatic and simplified approaches that facilitate bedside implementation. While many sub-phenotypes have been derived from complex, multimodal data, future efforts should focus on translating these into clinically feasible tools using routine clinical parameters or limited biomarker panels. This will allow clinicians to readily identify sub-phenotypes and tailor interventions without requiring extensive laboratory or computational resources. Another related issue is the integration of sub-phenotyping into precision medicine, where patients can be stratified for targeted interventions in both clinical trials and routine practice. Sub-phenotypes may guide therapeutic decisions, optimize treatment allocation, and improve the efficiency and success of critical care trials.[2,3]

Equity and inclusion must also guide future work. Underrepresentation of specific population subgroups such as racial and ethnic minorities, children, and pregnant women in existing trials limits generalizability and may perpetuate disparities in access to novel therapies. Future research should actively incorporate these populations and focus on patient-centered outcomes relevant across diverse groups. At the same time, the use of machine learning and artificial intelligence to define sub-phenotypes must become more transparent and interpretable. Clinicians should be able to understand and communicate the rationale behind model-derived treatment recommendations, ensuring informed decision-making and fostering trust in precision approaches.

Finally, there is considerable potential to refine sub-phenotypes by integrating multiomics data, including genomics, proteomics, metabolomics, and real-time physiologic parameters. Combining molecular and clinical data may identify mechanistic endotypes that not only predict outcomes but also reveal novel therapeutic targets. Ultimately, successful implementation will require developing clinical decision support systems and protocols that incorporate sub-phenotyping into routine care, alongside rigorous evaluation of their impact on patient outcomes, resource utilization, and cost-effectiveness. Through these efforts, sub-phenotyping can evolve from a research concept into a practical and equitable tool for personalized critical care.[7]

CONCLUSION

Sub-phenotyping is ushering in a new era of precision-based critical care medicine. By acknowledging and delineating patient heterogeneity, this approach holds promise for optimizing therapeutic strategies, enhancing trial efficiency, and ultimately improving patient prognostication and outcomes. While numerous methodological, practical, and ethical challenges remain, the combined advances in data science, diagnostics, and global collaboration highlight a future where individualized care is not only possible, but routine.

Transforming practice from a "one-size-fits-all" to a "personalized" approach in the ICU will require not just innovations in technology and science but also a commitment to equity, collaboration, and continuous learning. As the field progresses, clinicians are encouraged to remain engaged with emerging evidence, embrace data-driven care pathways, and contribute to collaborative efforts that will drive the next wave of progress in critical care.

REFERENCES

1. Gordon AC, Alipanah-Lechner N, Bos LD, Dianti J, Diaz JV, Finfer S, et al. From ICU Syndromes to ICU Subphenotypes: Consensus Report and Recommendations for Developing Precision Medicine in the ICU. Am J Respir Crit Care Med. 2024;210(2):155-66.

2. Antcliffe DB, Burrell A, Boyle AJ, Gordon AC, McAuley DF, Silversides J. Sepsis subphenotypes, theragnostics and personalized sepsis care. Intensive Care Med. 2025;51(4):756-68.
3. Reddy K, Sinha P, O'Kane CM, Gordon AC, Calfee CS, McAuley DF. Subphenotypes in critical care: translation into clinical practice. Lancet Respir Med. 2020;8(6):631-43.
4. Nasa P, Bos LD, Estenssoro E, van Haren FMP, Neto AS, Rocco PRM, et al. Defining and subphenotyping ARDS: insights from an international Delphi expert panel. Lancet Respir Med. 2025;13(7):638-50.
5. Kitsios GD, Yang L, Manatakis DV, Nouraie M, Evankovich J, Bain W, et al. Host-Response Subphenotypes Offer Prognostic Enrichment in Patients With or at Risk for Acute Respiratory Distress Syndrome. Crit Care Med. 2019;47(12):1724-34.
6. Nasa P, Bos LD, Estenssoro E, van Haren FM, Serpa Neto A, Rocco PR, et al. Consensus statements on the utility of defining ARDS and the utility of past and current definitions of ARDS-protocol for a Delphi study. BMJ Open. 2024;14(4):e082986.
7. Vaara ST, Bhatraju PK, Stanski NL, McMahon BA, Liu K, Joannidis M, et al. Subphenotypes in acute kidney injury: a narrative review. Crit Care. 2022; 26(1):251.
8. Xu Z, Mao C, Su C, Zhang H, Siempos I, Torres LK, et al. Sepsis subphenotyping based on organ dysfunction trajectory. Crit Care. 2022;26(1):197.
9. Sinha P, Kerchberger VE, Willmore A, Chambers J, Zhuo H, Abbott J, et al. Identifying molecular phenotypes in sepsis: an analysis of two prospective observational cohorts and secondary analysis of two randomised controlled trials. Lancet Respir Med. 2023;11(11):965-74.
10. Seymour CW, Kennedy JN, Wang S, Chang CH, Elliott CF, Xu Z, et al. Derivation, Validation, and Potential Treatment Implications of Novel Clinical Phenotypes for Sepsis. JAMA. 2019;321(20):2003-17.
11. Bhavani SV, Spicer A, Sinha P, Malik A, Lopez-Espina C, Schmalz L, et al. Distinct immune profiles and clinical outcomes in sepsis subphenotypes based on temperature trajectories. Intensive Care Med. 2024;50(12):2094-104.
12. Hao C, Hao R, Zhao H, Zhang Y, Sheng M, An Y. Identification and validation of sepsis subphenotypes using time-series data. Heliyon. 2024;10(7):e28520.
13. Das SK, Choupoo NS, Rochwerg B, Goswami D, Ray S, Gupta A, et al. The impact of inflammatory biomarker subphenotypes on acute respiratory distress syndrome prognosis: a systematic review and meta-analysis. Indian J Crit Care Med. 2025;29(7):597-603.
14. Constantin JM, Jabaudon M, Lefrant JY, Jaber S, Quenot JP, Langeron O, et al. Personalised mechanical ventilation tailored to lung morphology versus low positive end-expiratory pressure for patients with acute respiratory distress syndrome in France (the LIVE study): a multicentre, single-blind, randomised controlled trial. Lancet Respir Med. 2019;7(10):870-80.
15. Boumans MMA, Aerts W, Pisani L, Bos LDJ, Smit MR, Tuinman PR. Diagnostic accuracy of lung ultrasound in diagnosis of ARDS and identification of focal or non-focal ARDS subphenotypes: a systematic review and meta-analysis. Crit Care. 2024;28(1):224.
16. Sinnige JS, Smit MR, Ghose A, de Grooth HJ, Itenov TS, Ischaki E, et al. Personalized mechanical ventilation guided by ultrasound in patients with acute

respiratory distress syndrome (PEGASUS): study protocol for an international randomized clinical trial. Trials. 2024;25(1):308.

17. Bai Y, Chen S, Yang H, Huang X, Xia J, Zhan Q. Dynamic oxygenation subgroup bringing new insights in ARDS: more predictive of outcomes and response to PEEP than static PaO2/FiO2. Thorax. 2025;80(9):594-603.
18. Ma W, Tang S, Yao P, Zhou T, Niu Q, Liu P, et al. Advances in acute respiratory distress syndrome: focusing on heterogeneity, pathophysiology, and therapeutic strategies. Signal Transduct Target Ther. 2025;10(1):75.
19. Andrew BY, Pieper CF, Cherry AD, Pendergast JF, Privratsky JR, Mathew JP, et al. Identification of Trajectory-Based Acute Kidney Injury Phenotypes Among Cardiac Surgery Patients. Ann Thorac Surg. 2022;114(6):2235-43.
20. Smith TD, Soriano VO, Neyra JA, Chen J. Identifying KDIGO trajectory phenotypes associated with increased inpatient mortality. Proc (IEEE Int Conf Healthc Inform). 2019;2019:10.1109/ichi.2019.8904739.
21. Takkavatakarn K, Oh W, Chan L, Hofer I, Shawwa K, Kraft M, et al. Machine learning derived serum creatinine trajectories in acute kidney injury in critically ill patients with sepsis. Crit Care. 2024;28(1):156.
22. Molinari L, Del Rio-Pertuz G, Smith A, Landsittel DP, Singbartl K, Palevsky PM, et al. Utility of biomarkers for sepsis-associated acute kidney injury staging. JAMA Netw Open. 2022;5(5):e2212709.
23. Fiorentino M, Xu Z, Smith A, Singbartl K, Palevsky PM, Chawla LS, et al. Serial measurement of cell-cycle arrest biomarkers [timp-2] · [igfbp7] and risk for progression to death, dialysis, or severe acute kidney injury in patients with septic shock. Am J Respir Crit Care Med. 2020;202(9):1262-70.
24. Russell JA, Walley KR, Singer J, Gordon AC, Hébert PC, Cooper DJ, et al. Vasopressin versus norepinephrine infusion in patients with septic shock. N Engl J Med. 2008;358(9):877-87.

CHAPTER 10

Intensive Care in the Era of Molecular Targeted Therapies

Abhishek Pratap Singh, Rahul Harne, Deepak Govil

INTRODUCTION

Molecular targeted therapies (MTTs) represent a fundamental paradigm shift in modern medicine, signifying a departure from generalized treatments toward highly specific interventions. These therapies are meticulously designed to modulate discrete molecular pathways that are critically involved in disease pathogenesis. While MTTs have undeniably revolutionized oncology by specifically addressing cancer-driving mutations and pathways, their potential application is increasingly being explored across a broader spectrum of complex diseases, including those frequently encountered in critical care.

The compelling rationale for applying MTTs in critical care settings arises from a growing understanding that many critical illnesses, such as sepsis and acute respiratory distress syndrome (ARDS), are not merely direct consequences of infection or injury. Instead, they result from a dysregulated host response involving specific, identifiable molecular pathways. By precisely targeting these pathways, MTTs aim to restore physiological homeostasis, mitigate organ damage, and ultimately improve patient outcomes. However, the translation of this conceptually revolutionary approach into effective critical care interventions faces significantly greater hurdles compared to its success in oncology. This is primarily due to the dynamic, heterogeneous, and often rapidly evolving nature of critical illness, where the "target" is a dysregulated host response rather than a static, identifiable mutation. The complexity and multifactorial nature of critical care diseases necessitate a profound understanding of disease mechanisms and patient heterogeneity for successful implementation. Therefore, a comprehensive discussion of MTTs in intensive care must adopt a balanced perspective, articulating their immense promise while critically evaluating the substantial challenges inherent to the critical care environment.[1]

FOUNDATIONS OF MOLECULAR TARGETED THERAPIES: MECHANISMS AND PRINCIPLES

Molecular targeting fundamentally relies on the identification and precise modulation of specific molecules—such as proteins (e.g., cell surface receptors, intracellular enzymes), nucleic acids, or lipids—that play pivotal roles in the initiation or progression of disease. These targets are often integral components of complex cellular signaling cascades and interfering with their function aims to precisely halt or redirect pathological processes. The specificity of these interventions is a cornerstone of their design, aiming to minimize off-target effects and thereby reduce systemic toxicity.[1]

Classes of targeted agents relevant to critical care include:

- *Monoclonal antibodies (mAbs):* These are large protein molecules engineered to bind with high affinity and specificity to extracellular targets, such as cell surface receptors, circulating cytokines, or growth factors. Their high specificity generally translates to fewer off-target effects, making them attractive candidates for modulating specific immune or inflammatory responses. However, their large molecular weight can limit tissue penetration, particularly into intracellular compartments, and their relatively long half-lives can prolong both therapeutic and potential adverse effects.
- *Small molecule inhibitors (SMIs):* In contrast to mAbs, SMIs are low molecular weight compounds capable of penetrating cell membranes. This characteristic allows them to target intracellular proteins such as kinases, proteases, or transcription factors that are often involved in critical signaling pathways. However, their smaller size and potential for broader interactions across related protein families can sometimes lead to less specificity and a higher propensity for off-target effects compared to mAbs, necessitating careful design and evaluation.
- *Nucleic acid-based therapies:* This emerging class includes antisense oligonucleotides (ASOs) and small interfering RNAs (siRNAs). These therapies function by targeting messenger RNA (mRNA) to inhibit the synthesis of specific disease-causing proteins. By directly interfering with gene expression, they represent a promising avenue for targeting previously "unreachable" proteins and pathways that are implicated in critical illness. While still largely investigational in critical care, their potential to precisely control protein production offers a novel therapeutic dimension.

TARGETING SEPSIS AND SEPTIC SHOCK: A MOLECULAR APPROACH

Sepsis is a life-threatening syndrome characterized by a dysregulated host response to infection, leading to organ dysfunction.[2]

Its complex pathophysiology involves an initial hyperinflammatory phase that can lead to profound immunosuppression, along with widespread microcirculatory dysfunction and coagulopathy.[3]

The process begins with pattern recognition receptors (PRRs), such as Toll-like receptors (TLRs), identifying microbial pathogen-associated molecular patterns (PAMPs) or host damage-associated molecular patterns (DAMPs).[3] This triggers intracellular signaling pathways that converge on transcription factors such as nuclear factor-κB (NF-κB) and interferon regulatory factor (IRF). NF-κB and activator protein 1 (AP-1) activate inflammatory genes, while IRF promotes type I interferon (IFN) production. In sepsis, these pathways are overactivated, causing a massive release of cytokines and alarmins that fuel systemic inflammation and immune suppression.

A critical pathway is the STING-IRF3-NF-κB pathway, activated by cytosolic sensing of cell-free DNA (cfDNA), particularly mitochondrial DNA (mtDNA). The inability to degrade cfDNA due to deficient deoxyribonuclease (DNase) contributes to this inflammation. Administering DNase can improve survival by cleaving cfDNA and mitigating its pro-inflammatory effects. Key therapeutic targets in this cascade include PRRs, pro-inflammatory cytokines like TNF-alpha, IL-1, and IL-6, DAMPs such as HMGB1, and components of the coagulation cascade.[4]

Immunomodulation and Anti-inflammatory Targets

Early, broad attempts to block pro-inflammatory cytokines in sepsis generally failed, highlighting the complexity and dual roles of these mediators. Therapies such as infliximab and etanercept, designed to neutralize TNF-alpha, failed to improve outcomes in large sepsis trials and, in some cases, were associated with harm, likely due to TNF-alpha's crucial role in early host defense against infection.[5] Similarly, Eritoran, a TLR4 antagonist central to initiating inflammatory responses upon recognizing PAMPs, failed in clinical trials for sepsis, suggesting that broad inhibition of TLR signaling can be detrimental by impairing essential pathogen recognition and host defence.[6]

The repeated failures of these broad anti-inflammatory agents point to a critical understanding—the host immune response in sepsis is biphasic and dynamically evolving. An initial pro-inflammatory response is essential for pathogen clearance, while a later, dysregulated phase contributes significantly to organ damage. Administering a broad anti-inflammatory agent too early or too broadly risks suppressing beneficial immunity, potentially leading to worse outcomes.

In contrast, Anakinra, an IL-1 receptor antagonist, has shown some promise in specific subsets of septic patients, particularly those with features of macrophage activation syndrome (MAS) or significantly elevated IL-18 levels. This limited success underscores the critical need for precise patient stratification.[7]

Both tocilizumab and sarilumab, IL-6 receptor antagonists, have been explored, particularly in hyperinflammatory conditions such as COVID-19-associated cytokine storm. However, large-scale sepsis trials specifically targeting IL-6 have yielded mixed or inconclusive results, reflecting the challenges of broad cytokine blockade in heterogeneous populations.[8]

High mobility group box 1 (HMGB1) is a prototypic DAMP that acts as a late mediator of inflammation and organ damage in sepsis. Anti-HMGB1 antibodies have demonstrated preclinical promise in mitigating sepsis severity, with ongoing early-phase clinical trials exploring their efficacy.[9]

Targeting components of the complement cascade, such as C5a and C3a, which contribute significantly to inflammation, neutrophil activation, and organ damage in sepsis, is another active area of research. Challenges include the dual role of complement in both host defense and pathology, requiring highly precise modulation.[10]

Coagulation Pathway Modulation

The coagulation system is inextricably linked with inflammation in sepsis, forming a vicious cycle of thromboinflammation. Recombinant human activated protein C (rhAPC, drotrecogin alfa) was a pioneering targeted therapy aimed at modulating both coagulation and inflammation. Despite initial positive results, a large confirmatory trial failed to show benefit and led to its withdrawal from the market, highlighting the delicate balance of the coagulation system and the significant risks associated with broad interventions in critically ill patients.[11,12]

The angiopoietin-1/2 pathway is crucial for maintaining vascular integrity. Dysregulation of angiopoietins (Ang-1 and Ang-2) is a key contributor to endothelial dysfunction and vascular leak, which are hallmarks of septic shock. Research suggests that vascular leakage in sepsis-induced ARDS may be caused by disruptions in the angiopoietin/Tie2 signaling axis. Therapies designed to restore endothelial barrier function, such as Tie2 agonists or Ang-2 inhibitors, are currently under investigation.[13]

Nutritional and Metabolic Support Strategies

Sepsis frequently leads to mitochondrial dysfunction, impairing cellular energy production and contributing to organ failure. Nutritional and metabolic support strategies, including the administration of CoQ10, thiamine, and vitamin C, have been explored to restore mitochondrial function, though their "targeted" nature is more metabolic than molecular in the traditional sense **(Table 1)**.

MOLECULAR STRATEGIES AGAINST SEVERE INFECTIONS IN THE INTENSIVE CARE UNIT

The global crisis of antimicrobial resistance (AMR) necessitates the urgent development of novel antimicrobials that exploit unique bacterial vulnerabilities or overcome existing resistance mechanisms. Beyond direct pathogen targeting, modulating the host's response to infection has emerged as a complementary strategy. A more profound understanding suggests that host-directed therapies (HDTs) and novel antimicrobials are not mutually

TABLE 1: Key molecular targets and corresponding therapies in sepsis/septic shock.

Target pathway/ molecule	*Therapeutic agent*	*Mechanism of action*	*Clinical status/trial phase/outcome*
TNF-alpha	Infliximab, etanercept	Cytokine blockade	Failed Phase III, associated with harm
IL-1	Anakinra	IL-1 receptor antagonist	Limited use in specific subsets (MAS/IL-18 high)
IL-6	Tocilizumab	IL-6 receptor antagonist	Mixed/inconclusive results in sepsis trials
TLR4	Eritoran	TLR4 antagonist	Failed Phase III
HMGB1	• Anti-HMGB1 • Antibodies	DAMP neutralization	Early clinical trials, preclinical
Complement system (C5a, C3a)	Complement inhibitors	Complement cascade modulation	Active research, challenges with dual roles
Activated protein C	Drotrecogin alfa (rhAPC)	Coagulation modulator, anti-inflammatory	Withdrawn from market after confirmatory trial failure
Angiopoietin pathway	Tie2 agonists, Ang-2 inhibitors	Vascular stabilizer	Under investigation
Mitochondrial dysfunction	CoQ10, thiamine, vitamin C	Metabolic support, mitochondrial restoration	Being explored, more metabolic than molecular

exclusive; they have significant potential for synergy. While HDTs aim to optimize the host's ability to clear infection and mitigate damage, novel antimicrobials directly reduce the pathogen burden. For severe, resistant infections, a combined approach—reducing the microbial load while simultaneously fine-tuning the host's immune response—could be more effective than either strategy alone, especially given the rising threat of AMR.

Host-directed Therapies: Targeting Host Immune Response to Infection

Host-directed therapies represent a promising paradigm shift in managing severe infections, particularly in the context of rising AMR. Instead of directly targeting the pathogen, HDTs aim to modulate the host's immune response to enhance pathogen clearance, reduce infection-induced tissue damage, or restore immune homeostasis. Examples of HDTs include immunomodulators, such as granulocyte-macrophage colony-stimulating factor (GM-CSF) to enhance neutrophil function, or interferon-gamma (IFN-gamma) to activate macrophages. Other HDTs encompass anti-virulence strategies, which target bacterial toxins or quorum sensing pathways without directly killing the pathogen, and anti-inflammatory agents used specifically to mitigate excessive host-mediated damage. Challenges in developing and implementing HDTs include the need for precise targeting of specific host pathways, determining the optimal timing of administration (as immune responses evolve), and accurately identifying appropriate patient subsets (patient stratification) to ensure efficacy and avoid detrimental immunosuppression or other adverse effects.[14]

Novel Antimicrobials with Specific Molecular Targets

The escalating crisis of AMR has driven the development of novel antimicrobials that target unique bacterial vulnerabilities or circumvent established resistance mechanisms. This includes agents that:

- *Inhibit resistance mechanisms:* Such as efflux pump inhibitors (e.g., small molecules that block bacterial efflux pumps, thereby restoring susceptibility to existing antibiotics that would otherwise be expelled) or novel beta-lactamase inhibitors (e.g., avibactam, relebactam, vaborbactam, which protect beta-lactam antibiotics from enzymatic degradation by bacterial enzymes).
- *Disrupt biofilms:* Bacterial biofilms are structured communities of microbes encased in an extracellular matrix, rendering them highly resistant to both antibiotics and host immunity. Molecular strategies targeting biofilms include quorum sensing inhibitors (interfering with bacterial communication required for biofilm formation) and enzymes or small molecules that specifically disperse the biofilm matrix, making bacteria more susceptible to conventional antibiotics.
- *Target novel bacterial pathways:* Developing entirely new classes of antibiotics that target previously unexploited bacterial metabolic pathways, protein synthesis machinery, cell wall components, or DNA replication processes, thereby circumventing existing resistance mechanisms.
- *Nanotechnology-based interventions:* Nanotechnology is emerging as a powerful tool for sepsis management, offering both diagnostic and therapeutic solutions. Nanoparticle-based delivery of antimicrobials has shown promising results in overcoming drug resistance and improving treatment outcomes. These innovations highlight the potential of nanotechnology to provide more precise and effective solutions for sepsis, ultimately enhancing patient care.[15]

Antiviral and Antifungal Targeted Therapies in Critical Care

The recent COVID-19 pandemic underscored the critical importance of targeted antivirals in thc ICU. Examples include remdesivir, an RNA-dependent RNA polymerase inhibitor, and molnupiravir, a nucleoside analogue that induces lethal mutagenesis in viral RNA, both of which specifically target essential viral replication enzymes. Other targeted antivirals include those that inhibit viral proteases (e.g., nirmatrelvir/ritonavir for SARS-CoV-2) or block viral entry mechanisms into host cells. Targeted antifungals exploit unique fungal structures or metabolic pathways that are absent or significantly different in human cells, providing a selective therapeutic window. Examples include echinocandins, which target fungal cell wall synthesis by inhibiting beta-(1,3)-D-glucan synthase, and azoles, which inhibit ergosterol synthesis, a key component of fungal cell membranes, thereby disrupting membrane integrity.

Therapeutic Challenges

Targeted antimicrobials often rely on identifying unique microbial structures or metabolic pathways (e.g., ergosterol in fungi, RNA-dependent RNA polymerase (RdRp) in viruses, bacterial cell wall components) that are absent or significantly different in human cells. This provides a clear therapeutic window, allowing for selective toxicity to the microbe while minimizing harm to the host. In contrast, HDTs for sepsis often target host pathways essential for normal physiological function (e.g., inflammation, coagulation), making the therapeutic window much narrower and the risk of adverse effects higher (as evidenced by broad anti-inflammatory failures in sepsis). This highlights why, despite the challenges of resistance, targeted antimicrobial development conceptually offers a clearer path to specificity and safety than many HDTs. It reinforces the inherent complexity and higher risk associated with modulating host physiology in critical illness, underscoring the need for extremely precise patient selection and a profound mechanistic understanding to avoid iatrogenic harm.

MOLECULAR TARGETED INTERVENTIONS IN ACUTE RESPIRATORY DISTRESS SYNDROME

Acute respiratory distress syndrome is a severe form of acute lung injury characterized by widespread lung inflammation, increased alveolar-capillary membrane permeability leading to pulmonary edema, and impaired gas exchange, often progressing to pulmonary fibrosis in survivors. This cascade begins with PRRs sensing PAMPs and DAMPs, which activate a number of signaling pathways. Key mechanisms include NF-κB, JAK/STAT, RAGE, and MAPK, which lead to overwhelming inflammation. This is compounded by cellular stress pathways such as ER stress and TNF-α signaling. These events collectively lead to the breakdown of the alveolar-capillary barrier, causing pulmonary edema and impaired alveolar fluid clearance (AFC). This damage is further exacerbated by excessive reactive oxygen species (ROS), which also compromises the body's natural antioxidant defenses such as the Nrf2 pathway.[16]

TABLE 2: Key molecular targets and corresponding therapies in acute respiratory distress syndrome (ARDS).[16,17]

Mechanism	*Target pathway/molecule*	*Therapeutic agent*
Anti-inflammatory agents	PRR inhibitors	Cirsilineol, diacerein, and glibenclamide
	NF-κB inhibitors	Sivelestat and simvastatin
	JAK inhibitors	Baricitinib
	GM-CSF modulators/ antibodies	Lenzilumab and mavrilimumab
	Interleukin inhibitors	Anakinra and sarilumab
	Complement system inhibitors	Vilobelimab
	Other immunomodulators	Thymosin α1
Alveolar capillary barrier protection	Cell death inhibitors	Imatinib
	Tie2 agonist	Vasculotide
Enhancing alveolar fluid clearance	Ion channel modulators	B adrenergic agonists
Attenuating oxidative stress	Antioxidants	Vitamin C, N-acetylcysteine

Similar to sepsis, broad anti-inflammatory strategies have largely failed to improve outcomes in ARDS. Current research focuses on more precisely targeted approaches aimed at specific inflammatory mediators or pathways that are uniquely detrimental to lung integrity **(Table 2)**.

Emerging Therapies[16,17]

- *MicroRNAs (miRNAs):* These small noncoding RNAs are being investigated as potential therapeutic targets to modulate gene expression and inflammation.
- *Mesenchymal stromal cells (MSCs):* MSCs are being explored for their *immunomodulatory* and regenerative properties, although their clinical efficacy is still being determined.
- *Neutrophil extracellular traps (NETs) targeting:* Dornase alfa is being investigated for its potential to degrade NETs and reduce lung injury.

Despite these promising developments, challenges remain. The heterogeneity of ARDS makes it difficult to find a single target for all patients. The timing of treatment is crucial, and the risk of off-target effects and immune suppression must be carefully managed. Future directions include personalized medicine based on individual patient characteristics, and the use of combination therapies that target multiple pathways to improve treatment efficacy.

ACUTE KIDNEY INJURY: MOLECULAR APPROACHES TO MITIGATE INJURY AND PROMOTE REPAIR

Acute kidney injury (AKI) is a frequent and severe complication in critically ill patients, characterized by a rapid decline in kidney function. Its complex pathophysiology involves multiple mechanisms, including inflammation, oxidative stress, and various forms of cell death (e.g., apoptosis, necroptosis) within renal tubular cells. Similar to other critical conditions, anti-inflammatory strategies targeting cytokines such as IL-6 and TNF-alpha are under investigation to reduce the inflammatory component of kidney injury.

In a randomized controlled trial by Panacek et al., the monoclonal antibody fragment afelimomab, an anti-TNF agent, was tested in septic patients. Patients with elevated serum IL-6 levels (>1,000 pg/mL) who received afelimomab showed a 4% absolute risk reduction in 28-day mortality. While kidney failure rates were not detailed, there was a statistically significant improvement in the overall Sequential Organ Failure Assessment (SOFA) score starting 48 hours post-treatment.[18]

Alternative sepsis treatments using extracorporeal blood purification aim to broadly regulate the inflammatory response. In animal studies, hemadsorption has shown promise, improving bacterial clearance, hemodynamics, and survival while protecting against organ injury. However, its effectiveness in humans is unproven.[19,20]

The EUPHAS trial, though methodologically flawed, suggested that polymyxin B hemoperfusion could improve hemodynamics, organ function, and 28-day mortality in patients with severe sepsis from Gram-negative infections. Specifically, it showed improved renal SOFA scores and cardiovascular function. These preliminary results warrant larger clinical trials.[21]

While animal studies suggest that cytokine-reducing resins can broadly regulate cytokine levels, human studies using high-volume hemofiltration have not consistently demonstrated this effect or provided a clear clinical benefit. The VA/NIH Acute Renal Failure Trial Network study found no overall mortality benefit from more intense renal replacement in septic patients, but subsequent analysis suggested that patients with higher levels of inflammatory cytokines may have a worse prognosis. This supports the idea that targeting specific patient subgroups could be beneficial for both targeted therapies and broad modulation strategies.[22,23]

Antioxidants are being explored to counteract the excessive production of reactive oxygen species (ROS) that contribute significantly to renal tubular cell damage and dysfunction in AKI. Inhibitors of specific programmed cell death pathways, such as caspase inhibitors (for apoptosis) or RIPK1 inhibitors (for necroptosis), are being studied to prevent widespread kidney tubular cell death and promote renal recovery in AKI induced by cisplatin, ischemia-reperfusion injury and contrast.[24]

OTHER RELEVANT CONDITIONS WHERE TARGETED THERAPIES ARE EMERGING

Cardiogenic Shock

Molecular targets could include pathways involved in myocardial contractility such as calcium sensitizers, sarcoplasmic/endoplasmic reticulum Ca^{2+} ATPase (SERCA2a) activator (istaroxime),[25] vascular tone regulation, cardiac myosin activation (omecamtiv mecarbil) or inflammation-induced myocardial depression such as JAK inhibitors (ruxolitinib), neutralizing circulating dipeptidyl peptidase 3 (cDPP3) (procizumab).[26]

Neurological Emergencies (e.g., Ischemic Stroke, Traumatic Brain Injury)

Research focuses on neuroprotective strategies that target excitotoxicity (AMPA receptor antagonists like perampanel), neuroinflammation by IL-1β blockade (anakinra), caspase-1 inhibitors (belnacasan), statins (rosuvastatin), oxidative stress (by antioxidants like uric acid), and apoptosis to limit neuronal damage and promote neurological recovery[27] **(Table 3)**.

TABLE 3: Emerging molecular targets and therapies for other critical care syndromes.

Critical care syndrome	*Key pathophysiological process*	*Specific molecular target*	*Therapeutic agent (or class)*	*Status/trial phase*
AKI	Inflammation	IL-6, TNF-alpha	Anti-inflammatory agents and monoclonal antibodies	Investigational and preclinical
AKI	Oxidative stress	Reactive oxygen species (ROS)	Antioxidants	Preclinical and investigational
AKI	Cell death (apoptosis and necroptosis)	Caspases and RIPK1	Caspase inhibitors and RIPK1 inhibitors	Preclinical and investigational
Neurological emergencies (e.g., stroke, TBI)	Neuroprotection	Excitotoxicity, inflammation, and apoptosis	Neuroprotective agents. IL inhibitors and statins	Investigational, preclinical/ early clinical
Cardiogenic shock	Myocardial depression	Contractility pathways and vascular tone	Calcium sensitizers and vasodilators, monoclonal antibodies	Investigational and preclinical

CHALLENGES, CONSIDERATIONS, AND PATIENT SELECTION IN INTENSIVE CARE UNIT SETTINGS

The application of MTTs in the intensive care unit is fraught with unique challenges that extend beyond the identification of a relevant molecular target.

Pharmacokinetics/Pharmacodynamics in Critically Ill Patients

Critically ill patients exhibit profound and dynamic physiological alterations that significantly impact the pharmacokinetics (PK) and pharmacodynamics (PD) of administered drugs, including targeted therapies. These alterations encompass changes in drug absorption, altered volume of distribution (due to fluid shifts and capillary leak), impaired organ function (renal and hepatic clearance), altered protein binding, and changes in drug metabolism. Such variability can lead to sub-therapeutic drug concentrations, rendering the therapy ineffective, or, conversely, drug accumulation and toxicity. These complex physiological changes necessitate highly individualized dosing adjustments and often require therapeutic drug monitoring for targeted agents to ensure optimal exposure and minimize harm.

Biomarker-guided Therapy and Patient Stratification

The extreme heterogeneity of critical illness, where patients with the same clinical diagnosis can have vastly different underlying molecular pathologies, represents a major barrier to the successful implementation of targeted therapies. Biomarkers are therefore crucial for identifying specific patient "endotypes" or "sub-phenotypes" that are most likely to respond to a particular targeted intervention. This precision medicine approach aims to move away from a "one-size-fits-all" treatment paradigm that has historically proven ineffective in critical care. Beyond patient selection, biomarkers are also essential for real-time monitoring of treatment response, predicting outcomes, and identifying the optimal window for therapeutic intervention.

Adverse Effects, Drug Interactions, and Resistance Mechanisms

While MTTs are designed for specificity, they are not devoid of adverse effects, which can be particularly severe and unpredictable in critically ill patients whose physiological reserves are already compromised. These can include profound immune suppression (e.g., with certain anti-inflammatory agents), organ-specific toxicities, or paradoxical effects. Drug-drug interactions are a significant concern in the ICU, where polypharmacy is common. Targeted therapies can interact with other medications, altering their metabolism, increasing toxicity, or reducing efficacy. Furthermore, resistance mechanisms can emerge, particularly with antimicrobial targeted therapies or even HDTs that induce adaptive changes in pathogens or host cells, potentially limiting long-term efficacy.

Cost-effectiveness and Accessibility

The high cost of MTTs poses a significant challenge to their widespread use, particularly in resource-limited settings. To justify their high price and ensure the responsible allocation of healthcare resources, these therapies must demonstrate a clear and substantial clinical benefit in well-defined patient populations.

FUTURE DIRECTIONS AND EMERGING THERAPIES

The trajectory of critical care is undeniably moving toward personalized or precision medicine. This approach aims to tailor treatment decisions to the individual patient's unique biological characteristics, which include their genetic makeup, specific immune status, real-time physiological responses, and the molecular "endotype" of their critical illness.

Genomic and Proteomic Insights

Advanced "omics" technologies, including genomics (studying the entire genome), transcriptomics (gene expression), proteomics (protein expression and function), and metabolomics (metabolite profiles), will play an increasingly pivotal role. These technologies enable the identification of novel molecular targets, the discovery of predictive and prognostic biomarkers, and an unprecedented understanding of disease trajectories at a systems biology level. Emerging technologies such as single-cell RNA sequencing are revolutionizing our understanding of critical illness by revealing the profound heterogeneity of cellular responses within tissues.

Novel Drug Delivery Systems and Therapeutic Modalities

Nanoparticles and other advanced nanocarriers offer immense potential for targeted drug delivery. By encapsulating therapeutic agents within nanoscale vehicles, it is possible to achieve improved drug concentration at specific organs or cell types, enhance bioavailability, and simultaneously minimize systemic exposure and off-target toxicity. While still in nascent stages for acute critical care, sophisticated gene editing technologies (e.g., CRISPR-Cas9) or cell-based therapies (e.g., mesenchymal stem cells) could offer highly specific and potentially curative approaches. These modalities aim to directly modify disease-causing genes, introduce therapeutic genes, or leverage the regenerative and immunomodulatory properties of specific cell populations.

Artificial intelligence and machine learning (AI/ML) algorithms are poised to transform critical care by analyzing vast and complex datasets derived from omics, electronic health records, continuous physiological monitoring, and imaging. These computational tools can identify intricate patterns, predict patient trajectories, uncover novel drug targets, and optimize treatment strategies in ways that are impossible for human analysis alone.

CONCLUSION

Molecular targeted therapies are a crucial evolution in intensive care, offering a path beyond conventional treatments for critical illnesses such as sepsis, ARDS, and AKI. While initial trials have had setbacks, they have provided invaluable insights into the complex pathophysiology of these conditions.

The approach of precision medicine addresses patient heterogeneity, the dynamic nature of critical illness, and altered pharmacokinetics. Future advancements depend on developing robust biomarkers for patient stratification and therapeutic monitoring, integrating omics technologies and AI/machine learning, and exploring novel modalities such as gene and cell therapies. These innovations offer a hopeful path to improving patient outcomes in the ICU.

REFERENCES

1. Lee YT, Tan YJ, Oon CE. Molecular targeted therapy: Treating cancer with specificity. Eur J Pharmacol. 2018;834:188-96.
2. Singer M, Deutschman CS, Seymour CW, Shankar-Hari M, Annane D, Bauer M, et al. The Third International Consensus Definitions for Sepsis and Septic Shock (Sepsis-3). JAMA. 2016;315(8):801-10.
3. Huang M, Cai S, Su J. The pathogenesis of sepsis and potential therapeutic targets. Int J Mol Sci. 2019;20(21):5376.
4. Zhang YY, Ning BT. Signaling pathways and intervention therapies in sepsis. Signal Transduct Target Ther. 2021;6(1):407.
5. Sawoo R, Dey R, Ghosh R, Bishayi B. TLR4 and TNFR1 blockade dampen M1 macrophage activation and shifts them towards an M2 phenotype. Immunol Res. 2021;69(4):334-51.
6. Tidswell M, Tillis W, Larosa SP, Lynn M, Wittek AE, Kao R, et al. Phase 2 trial of eritoran tetrasodium (E5564), a Toll-like receptor 4 antagonist, in patients with severe sepsis. Crit Care Med. 2010;38(1):72-83.
7. Grimaldi D, Goicoechea Turcott EW, Taccone FS. IL-1 receptor antagonist in sepsis: new findings with old data? J Thorac Dis. 2016;8(9):2379-82.
8. Angus DC, Berry S, Lewis RJ, Al-Beidh F, Arabi Y, van Bentum-Puijk W, et al. The REMAP-CAP (Randomized Embedded Multifactorial Adaptive Platform for Community-acquired Pneumonia) Study. Rationale and Design. Ann Am Thorac Soc. 2020;17(7):879-91.
9. Deng C, Zhao L, Yang Z, Shang JJ, Wang CY, Shen MZ, et al. Targeting HMGB1 for the treatment of sepsis and sepsis-induced organ injury. Acta Pharmacol Sin. 2022;43(3):520-8.

10. Yan C, Gao H. New insights for C5a and C5a receptors in sepsis. Front Immunol. 2012;10(3):368.
11. Levi M, Levy M, Williams MD, Douglas I, Artigas A, Antonelli M, et al. Prophylactic heparin in patients with severe sepsis treated with drotrecogin alfa (activated). Am J Respir Crit Care Med. 2007;176(5):483-90.
12. Ranieri VM, Thompson BT, Barie PS, Dhainaut JF, Douglas IS, Finfer S, et al. Drotrecogin alfa (activated) in adults with septic shock. N Engl J Med. 2012;366(22):2055-64.
13. Chi Y, Yu S, Yin J, Liu D, Zhuo M, Li X. Role of Angiopoietin/Tie2 System in Sepsis: A Potential Therapeutic Target. Clin Appl Thromb Hemost. 2024;30:1-8.
14. Ono S, Tsujimoto H, Hiraki S, Aosasa S. Mechanisms of sepsis-induced immunosuppression and immunological modification therapies for sepsis. Ann Gastroenterol Surg. 2018;2(5):351-8.
15. Choudhary R. Sepsis management, controversies, and advancement in nanotechnology: a systematic review. Cureus. 2022;14(2):1-15.
16. Huang Q, Le Y, Li S, Bian Y. Signaling pathways and potential therapeutic targets in acute respiratory distress syndrome (ARDS). Respir Res. 2024;25(1):30.
17. Ma W, Tang S, Yao P, Zhou T, Niu Q, Liu P, et al. Advances in acute respiratory distress syndrome: focusing on heterogeneity, pathophysiology, and therapeutic strategies. Sig Transduct Target Ther. 2025;10(75):1-35.
18. Panacek EA, Marshall JC, Albertson TE, Johnson DH, Johnson S, MacArthur RD, et al. Efficacy and safety of the monoclonal anti-tumor necrosis factor antibody F(ab')2 fragment afelimomab in patients with severe sepsis and elevated interleukin-6 levels. Crit Care Med. 2004;32(11):2173-82.
19. Peng ZY, Wang HZ, Carter MJ, Dileo MV, Bishop JV, Zhou FH, et al. Acute removal of common sepsis mediators does not explain the effects of extracorporeal blood purification in experimental sepsis. Kidney Int. 2012;81(4):363-9.
20. Peng ZY, Carter MJ, Kellum JA. Effects of hemoadsorption on cytokine removal and short-term survival in septic rats. Crit Care Med. 2008;36(5):1573-7.
21. Cruz DN, Antonelli M, Fumagalli R, Foltran F, Brienza N, Donati A, et al. Early use of polymyxin B hemoperfusion in abdominal septic shock: the EUPHAS randomized controlled trial. JAMA. 2009;301(23):2445-52.
22. Cole L, Bellomo R, Journois D, Davenport P, Baldwin I, Tipping P. High-volume haemofiltration in human septic shock. Intensive Care Med. 2001;27(6):978-86.
23. Joannes-Boyau O, Honoré PM, Perez P, Bagshaw SM, Grand H, Canivet JL, et al. High-volume versus standard-volume haemofiltration for septic shock patients with acute kidney injury (IVOIRE study): a multicentre randomized controlled trial. Intensive Care Med. 2013;39(9):1535-46.
24. Wang JN, Liu MM, Wang F, Wei B, Yang Q, Cai YT, et al. RIPK1 inhibitor Cpd-71 attenuates renal dysfunction in cisplatin-treated mice via attenuating necroptosis, inflammation and oxidative stress. Clin Sci. 2019;133(14):1609-27.
25. Biegus J, Mebazaa A, Metra M, Pagnesi M, Chioncel O, Davison B, et al. Safety and efficacy intravenous istaroxime up to 60 hours for patients with pre-cardiogenic shock. J Heart Lung Transplant. 2025;44(10):1569-80.
26. Wenzl FA, Bruno F, Kraler S, Klingenberg R, Akhmedov A, Ministrini S, et al. Dipeptidyl peptidase 3 plasma levels predict cardiogenic shock and mortality in acute coronary syndromes. Eur Heart J. 2023;44(38):3859-71.
27. Chamorro Á, Dirnagl U, Urra X, Planas AM. Neuroprotection in acute stroke: targeting excitotoxicity, oxidative and nitrosative stress, and inflammation. Lancet Neurol. 2016;15(8):869-81.

CHAPTER 11

Frailty and Sarcopenia in Critically Ill Patients

Shilpushp Jagannath Bhosale, Malini Premkumar Joshi, Atul Prabhakar Kulkarni

INTRODUCTION

Frailty and sarcopenia have traditionally been associated with aging. Increasing life expectancy and advancements in critical care has led to larger proportion of elderly and physiologically vulnerable patients getting admitted to intensive care units.[1] The evolving demographics have highlighted the growing prevalence of frailty and sarcopenia amongst intensive care unit (ICU) patients.[2] Frailty is reported to be present in nearly 30–50% of older ICU patients, but is also increasingly recognized in younger individuals with chronic diseases.[3] Sarcopenia is observed in nearly 70% of ICU patients, particularly those with sepsis, prolonged mechanical ventilation, or malnutrition.[4] Both conditions are still underdiagnosed due to lack of routine screening and standardized diagnostic tools in ICU weightloss with risk of impairment of organ while sarcopenia is described as loss of muscle mass, they commonly have overlapping phenotypes.

Frailty is a syndrome characterized by decreased physiological reserve and increased vulnerability to stressors. It reflects a cumulative decline in multiple physiological systems, leading to a reduced ability to recover from acute illness.[5] Sarcopenia is a progressive and generalized skeletal muscle weakness involving the accelerated loss of muscle mass and function. It can be primary (age-related) or secondary (associated with disease, inactivity, or malnutrition). In critically ill patients, both frailty and sarcopenia may coexist or act synergistically, leading to profound muscle catabolism, functional decline, and higher risk of ICU-acquired weakness. It is also ironical that some elderly patients might display significant ability to tolerate stress, while some young individuals may lack significant physiologic reserve. This varying ability to recover from physiologic insults, independent of age best describes frailty.[6] Frailty is independently associated with prolonged hospital stay, longer ventilator days, delayed wound healing, infections, delirium, increased morbidity and mortality, length of stay and cost of treatment. Sarcopenia has been associated with increased mechanical ventilation duration and higher sepsis-related mortality. These patients often experience long-term disability, poor quality of life, and high rates of institutionalization post-discharge. Recognizing and managing frailty and sarcopenia is important for optimizing patient outcomes, resource utilization, and ethical decision-making.

MECHANISMS IN FRAILTY AND SARCOPENIA IN CRITICAL ILLNESS

Quite often critical illness strips away the normal compensatory mechanisms of the body and exposes frailty amongst vulnerable patients. It is very often seen that there is significant amount of muscle mass loss occurring within the first week of ICU admission and persistent neuromuscular impairments, commonly termed as prolonged ICU-acquired weakness.[7] Various mechanism and pathophysiological process exacerbate frailty and sarcopenia in ICU patients. The hypercatabolism and inflammatory cytokines (IL-6 and TNF-α) drive muscle protein breakdown which leads to loss of muscle mass.[8]

Prolonged immobilization leads to rapid muscle atrophy and insulin resistance. Most common contributing factor is inadequate nutrition or malnutrition due to various reasons such as gastrointestinal dysfunction or inappropriate nutrition supplementation or mitochondrial dysfunction in sepsis which leads to impaired energy metabolism or poor energy utilization which further exacerbates muscle loss.[9]

ASSESSMENT OF FRAILTY AND SARCOPENIA IN THE INTENSIVE CARE UNIT

Assessment of frailty in the ICU setting can be quite challenging. The commonly used tools to diagnose frailty are Fried's frailty phenotype scale and the Canadian Study of Health and Aging's, frailty index.[6,10]

The Fried's frailty phenotype scale consists of five components: unintentional weight loss, exhaustion, weakness (assessed by low hand grip strength), slow walking speed and low physical activity. The presence of any three or more can help diagnose frailty. A frailty index uses elaborate information regarding cumulative burden of health deficits and assesses physical, psychosocial, and medical deficits including disability, diseases, physical and cognitive impairment, psychosocial risk factors, and geriatric syndromes and calculates the frailty index. Several less common scales such as Groningen Frailty Indicator (GFI) or Morley FRAIL scale have been developed but not frequently used in ICU.[11,12] Simplified frailty scales such as clinical frailty scale (CFS) and modified frailty scale (MFI) are 9 point or 11 point scales and range patients from very fit to severely frail. These are simple and reproducible and hence better for use in critically ill patients.[13]

Assessing sarcopenia in ICU patients is also challenging due to limitations in measuring parameters such as muscle strength and physical performance. While there is currently no standard for assessing muscle function as part of sarcopenia in the ICU, the assessment of muscle mass is still possible and of clinical relevance.

The Sarcopenia Definitions and Outcomes Consortium (SDOC) described low muscle strength and poor function, assessed by grip strength and gait speed, as better predictors of outcomes than muscle mass.[14] It is also important to know that sarcopenia can occur in younger, inactive individuals. Sarcopenic obesity which combines obesity with impaired skeletal muscle mass and strength also needs to be identified.[15] For skeletal muscle strength, dynamometer handgrip strength or isometric torque methods are commonly advised.[16] Imaging modalities to assess muscle mass can be done using magnetic resonance imaging (MRI), computed tomography (CT) and dual X-ray absorptiometry but not always feasible in critically ill patients.[17] Ultrasonography and bio electrical impedance (BIA) are better alternatives to determine skeletal muscle thickness, cross-sectional area (CSA), or fat free mass but remain to be validated in ICU patients.[18]

IMPORTANCE OF ASSESSMENT OF FRAILTY AND SARCOPENIA IN INTENSIVE CARE UNIT PATIENTS

Evidence suggests that frailty at ICU admission is independently associated with increased mortality and a decline in health-related quality of life (QOL).[19]

Sarcopenia is an important determinant of clinical outcome during critical illness. This aspect is even more pronounced in female patients as they have lower muscle mass in relation to bodyweight. Withholding or withdrawal of life support therapies are discussed more frequently amongst patients in ICU.[20] Frail patients are more prone to falls while in the ICU or hospital.[21,22]

It has been observed that in ICU patients quadriceps muscle layer thickness decreased progressively with higher CFS scores suggesting frailty and sarcopenia often coexist.[23]

Although physical performance and muscle function can be evaluated through gait speed tests (6-meter walk test), sit-to-stand test, or short physical performance test, these assessments are often not feasible in critically ill patients.

MANAGEMENT OF FRAILTY AND SARCOPENIA IN INTENSIVE CARE UNIT PATIENTS

Adequacy of nutrition and mobilization have gained importance in recent years.

There are no specific nutrition guidelines or recommendations for patients with frailty or sarcopenia.[24,25] It may be better to achieve energy targets by use of indirect calorimetry compared to predictive equations. Evidence suggests use of isocaloric enteral nutrition (20–25 kcal/kg/day) and standard protein intake (1.3 g/kg/day) in mechanically ventilated ICU patients is reasonable. Targeting higher protein intake (2.0 g/kg/day) may be harmful.[26]

Use of amino acid leucine may activate the signaling pathways leading to protein synthesis. Testosterone supplementation may increase both muscle mass and strength in men but may cause serious adverse cardiovascular events. Studies on antioxidants, vitamin D supplements or drugs acting on renin-angiotensin system are ongoing but remain inconclusive.[27]

Early mobilization and physiotherapy may mitigate skeletal muscle loss, shorten ICU length of stay, and improve long-term functional outcomes, cognitive function, and QoL. Although no appropriate mobilization or rehabilitation regimen is recommended for frail and sarcopenic patients in ICU, protocol-based, step-wise mobilization for critical care patients within 72 hours may show benefit.[28]

Use of neuromuscular electrostimulation has reported positive effects on muscle mass, strength, and ICU-acquired weakness but evidence is still lacking.

CONCLUSION

Frailty and sarcopenia are emerging paradigms in the management of critically ill patients. Their presence significantly influences outcomes, resource utilization, and long-term survival and health-related quality of life (HRQOL). There is urgent need for standardized ICU-specific frailty and sarcopenia diagnostic criteria. Frailty and sarcopenia should not be used to deny ICU care, but rather to inform risk stratification, treatment proportionality, and resource allocation. Emerging need for ICU follow-up clinics for long-term functional recovery needs to be addressed.

REFERENCES

1. de Rooij SE, Govers A, Korevaar JC, Abu-Hanna A, Levi M, de Jonge E. Short-term and long-term mortality in very elderly patients admitted to an intensive care unit. Intensive Care Med. 2006;32(7):1039-44.
2. Bagshaw SM, Webb SA, Delaney A, George C, Pilcher D, Hart GK, et al. Very old patients admitted to intensive care in Australia and New Zealand: a multi-centre cohort analysis. Crit Care. 2009;13:R45.
3. Muscedere J, Waters B, Varambally A, Bagshaw SM, Boyd JG, Maslove D, et al. The impact of frailty on intensive care unit outcomes: a systematic review and meta-analysis. Intensive Care Med. 2017;43(8):1105-22.
4. Cruz-Jentoft AJ, Bahat G, Bauer J, Boirie Y, Bruyère O, Cederholm T, et al. Sarcopenia: revised European consensus on definition and diagnosis. Age Ageing. 2019;48(1):16-31. Erratum in: Age Ageing. 2019;48(4):601.
5. McDermid RC, Stelfox HT, Bagshaw SM. Frailty in the critically ill: a novel concept. Crit Care. 2011;15(1):301.
6. Rockwood K, Song X, MacKnight C, Bergman H, Hogan DB, McDowell I, et al. A global clinical measure of fitness and frailty in elderly people. CMAJ. 2005;173:489-95.

7. Griffiths RD, Hall JB. Intensive care unit-acquired weakness. Crit Care Med. 2010;38:779-87.
8. Winkelman C. The role of inflammation in ICU-acquired weakness. Crit Care. 2010;14:186.
9. Franceschi C, Capri M, Monti D, Giunta S, Olivieri F, Sevini F, et al. Inflammaging and anti-inflammaging: a systemic perspective on aging and longevity emerged from studies in humans. Mech Ageing Dev. 2007;128:92-105.
10. Fried LP, Tangen CM, Walston J, Newman AB, Hirsch C, Gottdiener J, et al. Frailty in older adults: evidence for a phenotype. J Gerontol A Biol Sci Med Sci. 2001;56:M146-56.
11. Steverink N, Slaets JPJ, Schuurmans H, van Lis M. Measuring frailty: Development and testing of the Groningen Frailty Indicator (GFI). Gerontologist. 2001;41(special issue 1):236-7.
12. Morley JE, Malmstrom TK, Miller DK. A simple frailty questionnaire (FRAIL) predicts outcomes in middle aged African Americans. J Nutr Health Aging. 2012;16(7):601-8.
13. Dent E, Kowal P, Hoogendijk EO. Frailty measurement in research and clinical practice: A review Eur J Intern Med. 2016;31:3-10.
14. Kirk B, Zanker J, Bani Hassan E, Bird S, Brennan-Olsen S, Duque G. Sarcopenia Definitions and Outcomes Consortium (SDOC) Criteria are Strongly Associated with Malnutrition, Depression, Falls, and Fractures in High-Risk Older Persons. J Am Med Dir Assoc. 2021;22(4):741-5.
15. Wei S, Nguyen TT, Zhang Y, Ryu D, Gariani K. Sarcopenic obesity: epidemiology, pathophysiology, cardiovascular disease, mortality, and management. Front Endocrinol. 2023;14:1185221.
16. Bohannon RW. Considerations and practical options for measuring muscle strength: a narrative review. Biomed Res Int. 2019;2019:8194537.
17. Kullberg J, Brandberg J, Angelhed JE, Frimmel H, Bergelin E, Strid L, et al. Whole-body adipose tissue analysis: comparison of MRI, CT and dual energy X-ray absorptiometry. Br J Radiol. 2009;82(974):123-30.
18. Isaka M, Sugimoto K, Akasaka H, Yasunobe Y, Takahashi T, Xie K, et al. The muscle thickness assessment using ultrasonography is a useful alternative to skeletal muscle mass by bioelectrical impedance analysis. Clin Interv Aging. 2022;17:1851-61.
19. Wozniak H, Beckmann TS, Dos Santos Rocha A, Pugin J, Heidegger CP, Cereghetti S. Long-stay ICU patients with frailty: mortality and recovery outcomes at 6 months. Ann Intensive Care. 2024;14(1):31.
20. McDermid RC, Bagshaw SM. Prolonging life and delaying death: the role of physicians in the context of limited intensive care resources. Philos Ethics Humanit Med. 2009;4:3.
21. Rivas-González N, López M, Martín-Gil B, Fernández-Castro M, Castro MJ, San Román JA. Relationship Between Frailty and Risk of Falls Among Hospitalised Older People with Cardiac Conditions: An Observational Cohort Study. Nurs Rep. 2025;15(3):100.
22. Bayer M, Krisinski H, Sak N, Sillevis R. A Cross-sectional pilot study on the impact of socioeconomic status on fall risk in older adults based on multiple outcome measures: 10MWT, 5TSIS, CTSIB-M, and 6MWT. J Rehab Pract Res. 2025;6(1):170.

23. Sundarsingh V, Manoj Kumar R, Kulkarni M, Pradhan D, Rodrigues PR, Baliga N, et al. Quadriceps muscle layer thickness and its association with frailty in critically ill patients: a prospective observational study. J Crit Care. 2025;85:154930.
24. Morley JE, Argiles JM, Evans WJ, Bhasin S, Cella D, Deutz NE, et al. Nutritional recommendations for the management of sarcopenia. J Am Med Dir Assoc. 2010;11(6):391-6.
25. Tohyama M, Shirai Y, Kokura Y, Momosaki R. Nutritional Care and Rehabilitation for Frailty, Sarcopenia, and Malnutrition. Nutrients. 2023;15(23):4908.
26. Studenski SA, Peters KW, Alley DE, Cawthon PM, McLean RR, Harris TB, et al. The FNIH sarcopenia project: rationale, study description, conference recommendations, and final estimates. J Gerontol A Biol Sci Med Sci. 2014;69(5):547-58.
27. Fenercioglu AK. The Anti-Inflammatory Roles of Vitamin D for Improving Human Health. Curr Issues Molecul Biol. 2024; 46(12):13514-25.
28. Vaidya AC, Kapre VM, Dobhal SP, Shukla MP, Mishra AS, Tiwari V. Effect of Early and Progressive Rehabilitation Protocol on Fatigue, Functional Outcome, and Kinesiophobia in Patients on Non-invasive Ventilation: A Randomized Controlled Trial. Indian J Crit Care Med. 2025;29(6):510-5.

CHAPTER 12

Renin: Biomarker of the Future?

Ashish Khanna, Kushal R Kalvit

INTRODUCTION

In this era of precision medicine, the field of intensive care is gradually drifting toward personalized therapy even in the setting of acutely ill patients with life-threatening organ dysfunction. Precision or personalized medicine warrants the identification of individual-specific disease pattern and response to therapies.[1] Biomarkers are a group of molecules that serve different purposes, one of them being identifying certain subsets of patients that would benefit from a tailored therapeutic approach as opposed to a blanket treatment protocol. An ideal biomarker would be one that is easy to measure, has a high sensitivity and specificity, minimally affected by other confounding factors, reflects real-time pathophysiological changes and, of course, is cost-effective.[2]

Shock is one of the most common life-threatening reasons for ICU admissions worldwide. Despite its varied etiopathogenesis, untreated shock eventually leads to organ failure and death. Hence, it has become essential to prioritize the identification of shock and initiate prompt treatment.[3] Moreover, identifying early organ failure and optimizing the hemodynamics as per the clinical condition is equally important to improve the survival. A battery of biomarkers has been extensively evaluated in the setting of shock, few of which have become standard of care (e.g., lactate).[4] Renin is one such novel biomarker that shows promising role in a hemodynamically unstable patient.[5]

RENIN–ANGIOTENSIN–ALDOSTERONE SYSTEM

The systems that regulate blood pressure and work in harmony (under physiological conditions) are sympathetic nervous system (SNS), vasopressinergic system, and RAAS (renin-angiotensin-aldosterone system). Among these, RAAS is unique as it exhibits a classical pathway as well as an alternate pathway that work in opposite directions. The RAAS pathway consists of angiotensinogen that is produced by the liver and is then converted to angiotensin-I (Ang-I) due to the action of renin, a peptide released from the juxtaglomerular apparatus in the kidneys. Ang-I is almost immediately converted into Ang-II in the presence of circulating as well as vascular angiotensin-converting enzyme (ACE). Ang-II, thus, acts as the main effector of the RAAS pathway and results in vasoconstriction (via AT1R receptor), sodium and water retention as well as pro-inflammatory and profibrotic actions to some extent.[6]

The alternate pathway of RAAS has Ang-(1–7) as its key player. Ang-(1–7) is formed by:

- Conversion of Ang-II to Ang-(1–7) by ACE2 enzyme
- Direct conversion of Ang-I to Ang-(1–7) by neprilysin.

Angiotensin-(1–7), in turn, acts via its Mas receptor and leads to vasodilatation, natriuresis, anti-inflammatory, and antifibrotic effects.[7] Under normal conditions, the affinity of AT1R is much higher for Ang-I as compared to that of ACE2; hence tilting the balance toward the classical pathway and its actions. However, pathological conditions such as septic shock leads to changes such as reduced expression of AT1R, increased expression of ACE2 and even reduced levels of ACE making the alternate pathway more pronounced.[8]

The importance of RAAS and its dysfunction in shock states has recently garnered attention in the field of intensive care medicine. Hypotension, reduced organ perfusion, and activation of the SNS are the most important triggers for the secretion of renin in critically ill patients.[9] Hence, it has been postulated that the measurement of renin levels and its trajectory can be exploited to identify shock states, assess response to treatment, use as a target for an intervention, and even predict outcomes. Moreover, owing to its short half-life of 10 minutes,[10] renin is also being viewed as a better perfusion marker than lactate.

RENIN AS AN OUTCOME PREDICTOR

The primary goal of the ATHOS3 trial was to assess whether Ang-II could effectively raise the mean arterial pressure (MAP) in patients with vasodilatory shock that was resistant to high-dose vasopressors. The main measure of success was increasing the MAP to 75 mm Hg or by at least 10 mm Hg within 3 hours, without the need to increase the existing vasopressor dose. Patients receiving Ang-II showed a significant improvement in blood pressure, with nearly 70% meeting the MAP target, compared to 23% in the placebo group. A secondary analysis of the trial revealed that although the renin levels in both arms were similar at baseline, there was statistically significant reduction in the renin levels at 3 hours post-randomization in the Ang-II group. It was also observed that the 28-day mortality in the Ang-II group was significantly reduced in patients with high baseline renin values (cutoff value being 172.7 pg/mL). Thus, it can be safely deduced that a higher baseline renin level indicates benefit from administration of exogenous Ang-II in vasodilatory shock. It is also interesting to note that the subset of patients who had more severe shock (noradrenaline equivalence >0.25 μg/kg/min) did not show any mortality reduction with receipt of Ang-II as compared to those who were receiving noradrenaline equivalence between 0.2 and 0.25 μg/kg/min. Ang-II administration may, therefore, confer benefit to a very niche subset of patients with septic shock. However, further studies are needed to validate these observations.[11]

Of the multiple studies done in critically ill patients, few have found renin to be an independent predictor of mortality. A study conducted among 20 patients (with and without shock) not only showed renin as a reliable marker of tissue perfusion based on the change in its levels over time but also as a marker that outperformed lactate. A direct comparison of the kinetics and absolute concentration of renin and lactate showed that renin kinetics performed better in the prediction of mortality, whereas the discriminative ability of their absolute values did not differ significantly. They also observed a cutoff value of 40 pg/mL for renin similar to the 2 mmol/L cutoff for lactate in the identification and prognostication of shock.[12] An interesting analysis of 103 biorepository samples of patients from the VICTAS trial revealed that baseline higher renin activity was associated with increased mortality in the study group. It also showed that an elevation of renin over 3 days was an independent predictor of mortality while this association was not found with change in the levels of Ang-II, ACE, ACE2, and Ang-(1–7).[13] Renin–Ang-II disconnection was obvious in this analysis where renin was elevated to up to 60 times normal in the most severe strata of septic shock, but consequent change in Ang-II was essentially flat and only up to 2 times normal. Other work has shown renin as not only a predictor of mortality but also of adverse renal outcomes, especially in the context of postoperative acute kidney injury (AKI).[14]

WHY IS RENIN NOT THE IDEAL BIOMARKER YET?

Although it looks very promising, renin must overcome many practical hurdles before being labeled as the go-to marker of shock states. Firstly, a point-of-care renin assay needs to be devised that would have a short turnaround time and can differentiate renin from prorenin efficiently.[15] Secondly, measuring the plasma renin activity (PRA) is influenced by sample handling, and angiotensinogen and prorenin levels. Thus, focusing on the standardization of method of measuring the active renin concentration instead of PRA is of utmost importance to reduce the heterogeneity among different studies being conducted.[16] Thirdly, owing to the widespread use of ACE inhibitors and angiotensin receptor blockers (ARBs), their effect on the baseline renin levels and its kinetics need to be taken into consideration before interpreting the results. It has been shown that the use of ACE inhibitors increases the baseline renin levels whereas the use of exogenous Ang-II reduces its levels.[17] A cost–benefit analysis is crucial before being advocated and/or implemented in the national and international guidelines as it has profound effect on the resource-limited countries. Lastly, renin cannot take the place of lactate which is a universally available and acceptable screening tool for sepsis, rather renin will add specificity to prognostication of shock and a personalized choice of vasopressors in these clinical scenarios.

CONCLUSION

Renin certainly has many potential applications in the field of intensive care medicine, but better and bigger studies are needed to validate its role. In addition to being an initiation criterion and the target for exogenous angiotensin therapy, it would not be surprising to find renin replace lactate as a biomarker for identification and prognostication of shock states, AKI, and mortality.

REFERENCES

1. Shankar-Hari M, Summers C, Baillie K. In pursuit of precision medicine in the critically ill. Annual Update in Intensive Care and Emergency Medicine 2018. 2018:649-58.
2. Méndez Hernández R, Ramasco Rueda F. Biomarkers as prognostic predictors and therapeutic guide in critically ill patients: clinical evidence. J Pers Med. 2023;13(2):333.
3. Sakr Y, Jaschinski U, Wittebole X, Szakmany T, Lipman J, Ñamendys-Silva SA, et al; ICON Investigators. Sepsis in intensive care unit patients: worldwide data from the intensive care over nations audit. Open Forum Infect Dis. 2018;5(12):ofy313.
4. Lee JH, Kim SH, Jang JH, Park JH, Jo KM, No TH, et al. Clinical usefulness of biomarkers for diagnosis and prediction of prognosis in sepsis and septic shock. Medicine (Baltimore). 2022;101(48):e31895.
5. Kotani Y, Chappell M, Landoni G, Zarbock A, Bellomo R, Khanna AK. Renin in critically ill patients. Ann Intensive Care. 2024;14(1):79.
6. Chappell MC. Biochemical evaluation of the renin-angiotensin system: the good, bad, and absolute? Am J Physiol Heart Circ Physiol. 2016;310(2):H137-52.
7. Donoghue M, Hsieh F, Baronas E, Godbout K, Gosselin M, Stagliano N, et al. A novel angiotensin-converting enzyme-related carboxypeptidase (ACE2) converts angiotensin I to angiotensin 1-9. Circ Res. 2000;87(5):E1-9.
8. Steckelings UM, Widdop RE, Sturrock ED, Lubbe L, Hussain T, Kaschina E, et al. The angiotensin AT_2 receptor: from a binding site to a novel therapeutic target. Pharmacol Rev. 2022;74(4):1051-135.
9. Leisman DE, Fernandes TD, Bijol V, Abraham MN, Lehman JR, Taylor MD, et al. Impaired angiotensin II type 1 receptor signaling contributes to sepsis-induced acute kidney injury. Kidney Int. 2021;99(1):148-60.
10. Basso N, Kurnjek ML, Taquini AC. Vascular renin-like activity and blood pressure. Mayo Clin Proc. 1977;52(7):437-41.
11. Bellomo R, Forni LG, Busse LW, McCurdy MT, Ham KR, Boldt DW, et al. Renin and Survival in Patients Given Angiotensin II for Catecholamine-Resistant

Vasodilatory Shock. A Clinical Trial. Am J Respir Crit Care Med. 2020;202(9):1253-61.

12. Gleeson PJ, Crippa IA, Mongkolpun W, Cavicchi FZ, Van Meerhaeghe T, Brimioulle S, et al. Renin as a marker of tissue-perfusion and prognosis in critically ill patients. Crit Care Med. 2019;47(2):152-8.
13. Busse LW, Schaich CL, Chappell MC, McCurdy MT, Staples EM, Ten Lohuis CC, et al; Vitamin C, Thiamine, and Steroids in Sepsis (VICTAS) Investigators. Association of Active Renin Content With Mortality in Critically Ill Patients: A Post hoc Analysis of the Vitamin C, Thiamine, and Steroids in Sepsis (VICTAS) Trial. Crit Care Med. 2024;52(3):441-51.
14. Nguyen M, Denimal D, Dargent A, Guinot PG, Duvillard L, Quenot JP, et al. Plasma renin concentration is associated with hemodynamic deficiency and adverse renal outcome in septic shock. Shock. 2019;52(4):e22-e30.
15. Khanna AK. Tissue perfusion and prognosis in the critically ill-is renin the new lactate? Crit Care Med. 2019;47(2):288-90.
16. Kotani Y, Belletti A, Maiucci G, Lodovici M, Fresilli S, Landoni G, et al. Renin as a prognostic marker in intensive care and perioperative settings: a scoping review. Anesth Analg. 2024;138(5):929-36.
17. Leisman DE, Handisides DR, Busse LW, Chappell MC, Chawla LS, Filbin MR, et al; ATHOS-3 Investigators. ACE inhibitors and angiotensin receptor blockers differentially alter the response to angiotensin II treatment in vasodilatory shock. Crit Care. 2024;28(1):130.

CHAPTER 13

Sodium-glucose Transporter 2 Inhibitors in Intensive Care Unit

Amit Srivastava, Devansh Gupta, Afzal Azim

INTRODUCTION

The discovery of phlorizin, a natural compound found in apple trees, in the early 19th century marked the beginning of sodium-glucose cotransporter 2 (SGLT2) inhibitor research. Although its ability to induce glucosuria and lower blood glucose was identified later, its instability and nonselective action limited clinical use. Ongoing pharmaceutical research eventually produced more targeted molecules. Dapagliflozin, developed in 2008, emerged as the first clinically viable SGLT2 inhibitor with enhanced selectivity, metabolic stability, and extended half-life, paving the way for a new class of treatments in cardiometabolic disease.[1] Additional agents in this class include *canagliflozin, empagliflozin, ertugliflozin, bexagliflozin, and sotagliflozin.*

Sodium-glucose cotransporter 2 inhibitors have emerged as multifunctional agents that extend well beyond their foundation in glycemic control. While initially approved for the treatment of type 2 diabetes mellitus, these agents have demonstrated a robust capacity to mitigate heart failure progression, delay chronic kidney disease (CKD) events, and improve cardiovascular outcomes independent of glucose-lowering effects. Rapidly evolving trial evidence and mechanistic data have prompted reassessment of their clinical utility across a broader continuum of illness severity.[2,3]

In the contemporary landscape of critical care medicine, therapeutic strategies that offer pleiotropic benefits without compromising hemodynamic stability are both desirable and scarce. The intensive care unit (ICU) presents a unique biological milieu: marked by oxidative stress, endothelial dysfunction, multiorgan cross-talk, altered pharmacokinetics, and a high burden of immunometabolic derangement.[4] In this complex environment, traditional therapies often yield limited survival benefit or carry prohibitive risks. Early phase investigations suggest that SGLT2 inhibitors may offer novel adjunctive capabilities to enhance cardiorenal performance, restrain inflammation, and conserve mitochondrial energetics, all without precipitating hypovolemia or derangements in serum electrolytes.[5]

Recent randomized controlled trials and observational cohorts have consistently demonstrated that SGLT2 inhibitors improve outcomes in patients with heart failure, renal impairment, and atherosclerotic cardiovascular disease, populations frequently represented in the critically ill.[1,3] In parallel, mechanistic studies have elucidated downstream effects of SGLT2 inhibition, including augmentation of ketone body metabolism, downregulation of inflammatory cytokines, stabilization of endothelial barrier function, and suppression of sympathetic overdrive.[6] These properties align closely with the pathophysiologic targets in many ICU patients, particularly those with septic shock, type 2 diabetes mellitus, acute kidney injury, and circulatory failure. Importantly, their favorable pharmacodynamic profile, defined by glucose and glomerular filtration rate-dependent action, insulin independence, and preserved efficacy in transient renal dysfunction, offers additional rationale for consideration in acute care. Unlike insulin, SGLT2 inhibitors exert minimal risk for hypoglycemia in fasting states, a frequent metabolic concern in critically ill populations undergoing variable nutritional support. Moreover, their renal and cardiovascular safety profiles have been substantiated in diverse patient subgroups, including those recovering from acute myocardial infarction, respiratory failure, and septic syndromes.[2,7]

This chapter synthesizes mechanistic evidence, pharmacokinetics, clinical efficacy, and safety considerations to explore the evolving position of SGLT2 inhibitors in intensive care medicine. Special emphasis is placed on their application in complex scenarios such as septic shock, acute heart failure, steroid-resistant inflammation, and organ support transition periods. By examining both translational biology and emerging clinical data, we aim to define the contemporary relevance and future potential of SGLT2 inhibition in critically ill patient populations.

MECHANISM OF ACTION OF SODIUM-GLUCOSE COTRANSPORTER 2 INHIBITORS

The mechanism of action of these drugs are enumerated below and summarized in **Figure 1**.

- Inhibit SGLT2 in the proximal renal tubule, reducing glucose and sodium reabsorption.
- Induce glycosuria and natriuresis, leading to modest osmotic diuresis without significant intravascular volume depletion.
- Lower plasma glucose levels independent of insulin, reducing glucotoxicity.
- Elevate circulating ketone bodies, enhancing myocardial metabolic efficiency under stress.
- Improve endothelial function and reduce oxidative stress via nitric oxide modulation and cytokine suppression.
- Mitigate glomerular hyperfiltration and intraglomerular hypertension, preserving renal function.
- Attenuate inflammation and cellular injury through downregulation of proinflammatory mediators.

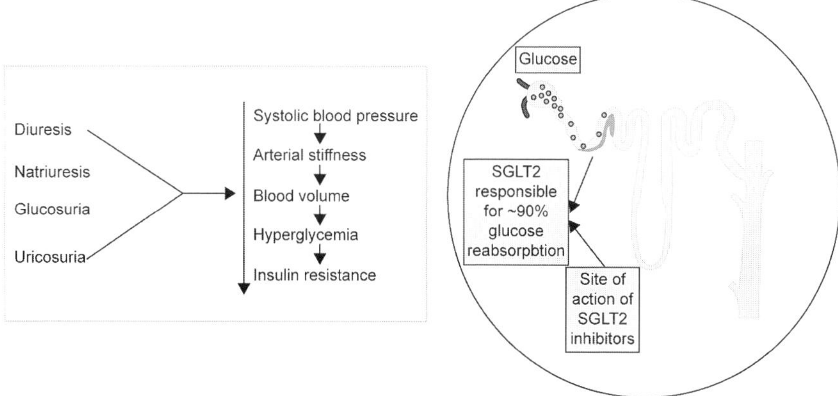

Fig. 1: Mechanism of action of sodium-glucose cotransporter 2 (SGLT2) inhibitors.

TABLE 1: FDA-approved indications for SGLT2 inhibitors.

Clinical indication	*Approved agents*
T2DM	All (e.g., dapagliflozin and empagliflozin)
Reduction in major adverse cardiovascular events (patients with T2DM and ASCVD)	Empagliflozin and canagliflozin
HFrEF	Dapagliflozin and empagliflozin
HFpEF	Dapagliflozin and empagliflozin
Chronic kidney disease with albuminuria	Dapagliflozin and empagliflozin

(ASCVD: atherosclerotic cardiovascular disease; HFpEF: heart failure with preserved ejection fraction; HFrEF: heart failure with reduced ejection fraction; T2DM: type 2 diabetes mellitus)

- Maintain hemodynamic stability without causing hypotension or major electrolyte imbalance.[1]

Food and Drug Administration (FDA)-approved indications for SGLT2 inhibitors, with key research trials, are enumerated here, as well as in ***Table 1****.*

- *Adjunct to diet and exercise for glycemic control*: They have been approved for improving glycemic control in adults with type 2 diabetes mellitus alongside diet and exercise.
- *Reduction of major adverse cardiovascular events (MACE):* Approved to reduce the risk of MACE—including nonfatal myocardial infarction, nonfatal stroke, and cardiovascular death—in patients with type 2 diabetes mellitus and established cardiovascular disease.
- *Heart failure reduced ejection fraction (HFrEF):* To reduce the risk of cardiovascular death and hospitalizations for heart failure, specifically in patients with heart failure with reduced ejection fraction [New York Heart Association Functional Classification (NYHA) class II–IV].

- *CKD:* They have been approved for kidney disease, and hospitalizations in patients with CKD and at risk of progression to lower the risk of significant decline in estimated glomerular filtration rate (eGFR) and progression to end-stage.
- *Heart failure preserved ejection fraction (HFpEF):* Certain SGLT-2 inhibitors are now indicated for improving cardiovascular outcomes in heart failure patients with preserved ejection fraction.
- *Broad coverage of heart failure:* Dapagliflozin is specifically FDA-approved for treating heart failure across the full spectrum of left ventricular ejection fraction (LVEF), including heart failure with reduced, mildly reduced, and preserved ejection fraction [(HFrEF, heart failure with mildly reduced ejection fraction (HFmrEF), and HfpEF].[8]

PHARMACOKINETICS AND PHARMACODYNAMICS

Sodium-glucose cotransporter 2 inhibitors possess favorable pharmacokinetic properties conducive to ICU use. These agents have high oral bioavailability (75–90%), reach peak plasma concentration within 1–2 hours, and demonstrate a half-life ranging from 10 to 15 hours, enabling once-daily dosing. They are extensively protein-bound (>90%) and undergo minimal hepatic metabolism through uridine 5'-diphospho-glucuronosyltransferase (UGT) enzymes, with primary renal elimination.[6,8]

Their pharmacodynamics are notably glucose- and glomerular filtration rate (GFR)-dependent. The efficacy of SGLT2 inhibitors declines as estimated glomerular filtration rate (eGFR) drops below 45 mL/min/1.73 m^2.[9] However, in many ICU patients with transient renal dysfunction, glycemic control and organ-protective effects may persist, though it needs to be substantiated by clinical trials. Importantly, SGLT2 inhibitors do not augment insulin secretion, thus posing minimal risk of hypoglycemia when used in monotherapy, an essential safety attribute in the critically ill with fluctuating nutritional and metabolic states.[8] The summary is presented below in **Table 2**.

CLINICAL BENEFITS IN CRITICAL ILLNESS

Hemodynamic Stabilization and Tissue Perfusion

Sodium-glucose cotransporter 2 inhibitors reduce interstitial volume via osmotic diuresis while sparing intravascular volume, thereby alleviating congestion of organs, reducing third-space extravasation of fluid without precipitating hypotension.[10] Erythropoietin-mediated hematocrit elevation and enhanced oxygen delivery can further contribute to improved organ perfusion. Moreover, their effect on enhanced myocardial ketone oxidation may optimize cardiac efficiency in shock states.[2,6]

TABLE 2: Pharmacokinetics and pharmacodynamics of SGLT2 inhibitors in ICU-relevant contexts.

Parameter	*Pharmacokinetic/ pharmacodynamic feature*	*Clinical relevance in the ICU*
Bioavailability	High (75–90%) oral bioavailability	Reliable absorption in stable enteral-fed ICU patients
Time to peak plasma concentration	1–2 hours after oral administration	Rapid onset may support early stabilization in step-down settings
Half-life	10–15 hours	Supports once-daily dosing; ideal for low-intervention environment
Protein binding	Extensive (>90%)	Low free drug in circulation minimizes variable effects
Metabolism	Minimal hepatic metabolism (via UGT enzymes)	Safer in hepatic dysfunction, common in sepsis or MODS
Elimination	Mainly renal	Dose adjustments may be needed in severe renal impairment
eGFR dependence	Efficacy declines if eGFR <45 mL/min/1.73 m^2	May retain some benefit in ICU patients with transient AKI
Insulin independence	No stimulation of insulin secretion	Minimal hypoglycemia is risked even in patients with intermittent feeding
Glucose threshold dependence	Effects diminish at low plasma glucose	Built-in metabolic safety check in fasting or catabolic states

[AKI: acute kidney injury; eGFR: estimated glomerular filtration rate; MODS: multiple organ dysfunction syndrome; UGT: uridine 5′-diphospho-glucuronosyltransferase; mL/min/1.73 m^2: milliliters per minute per 1.73 square meters (body surface area)]

Renal Protection in Acute Illness

By mitigating glomerular hyperfiltration, decreasing albuminuria, and attenuating oxidative stress, SGLT2 inhibitors preserve renal function, even following an initial eGFR dip. Their modest natriuretic effects minimize electrolyte losses, making them attractive adjuncts in AKI-prone ICU patients.[2,11] Similarly, Empagliflozin in Patients with Chronic Kidney Disease (EMPA-KIDNEY) trial demonstrated that empagliflozin significantly slowed kidney disease progression and reduced cardiovascular and kidney events in a broad range of CKD patients, regardless of diabetes status.[12] Though not yet established as a standard in ICU algorithms, evidence from Empagliflozin Outcome Trial in Patients with Chronic Heart Failure with Preserved Ejection

Fraction (DAPA-HF), Empagliflozin in Heart Failure with a Preserved Ejection Fraction (EMPEROR-Preserved), and Dapagliflozin Evaluation to Improve the Lives of Patients with Preserved Ejection Fraction Heart Failure (DELIVER) trials, and expert consensus statements, supports individualized use in hemodynamically stable ICU patients with cardiorenal dysfunction.[13-15]

Septic Shock

Emerging data indicates a potential role for SGLT2 inhibitors in septic shock. In a retrospective analysis by Ashcherkin et al. (2024), diabetic ICU patients with septic shock who had prior exposure to SGLT2 inhibitors demonstrated significantly lower 28-day mortality, reduced vasopressor needs, and shorter ICU stays.[16]

These benefits may be attributed to the effects of these drugs, which include enhanced endothelial integrity, improved mitochondrial efficiency, and attenuation of systemic inflammation. Furthermore, their capacity to reduce interstitial edema without compromising intravascular volume may support hemodynamic stability in septic states. While causality remains to be established, these findings highlight the therapeutic promise of SGLT2 inhibitors in select critically ill populations.[2]

Anti-inflammatory and Metabolic Modulation

The cardiometabolic benefits of SGLT2 inhibitors may be partially mediated by attenuation of inflammatory cascades and favorable shifts in myocardial substrate utilization, as evidenced in post hoc analyses of cardiovascular outcome trials and large-scale meta-analyses. By promoting ketone body oxidation and reducing accumulation of toxic lipid intermediates, these agents may alleviate cardiac steatosis and support reverse ventricular remodeling, mechanisms particularly relevant in the setting of metabolic stress and cardiac dysfunction frequently seen in sepsis.[17,18]

Cardiovascular Outcomes in Acute Heart Failure and Shock

In trials such as DAPA-HF and Empagliflozin, Cardiovascular Outcomes, and Mortality in Type 2 Diabetes (EMPA-REG OUTCOME) and Cardiovascular and Renal Outcomes with Empagliflozin in Heart Failure (EMPEROR-Reduced), early initiation of SGLT2 inhibitors resulted in significant reductions in heart failure hospitalizations and cardiovascular mortality.[3,13,17] The Empagliflozin in Patients Hospitalized for Acute Heart Failure-EMPULSE (EMPULSE) trial confirmed that initiating empagliflozin during acute heart failure hospitalization improves clinical outcomes, including symptom burden and biomarker trajectories[19] **(Tables 3 and 4)**.

TABLE 3: Major randomized controlled trials supporting SGLT2 use in ICU/acute hospital setting trials.

Trial name	*Population*	*Setting*	*Intervention*	*Dose*	*Primary outcome*
EMPULSE	Acute heart failure hospitalization	Hospitalized/ ICU-capable	Empagliflozin	10 mg once daily	Hierarchical clinical benefit at day 90
SOLOIST-WHF	T2DM + recent worsening HF	Recently hospitalized/ Acute	Sotagliflozin	200 mg then 400 mg once daily	CV death + HF hospitalization + urgent HF visits
DARE-19	COVID-19 + cardiometabolic risk	Hospitalized (including critical illness)	Dapagliflozin	10 mg once daily	Organ failure + all-cause death

(COVID-19: coronavirus disease of 2019; CV: cardiovascular; DARE-19: Dapagliflozin in Respiratory Failure in Patients with COVID-19; SOLOIST-WHF: Sotagliflozin in Patients with Diabetes and Recent Worsening Heart Failure)

TABLE 4: Major randomized controlled trials supporting SGLT2 Use in non-ICU/ chronic disease trials.

Trial name	*Population*	*Setting*	*Intervention*	*Dosage*	*Primary outcome*
DAPA-HF	HFrEF ± T2DM	Ambulatory/ chronic	Dapagliflozin	10 mg once daily	CV death + HF hospitalization
EMPEROR-Reduced	HFrEF ± T2DM	Ambulatory/ chronic	Empagliflozin	10 mg once daily	CV death + HF hospitalization
EMPEROR-Preserved	HFpEF ± T2DM	Ambulatory/ Chronic	Empagliflozin	10 mg once daily	CV death + HF hospitalization
EMPA-KIDNEY	Chronic Kidney Disease (CKD) ± T2DM	Ambulatory/ Chronic	Empagliflozin	10 mg once daily	CKD progression or CV death

(DAPA-HF: Dapagliflozin and Prevention of Adverse Outcomes in Heart Failure; EMPEROR-Reduced: Empagliflozin Outcome Trial in Patients with Chronic Heart Failure with Reduced Ejection Fraction; EMPEROR-Preserved: Empagliflozin Outcome Trial in Patients With Chronic Heart Failure With Preserved Ejection Fraction; HFrEF: heart failure with reduced ejection fraction; HFpEF: heart failure with preserved ejection fraction)

Frailty and Endothelial Dysfunction

Recent investigations demonstrate that empagliflozin exerts beneficial effects on both frailty and endothelial health in patients with diabetes and heart failure. Empagliflozin improved cognitive function and physical performance by attenuating mitochondrial calcium overload and reducing oxidative stress in endothelial cells. Another study reported significant downregulation of endothelial-specific microribonucleic acid (miRNAs), including miR21, miR92, and miR221, all implicated in vascular aging, angiogenesis, and inflammation. These findings suggest that empagliflozin may simultaneously target the molecular underpinnings of frailty and vascular dysfunction, offering dual protection in critically ill patients, particularly those vulnerable to age-associated decline during intensive care.[20]

Coronavirus Disease of 2019 and Critical Illness

The Dapagliflozin in Patients with Cardiometabolic Risk Factors Hospitalised with COVID-19 (DARE-19) trial (Kosiborod et al.) was a multicenter, double-blind, placebo-controlled phase 3 study that evaluated dapagliflozin in hospitalized COVID-19 patients with cardiometabolic risk factors. Although the trial did not achieve statistical significance for its primary endpoints—organ dysfunction and all-cause mortality, dapagliflozin was found to be safe and well-tolerated in the acute setting. Importantly, the rate of adverse renal events and hypotension was not increased, and a numerically lower rate of complications was observed in the treatment arm. These findings affirm the hemodynamic and renal safety of SGLT2 inhibitors in acutely ill patients and provide the first randomized trial data supporting their potential use in a heterogeneous critically ill population, including those with respiratory failure and systemic inflammation. The DARE-19 trial lays the groundwork for future studies exploring SGLT2 inhibitors in broader ICU contexts beyond COVID-19.[6]

Potential Role in Sepsis and Multiorgan Dysfunction

Animal studies suggest SGLT2 inhibition may modulate mitochondrial dysfunction, enhance endothelial barrier function, and blunt hyperinflammation in sepsis. These properties, together with renal and cardiovascular benefits, make SGLT2 inhibitors promising agents in septic shock and MODS.[2,7] The target ICU population with the potential benefits and clinical considerations are enumerated in **Table 5**.

CLINICAL GUIDELINES AND POSITION STATEMENTS

Multiple Guidelines Endorse Sodium-glucose Cotransporter 2 Inhibitors Beyond Glycemic Control

- The 2022 American Heart Association (AHA)/American College of Cardiology (ACC)/Heart Failure Society of America (HFSA) Heart Failure Guidelines recommend SGLT2 inhibitors as first-line agents for both HFrEF and HFpEF, irrespective of diabetic status.[21]

TABLE 5: ICU Populations for SGLT2 inhibitor use.

Population	*Potential benefit*	*Primary considerations*
ICU patients with HfrEF	Improved hemodynamics, reduced congestion	Ensure volume status, monitor BP
Type 2 diabetes + AKI-prone profile	Renal protection, reduced albuminuria	Avoid in active renal hypoperfusion
Postseptic shock recovery	Hemodynamic stabilization, endothelial protection	Initiate only after stabilization
COVID-19 with cardiometabolic risk	Safe profile, trend toward reduced complications (DARE-19)	Requires more trial data for ICU-specific protocols
Patients with MODS and inflammation	Anti-inflammatory, mitochondrial protection	Monitor lactate, ketones, and perfusion markers
Recently stabilized acute heart failure patients	Earlier post-ICU SGLT2 initiation reduces HF readmission (SOLOIST-WHF)	Start in step-down under close supervision
ICU patients with HFrEF	Improved hemodynamics, reduced congestion	Ensure volume status, monitor BP

(AKI: acute kidney injury; BP: blood pressure; COVID-19: coronavirus disease of 2019; DARE-19: Dapagliflozin in Respiratory Failure in Patients with COVID-19; ICU: intensive care unit; HfrEF: heart failure with reduced ejection fraction; MODS: multiorgan dysfunction score; SOLOIST-WHF: Sotagliflozin in Patients with Diabetes and Recent Worsening Heart Failure)

- The 2022 Canadian Cardiovascular Society Guideline recommends SGLT2 inhibitors for adults with type 2 diabetes mellitus and established atherosclerotic cardiovascular disease, heart failure, or CKD, citing a relative risk reduction of approximately 30–35% in heart failure hospitalization and 30–40% in progression of renal disease. In patients with heart failure with reduced ejection fraction (LVEF ≤40%), SGLT2 inhibitors reduced all-cause mortality by 13% and heart failure hospitalization by 26%, regardless of diabetes status.[22]
- *The 2022 Kidney Disease:* Improving Global Outcomes (KDIGO) CKD Guidelines advocate their use in patients with CKD and albuminuria, including those without diabetes (KDIGO Work Group).[23]
- 2021 Guidelines for Heart Failure states SGLT2 inhibitors (dapagliflozin or empagliflozin) are recommended (Class I, Level A) for all patients with HFrEF (LVEF ≤40%) to reduce heart failure hospitalization and mortality, irrespective of diabetes status. These agents are considered one of the four pillars of foundational therapy for HFrEF alongside angiotensin-converting enzyme inhibitor (ACEi)/angiotensin receptor-neprilysin inhibitor (ARNI), beta-blockers, and mineralocorticoid receptor antagonists (MRAs).[24]

RISKS AND CONTRAINDICATIONS

Absolute contraindications for SGLT2 inhibitors include:[1]

- Severe renal impairment (generally defined as eGFR <30 mL/min/1.73 m^2) or patients on dialysis.
- History of serious hypersensitivity reaction to the drug.
- Type 1 diabetes, due to the increased risk of diabetic ketoacidosis.
- Pregnancy or breastfeeding.
- History of diabetic ketoacidosis.
- End-stage renal disease (ESRD)

Despite strong efficacy signals, SGLT2 inhibitors have risks relevant to ICU patients:[4]

- *Volume Depletion:* Osmotic diuresis may exacerbate hypovolemia, and hence careful fluid management is essential.
- *Euglycemic DKA:* Particularly in fasting or catabolic states, requires high suspicion and prompt ketone monitoring.
- *Acute Kidney Injury:* A transient eGFR dip may be misclassified as AKI. Initiation of these drugs should be avoided during active hypoperfusion.
- *Genital Infections:* Common in ambulatory patients, less so in ICU settings.
- *Hypoglycemia:* Rare unless combined with insulin or sulfonylureas.

PRACTICAL ASPECTS AND GUIDELINES FOR USE

Patient Selection: Comorbidities, Risk Stratification, and Contraindications

Appropriate patient selection is critical when considering SGLT2 inhibitors in the ICU setting. Candidates likely to benefit include those with cardiometabolic risk factors such as type 2 diabetes mellitus, heart failure (especially with preserved ejection fraction), and early-stage acute kidney injury. Clinical judgment should guide risk-benefit evaluation in each case. SGLT2 inhibitors are best avoided in patients with active diabetic ketoacidosis, hypotension, severe volume depletion, or advanced renal failure (eGFR <20 mL/min/1.73 m^2). Special caution is warranted in patients with recent amputations, active foot ulcers, or necrotizing infections due to potential associations with Fournier's gangrene.[2]

INITIATION, TITRATION, AND MONITORING IN THE INTENSIVE CARE UNIT

When initiating therapy in critically ill patients, a conservative approach is advised. Begin with the lowest available dose (e.g., dapagliflozin 5 mg or empagliflozin 10 mg once daily) and monitor closely for signs of hypovolemia, hypotension, ketoacidosis, and electrolyte disturbances. Daily assessments of serum creatinine, ketones, bicarbonate, and glucose are essential. Glycemic control should be individualized based on the patient's nutritional status and concurrent insulin therapy.[22]

STOPPING RULES AND CRITERIA FOR WITHDRAWAL

- Discontinuation of SGLT2 inhibitors is warranted under the following circumstances: Recurrent or refractory of ketoacidosis.
- Sustained hypotension despite volume resuscitation.
- Progressive renal failure, or
- Suspected drug-related adverse effects such as genitourinary infections or dehydration.
- Clinical deterioration despite therapy should prompt reevaluation.[2]

Regular interdisciplinary reviews involving intensivists, nephrologists, and endocrinologists can help refine ongoing risk assessment and guide appropriate therapy cessation.

PERIOPERATIVE MANAGEMENT AND TRANSITION OF CARE

Sodium-glucose cotransporter 2 inhibitors should generally be withheld 3–4 days prior to major surgery or procedures requiring prolonged fasting, to mitigate the risk of euglycemic diabetic ketoacidosis. Resumption postoperatively should be based on stable hemodynamics, adequate oral intake, and the absence of surgical complications. During transitions from ICU to ward care or from hospital to home, communication between teams is vital to ensure appropriate continuation, discontinuation, or substitution.[22,23]

PITFALLS AND BEST PRACTICES

These vignettes emphasize the need for individualized SGLT2 inhibitor use based on patient-specific factors such as volume status, renal function, and frailty. Key pitfalls include initiating therapy in patients with ongoing hypoperfusion, critical ketoacidosis, or those at high risk of genitourinary infections. Best practices include close monitoring of fluid balance, renal markers, and glycemic status, with collaborative multidisciplinary decision-making. Timing, reinitiation post-stabilization, and attention to transitions of care are essential to optimize outcomes.

FUTURE DIRECTIONS AND RESEARCH GAPS

Unresolved questions remain regarding ICU use of SGLT2 inhibitors:

- *Initiation timing*: Best timing in acute illness—post-stabilization vs early intervention—requires exploration.
- *Target populations*: Efficacy in sepsis, acute respiratory distress syndrome (ARDS), and noncardiogenic AKI is under-researched.

- *Comparative studies*: Head-to-head ICU trials vs traditional diuretics or vasodilators are lacking.
- *Biomarker development*: Predictive indicators of therapeutic response are needed.
- *Safety in MODS*: Data on hepatic dysfunction, coagulopathy, and electrolyte abnormalities are sparse.
- Newer SGLT2 inhibitors and their role in critical illness.[25]

CONCLUSION

Sodium-glucose cotransporter 2 inhibitors represent a novel pharmacologic paradigm in critical care. Beyond glycemic modulation, they deliver multifaceted cardiorenal-metabolic benefits that address key pathophysiologic mechanisms in acute illness. Hemodynamic stabilization, renal protection, anti-inflammatory effects, and metabolic optimization support their emerging role in selecting ICU settings.

While caution is warranted in unstable or hypovolemic patients, data from randomized trials and guideline endorsements validate their safe use in appropriately selected cases. As ongoing research expands our understanding, SGLT2 inhibitors may increasingly become core components of intensive care pharmacotherapy.

REFERENCES

1. Morillas H, Galcerá E, Alania E, Seller J, Larumbe A, Núñez J, et al. Sodium-glucose Co-transporter 2 Inhibitors in Acute Heart Failure: A Review of the Available Evidence and Practical Guidance on Clinical Use. Rev Cardiovasc Med. 2022;23(4):139.
2. Hasan I, Rashid T, Jaikaransingh V, Heilig C, Abdel-Rahman EM, Awad AS. SGLT2 inhibitors: Beyond glycemic control. J Clin Transl Endocrinol. 2024;35:100335.
3. Packer M, Anker SD, Butler J, Filippatos G, Pocock SJ, Carson P, et al. Cardiovascular and Renal Outcomes with Empagliflozin in Heart Failure. N Engl J Med. 2020;383(15):1413-24.
4. Padda IS, Mahtani AU, Parmar M. Sodium-Glucose Transport Protein 2 (SGLT2) Inhibitors. In: Stat Pearls [Internet]. Treasure Island (FL): StatPearls Publishing; 2025.
5. Malyszko J, de Seigneux S, Cantaluppi V, Faguer S, Gameiro J, Lopes JA, et al. DEFENDER trial: dapagliflozin for critically ill patients with acute organ dysfunction-implications for clinicians. Nephrol Dial Transplant. 2025;40(7):1267-9.
6. Kosiborod MN, Esterline R, Furtado RHM, Oscarsson J, Gasparyan SB, Koch GG, et al. Dapagliflozin in patients with cardiometabolic risk factors hospitalised with COVID-19 (DARE-19): a randomised, double-blind, placebo-controlled, phase 3 trial. Lancet Diabetes Endocrinol. 2021;9(9):586-94.
7. Wright EM. SGLT2 Inhibitors: Physiology and Pharmacology. Kidney360. 2021;2(12):2027-37.

8. Butler J, Jones WS, Udell JA, Anker SD, Petrie MC, Harrington J, et al. Empagliflozin after Acute Myocardial Infarction. N Engl J Med. 2024; 390(17):1603-13.
9. Neal B, Perkovic V, Matthews DR. Canagliflozin and Cardiovascular and Renal Events in Type 2 Diabetes. N Engl J Med. 2017;377(7):644-57.
10. Heerspink HJL, Stefánsson BV, Correa-Rotter R, Chertow GM, Greene T, Hou FF, et al. Dapagliflozin in patients with chronic kidney disease. N Engl J Med. 2020;383(15):1436-46.
11. Mårtensson J, Cutuli SL, Osawa EA, Yanase F, Toh L, Cioccari L, et al. Sodium glucose co-transporter-2 inhibitors in intensive care unit patients with type 2 diabetes: a pilot case control study. Crit Care. 2023;27(1):189.
12. The EMPA-KIDNEY Collaborative Group; Herrington WG, Staplin N, Wanner C, Wanner C, Green JB, Hauske SJ, et al. Empagliflozin in Patients with Chronic Kidney Disease. N Engl J Med. 2023;388(2):117-27.
13. McMurray JJV, Solomon SD, Inzucchi SE, Køber L, Kosiborod MN, Martinez FA, et al. DAPA-HF Trial Committees and Investigators. Dapagliflozin in Patients with Heart Failure and Reduced Ejection Fraction. N Engl J Med. 2019; 381(21):1995-2008.
14. Anker SD, Butler J, Filippatos G, Ferreira JP, Bocchi E, Böhm M, et al. EMPEROR-Preserved Trial Investigators. Empagliflozin in Heart Failure with a Preserved Ejection Fraction. N Engl J Med. 2021;385(16):1451-61.
15. Solomon SD, McMurray JJV, de Boer RA, DeMets D, Hernandez AF, et al. DELIVER Trial Committees and Investigators. Dapagliflozin in Heart Failure with Mildly Reduced or Preserved Ejection Fraction. N Engl J Med. 2022;387(12):1089-98.
16. Ashcherkin N, Abdalla AA, Gupta S, Bhatt S, Yee CI, Cartin-Ceba R. Are sodium-glucose co-transporter-2 inhibitors associated with improved outcomes in diabetic patients admitted to intensive care units with septic shock? Acute Crit Care. 2024;39(2):251-56.
17. Zinman B, Wanner C, Lachin JM, Fitchett D, Bluhmki E, Hantel S, et al. Empagliflozin, cardiovascular outcomes, and mortality in type 2 diabetes. N Engl J Med. 2015;373(22):2117-28.
18. Shrestha DB, Budhathoki P, Sedhai YR, Karki P, Gurung S, Raut S, et al. Sodium-glucose cotransporter-2 Inhibitors in Heart Failure: An Updated Systematic Review and Meta-analysis of 13 Randomized Clinical Trials Including 14,618 Patients With Heart Failure. J Cardiovasc Pharmacol. 2021;78(4):501-14.
19. Voors AA, Angermann CE, Teerlink JR, Collins SP, Kosiborod M, Biegus J, et al. The SGLT2 inhibitor empagliflozin in patients hospitalized for acute heart failure: a multinational randomized trial. Nat Med. 2022;28(3):568-74.
20. Calila H, Bălășescu E, Nedelcu RI, Ion DA. Endothelial Dysfunction as a Key Link between Cardiovascular Disease and Frailty: A Systematic Review. J Clin Med. 2024;13(9):2686.
21. Heidenreich PA, Bozkurt B, Aguilar D, Allen LA, Byun JJ, Colvin MM, et al. 2022 AHA/ACC/HFSA guideline for the management of heart failure: a report of the American College of Cardiology/American Heart Association Joint Committee on Clinical Practice Guidelines. J Am Coll Cardiol. 2022;79(17):e263-421.
22. Mancini GBJ, O'Meara E, Bernier M, Cheng AYY, Cherney DZI, et al. 2022 Canadian Cardiovascular Society Guideline for Use of GLP-1 Receptor Agonists and SGLT2 Inhibitors for Cardiorenal Risk Reduction in Adults. Can J Cardiol. 2022;38(8):1153 67.

23. Kidney Disease: Improving Global Outcomes (KDIGO) CKD Work Group. KDIGO 2022 Clinical Practice Guideline for Diabetes Management in Chronic Kidney Disease. Kidney Int. 2022; 102(4S):S1-27.
24. McDonagh TA, Metra M, Adamo M, Gardner RS, Baumbach A, Böhm M, et al. ESC Scientific Document Group. 2021 ESC Guidelines for the diagnosis and treatment of acute and chronic heart failure. Eur Heart J. 2021;42(36):3599-726.
25. Bhatt DL, Szarek M, Steg PG, Cannon CP, Leiter LA, McGuire DK, et al. Sotagliflozin in Patients with Diabetes and Recent Worsening Heart Failure. N Engl J Med. 2021;384(2):117-28.

CHAPTER 14

Sovateltide

Prem Prakeerth P, Bhuvana Krishna

INTRODUCTION

Stroke remains one of the most formidable health challenges worldwide, contributing to high mortality, devastating disability, and significant socioeconomic burden. In recent decades, focus has shifted from merely limiting the extent of damage to restoring brain function through neuroregeneration and repair. Among novel therapeutic approaches, sovateltide- a first-in-class, highly selective endothelin-B (ETB) receptor agonist—has emerged as a promising neuroregenerative therapy for acute cerebral ischemic stroke (ACIS). This chapter provides a comprehensive overview of sovateltide, encompassing its molecular mechanisms of action, clinical efficacy, regulatory considerations, and potential future applications.

Stroke is defined as a neurological deficit resulting from an acute focal injury to the central nervous system due to a vascular cause. This includes cerebral infarction, intracerebral hemorrhage (ICH), and subarachnoid hemorrhage (SAH).[1] It is the second leading cause of death and the third highest cause of disability-adjusted life years (DALYs) globally.[2,3] In 2016, the global lifetime risk of stroke for individuals aged 25 years and older was estimated at nearly 1 in 4, highlighting its immense health impact. Stroke caused 5.5 million deaths in 2016 and accounted for a major share of DALYs globally. The prevalence of ischemic stroke is higher than that of hemorrhagic stroke. It is estimated that by the year 2050, low and middle-income countries (LMICs) will account for over 90% of all stroke-related deaths globally.[4] In India, the incidence of stroke is estimated to range between 116 and 163 cases per 100,000 population, making it a significant contributor to disability.[5]

Ischemic stroke is precipitated by a sudden reduction or cessation of cerebral blood flow, typically due to thrombotic or embolic occlusion of cerebral arteries that initiate energy failure and loss of ionic gradients, excitotoxicity, free radical and oxidative damage, inflammation, Disruption of the blood-brain barrier, apoptosis, and necrosis of neurons and subsequent neurological deficits.[6-9]

The area immediately surrounding the infarct (ischemic penumbra) is particularly vulnerable. Preservation and recovery in this area form the theoretical basis for neuroprotective and neurorestorative strategies.

Stroke occurrence is shaped by a complex interplay of risk factors, such as hypertension, hypercholesterolemia, diabetes, smoking, alcohol, sedentary lifestyle, and genetic factors, and recognition of these diverse factors is crucial for effective preventive strategies.

Timely recanalization with intravenous tissue plasminogen activator (tPA) and mechanical thrombectomy remains the mainstay of acute ischemic stroke treatment. However, each has significant limitations. *Tissue plasminogen activator*: Narrow therapeutic window (<4.5 hours); risk of intracranial hemorrhage (~4.9%). *Mechanical thrombectomy*: Limited to large vessel occlusions, with eligibility determined by timing and advanced imaging. Only 3–8% of all patients with ischemic stroke are eligible for thrombolysis, and less than one-third achieve full functional recovery.[1] Given these constraints, a significant unmet need exists for therapies that go beyond acute recanalization, especially those that promote neurorestoration beyond the conventional time window.

SOVATELTIDE: RATIONALE FOR DEVELOPMENT

Endothelins are a family of vasoactive peptides that play an important role in stroke physiology.[10]

In the 24 hours following a stroke, plasma endothelin levels increase to almost fourfold their normal levels. The binding of endothelin to the endothelin A (ETA) receptor can increase ischemic injury by promoting vasoconstriction, excitotoxicity, activation and recruitment of inflammatory cells, and cerebral edema. In contrast, binding of endothelin to the endothelin B (ETB) receptor, which is highly expressed in the cerebrum and is upregulated after ischemic injury,[10] can oppose the activity of ETA receptor activation by facilitating clearance of endothelin from circulation.[11] Sovateltide is a synthetic and highly selective endothelin B (ETB) receptor agonist, structurally analogous to endothelin-1 (ET-1), developed to enhance neuroprotective and neurorestorative effects while reducing vasoconstrictive activity.[6]

Sovateltide promoted differentiation/maturation of neuronal precursors (NPs) to generate a mature neuronal cell population, which would heal the stroke-damaged brain more efficiently. These findings have demonstrated a novel mechanism of action of sovateltide, which promotes differentiation of neuronal progenitors in the ischemic stroke brain and helps in neural regeneration and repair.[5]

Sovateltide treatment in rodent stroke models resulted in significant neuroprotection with notable reductions in infarct volume, increased neural differentiation, improved mitochondrial function, and enhanced functional recovery.[7] Unlike ETA antagonists or mixed antagonists—which have yielded mixed or disappointing results—ETB stimulation by sovateltide uniquely activates innate repair pathways.[8]

MECHANISM OF ACTION

Promotes differentiation/maturation of neural progenitor cells, thus fostering regeneration of mature neurons. It increases cerebral blood flow via ETB-mediated vasodilation. It also stimulates angiogenesis and neurogenesis through upregulation of VEGF and NGF. It has been shown to reduce infarct size by limiting apoptosis and promoting mitochondrial health, and enhances synaptic repair and neurovascular remodeling.[1,2,5]

INDICATIONS

The only approved indication is in the treatment of cerebral ischemic stroke within 24 hours of stroke onset.[12]

Research and early-phase clinical evaluation suggest sovateltide's unique neuroregenerative action may extend benefit to other neurological conditions such as hypoxic-ischemic encephalopathy (HIE), spinal cord injury, Alzheimer's disease, and other neurodegenerative diseases.

PHARMACOKINETICS AND SAFETY[13-16]

Available as "Tyvalzi™," as a sterile lyophilized powder (30 µg per vial) for reconstitution.

- *Administration:* Intravenous bolus over 1 minute.
- *Dosing:* 0.3 µg/kg per dose, three doses a day, 3 hours apart, administered on days 1, 3, and 6 (up to 0.9 µg/kg/day) (total nine doses).[12,14]
- *Pharmacokinetics:* Cmax increases dose-proportionally; short half-life (t1/2 ~4–8 minutes),[13] 83–85% plasma protein binding;[14] not a cytochrome P450 (CYP) substrate or significant CYP inducer/inhibitor.
- *Contraindications:* Hypersensitivity to sovateltide or any of its excipients (trisodium citrate dihydrate and mannitol).[14]
- *Safety profile:* Extensive preclinical and early-phase human studies demonstrate excellent tolerability, with no significant drug-related adverse events in multiple clinical trials.[8]

There is no clinical data on the use of the drug in pregnant women, although animal studies have shown no evidence of maternal or fetal toxicity or teratogenic effects. Information on use during lactation is lacking, so caution is advised in breastfeeding individuals. Similarly, data on pediatric patients is unavailable. In geriatric patients, no drug-related adverse events have been reported.[12]

EVIDENCE FOR USE

A phase 3 trial enrolled adults (18–78 years) within 24 hours of radiologically confirmed ischemic stroke, with mRS 3–4 and NIHSS >5. Patients with prior stroke were eligible if fully recovered; those receiving or eligible for endovascular/surgical intervention were excluded. Participants received

TABLE 1: Comparison of sovateltide with alteplase and mechanical thrombectomy.

Feature	*Sovateltide*	*tPA (alteplase)*	*Mechanical thrombectomy*
Mechanism	Neurorestorative (ETB agonist)	Thrombolysis	Clot retrieval
Time window	≤24 hours	≤4.5 hours	Up to 24 hours
Eligibility	Broad (ischemic stroke and imaging)	Exclusion in ICH/bleeds	Large vessel occlusion only
Mode of action	Promotes neurogenesis, angiogenesis	Fibrinolysis	Mechanical recanalization
Risk of symptomatic ICH	Very low	~4.9%	Modest
Tolerability	High	Modest	Procedural risks
Approved in	India	Worldwide	Worldwide (selected centers)

(ETB: endothelin-B; ICH: intracerebral hemorrhage; tPA: tissue plasminogen activator)

either sovateltide (0.3 μg/kg IV, three doses/day on days 1, 3, and 6) or placebo plus standard care, with the first dose within 24 hours of symptom onset. Baseline characteristics were similar between groups. At day 90, the sovateltide group showed significantly greater improvements in NIHSS, mRS, and Barthel Index scores, with more patients achieving NIHSS ≥6-point and mRS ≥2-point improvements compared to placebo **(Table 1)**.

COMPARISON WITH OTHER THERAPEUTIC MODALITIES

The **Table 1** shows the comparison of sovateltide with alteplase and mechanical thrombectomy.

CONCLUSION

In patients who present within 24 hours of the onset of ischemic stroke, the addition of sovateltide to standard treatment regimens has demonstrated enhancement in neurological recovery and improved functional outcomes. While thrombolytic agents remain a cornerstone of acute ischemic stroke management in India,[14] their use is strictly restricted to the first 4.5 hours after symptom onset, beyond which the risk of bleeding complications are very high. Furthermore, their administration is contraindicated in individuals with active internal bleeding, including intracranial hemorrhage, or in those with a high chance for bleeding, which restricts their applicability to only about 3–8% of all ischemic stroke patients.[16]

Sovateltide, in contrast, can be administered up to 24 hours after stroke onset, providing a valuable treatment alternative for patients who are ineligible for thrombolysis due to delayed presentation or contraindications. Importantly, it does not have intrinsic thrombolytic properties, nor does it interfere with the action of thrombolytic drugs, making it suitable for combined therapy.[12]

Despite promising early results, additional large-scale and long-term studies are warranted to establish a more comprehensive understanding of sovateltide's therapeutic profile. This includes its influence on a broader range of stroke outcomes, durability of neurological improvements, and potential benefits in diverse patient subgroups. Of particular interest would be trials assessing their use in patients eligible for endovascular interventions and in those with intracranial hemorrhage, both of whom were excluded from the pivotal phase 3 trial. Such research could further define its place in stroke management protocols and potentially expand its clinical indications.[12]

REFERENCES

1. Sacco RL, Kasner SE, Broderick JP, Caplan LR, (Buddy) Connors JJ, Culebras A, et al. An Updated Definition of Stroke for the 21st Century: A Statement for Healthcare Professionals From the American Heart Association/American Stroke Association. Stroke. 2013;44(7):2064-89.
2. Pacheco-Barrios K, Giannoni-Luza S, Navarro-Flores A, Rebello-Sanchez I, Parente J, Balbuena A, et al. Burden of Stroke and Population-Attributable Fractions of Risk Factors in Latin America and the Caribbean. J Am Heart Assoc. 2022;11(21):e027044.
3. GBD 2019 Stroke Collaborators. Global, regional, and national burden of stroke and its risk factors, 1990-2019: a systematic analysis for the Global Burden of Disease Study 2019. Lancet Neurol. 2021;20(10):795-820.
4. Feigin VL, Owolabi MO, Feigin VL, Abd-Allah F, Akinyemi RO, Bhattacharjee NV, et al. Pragmatic solutions to reduce the global burden of stroke: a World Stroke Organization–Lancet Neurology Commission. Lancet Neurol. 2023;22(12):1160-206.
5. Ranjan AK, Gulati A. Sovateltide Mediated Endothelin B Receptors Agonism and Curbing Neurological Disorders. Int J Mol Sci. 2022;23(6):3146.
6. Keam SJ. Sovateltide: First Approval. Drugs. 2023;83(13):1239-44.
7. Gulati A. Abstract TP17: Discovery and development of sovateltide, an endothelin-B receptor agonist to treat cerebral stroke patients. Stroke. 2025;56(Suppl_1).
8. Gulati A, Agrawal N, Vibha D, Misra UK, Paul B, Jain D, et al. Safety and Efficacy of Sovateltide (IRL-1620) in a Multicenter Randomized Controlled Clinical Trial in Patients with Acute Cerebral Ischemic Stroke. CNS Drugs. 2021;35(1):85-104.
9. Gulati A, Adwani SG, Vijaya P, Agrawal NR, Ramakrishnan TCR, Rai HP, et al. Efficacy and Safety of Sovateltide in Patients with Acute Cerebral Ischaemic Stroke: A Randomised, Double-Blind, Placebo-Controlled, Multicentre, Phase III Clinical Trial. Drugs. 2024;84(12):1637-50.
10. Kaundal RK, Deshpande TA, Gulati A, Sharma SS. Targeting endothelin receptors for pharmacotherapy of ischemic stroke: current scenario and future perspectives. Drug Discov Today. 2012;17(13):793-804.

11. Fukuroda T, Fujikawa T, Ozaki S, Ishikawa K, Yano M, et al. Clearance of circulating endothelin-1 by ETB receptors in rats. Biochem Biophys Res Commun. 1994;199(3):1461-5.
12. Fung S, Syed YY. Sovateltide in cerebral ischaemic stroke: a profile of its use. Drugs Ther Perspect. 2024;40(9):250-55.
13. Reddy G, Tolcher A, Gulati A, Chawla S. Pharmacokinetics of SPI-1620 in a phase I, open label, ascending dose study of the safety, tolerability, pharmacokinetics and pharmacodynamics of the endothelin B receptor agonist, SPI-1620, in recurrent or progressive carcinoma. Life Sci. 2013;93(25-26):e9.
14. Pharmazz Inc. (2023). Sovateltide injection 30 μg lyophilized injection for intravenous use only: Indian product information. [Online] Available from https://cdsco.gov.in/opencms/resources/UploadCDSCOWeb/2018/UploadCTApprovals/Pharmazz%20Solvateltide%20CT-06.pdf [Last accessed January, 2026].
15. ClinicalTrials.gov. (2023). Efficacy of Sovateltide (PMZ-1620) in Patients of Acute Ischemic Stroke. [Online] Available from http://clinicaltrials.gov/study/NCT04047563 [Last accessed January, 2026].
16. Ghozy S, Reda A, Varney J, Elhawary AS, Shah J, Murry K, et al. Neuroprotection in acute ischemic stroke: a battle against the biology of nature. Front Neurol. 2022;13: 870141.

CHAPTER 15

Newer Therapeutic Options for Myasthenia Gravis

Abhishek Rajput, Keyur Shah, Shilpushp Jagannath Bhosale

INTRODUCTION

Myasthenia gravis (MG) is an autoimmune disorder of the neuromuscular junction causing weakness of limb, ocular, facial, bulbar, and respiratory muscles.[1]

The traditional treatment of MG includes cholinesterase inhibitors, immunosuppressants (corticosteroids, azathioprine, and mycophenolate mofetil) and or IV immunoglobin/plasmapheresis (PLEX).[2]

The cholinesterase inhibitors transiently improve neuromuscular transmission but do not alter the underlying autoimmune process and may even precipitate a life-threatening cholinergic crisis. Corticosteroids may lead to paradoxical worsening necessitating rescue therapy in the form of intravenous immunoglobulin (IVIg) or PLEX.[3] These measures can temporarily suppress circulating antibodies but the autoimmune condition causing pathogenic B-cell and plasma-cell memory remain persistent. These patients with refractory and uncontrolled clinical symptoms warrant targeted therapy.[4]

Our understanding of the pathophysiology of MG has helped with targeted therapy with improved outcomes. The newer targeted therapy such as complements C5 inhibitors, neonatal Fc-receptor (FcRn) blockers and B cell/plasma cell depleters have significantly revolutionized the treatment of refractory MG.[5]

PATHOPHYSIOLOGY OF MYASTHENIA GRAVIS

Over the last decade, immunological studies have revealed various mechanisms causing MG such as

- Complement-mediated membrane attack triggered by acetylcholine receptor (AChR) antibodies
- Pathologic IgG persistence via FcRn recycling.
- Autoreactive B cell and plasma cell survival niches sustaining muscle-specific kinase (MuSK) and lipoprotein receptor-related protein 4 (LRP4) autoantibodies.[6]

The pathophysiology is presence of AChR autoantibodies directed against AChR on the postsynaptic membrane of the neuromuscular junction (NMJ). Thymus dysfunction commonly causes immune intolerance in MG.[7]

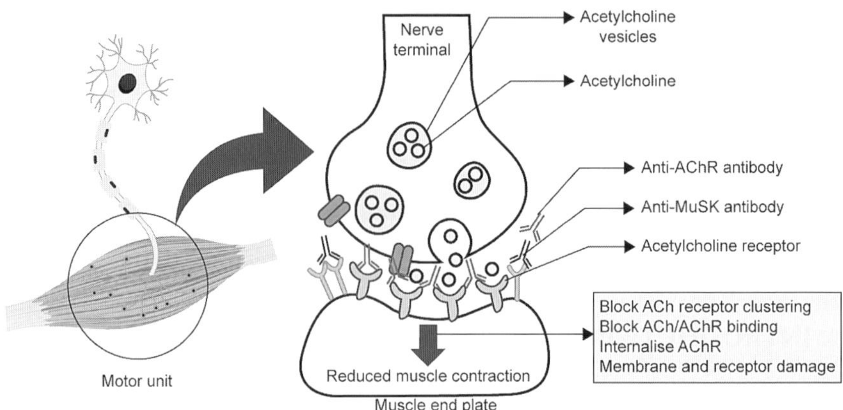

Fig. 1: Pathophysiology of myasthenia gravis.

IgG1/3 antibody against AChR binds to acetylcholine receptor, and inhibits the binding of acetylcholine to these receptors **(Fig. 1)**.[2] The antibody receptor complex activates the complement cascade to form the membrane attack complex that destroys postsynaptic membrane folds. Blocking C5 cleavage can halt this final cytolytic step.[8]

Around 10% of MG patients have autoantibodies directed against muscle specific tyrosine kinase (MuSK) and low-density lipoprotein receptor related protein 4.

The MuSK-IgG4 antibody interferes with agrin-LRP4-MuSK clustering, which is responsible for clustering of AChR, to the muscle endplate membrane and blocks AChR clustering.[6] Unlike IgG1 or IgG3 antibodies, IgG4 antibodies do not activate the complement cascade and thus complement inhibition does not help in this type of MG but respond well to rituximab.[4] MuSK-MG often requires deeper plasma cell targeting because IgG4 antibodies arise from long lived plasma cells that escape CD20 depletion.[9]

The FcRn, present on the surface of endothelial cells and some immune cells, salvages IgG from lysosomal destruction. Engineered Fc fragments or antibodies that compete endogenous IgG for FcRn binding leads to accelerated bulk IgG catabolism within 48–72 hours.[10] This leads to rapid reduction in pathogenic autoantibody titers, without plasma exchange.

FcRn inhibitors are anti-FcRn monoclonal antibodies that compete with IgG for binding to FcRn, and prevent IgG from binding to FcRn and thus IgG is transported to lysosome and degraded which leads to decrease in circulating IgG levels.[10]

TREATMENT OF MYASTHENIA GRAVIS

Traditionally treatment of MG comprises acetylcholinesterase inhibition, corticosteroids, immunosuppressants, and rapid immunomodulation using IVIg and PLEX.[11,12] Significant proportions of these patients are

Flowchart 1: Management of myasthenia gravis.

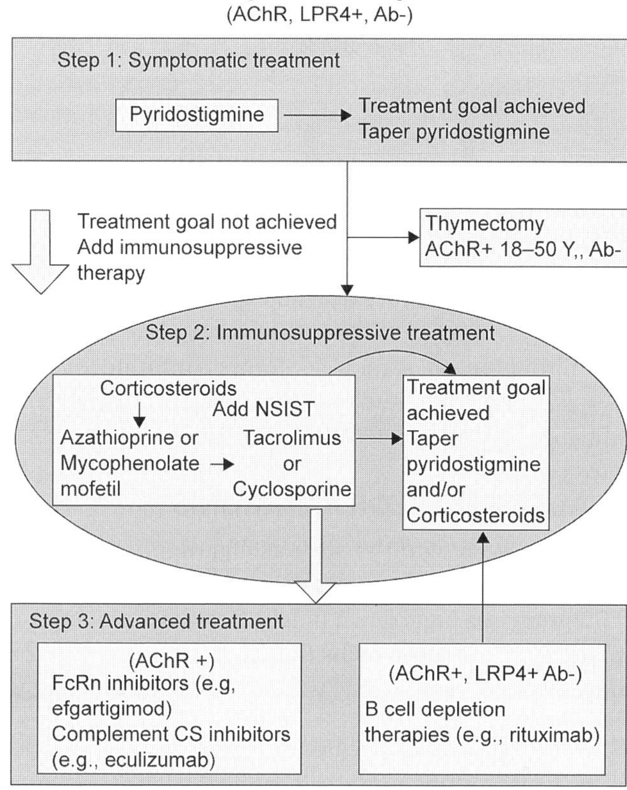

(AChR: acetylcholine receptor; gMG: generalized myasthenia gravis; LRP4: lipoprotein receptor-related protein 4)

refractory to this standard therapy and this led to the pursuit of newer targeted options.[13,14]

Various newer targeted agents such as complement C5 inhibitors, FcRn antagonists or the B-/plasma cell antagonists have significant advantage.[15] They help in rapid and prolonged autoantibody clearance with significant steroid sparing effect and dramatic improvement in quality of life.[16] This targeted therapy needs matching therapy to specific immune serotype (e.g., C5 for AChR+, B cell directed therapy for MuSK+ etc.) (**Flowchart 1**).

Complement C5 Inhibitors

Eculizumab is a recombinant monoclonal antibody that binds to C5 and prevents formation of the membrane attack complex **(Fig. 2)**. Since C5 inhibition neutralizes the final cytolytic step the upstream immune functions remain intact. In clinical studies, eculizumab have shown to improve muscle strength, functional ability, and quality of life.[17]

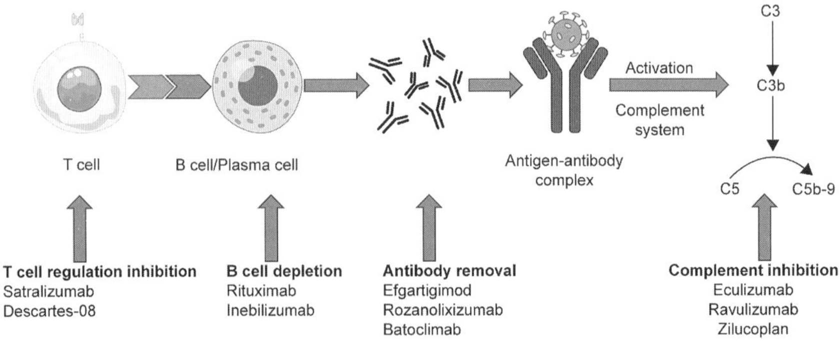

Fig. 2: Target sites of action by newer drugs.

It is recommended to screen for other immune or complement deficiencies, splenectomy, etc. and vaccinate against encapsulated organisms such as meningococcal, pneumococcal, or *Neisseria* infections.[18]

NEONATAL FC-RECEPTOR ANTAGONISTS

Neonatal Fc-receptor antagonists such as efgartigimod, rozanolixizumab binds to IgG antibodies and protect them from lysosomal degradation. Blocking FcRn promotes breakdown of IgG antibodies and is a prime target to reduce pathogenic autoantibodies in MG. It is observed that serum IgG auto antibody levels fall significantly within 3–7 days producing a PLEX like effect.[14,19,20]

T-CELL, B-CELL, AND PLASMA CELL DIRECTED THERAPIES

Since T cells promote B cell proliferation and also help them differentiate into plasma cells, inhibiting T cells can also help improve symptoms.

Chimeric antigen receptor T cells enable T cells to effectively destroy cells targeting the B cell maturation antigen found on antibody producing plasma cells.[21,22]

Rituximab targets CD20 B cells and can be used for targeted therapy in MG. There is insufficient evidence for rituximab in anti-AChR antibody-positive MG.[23,24]

The 2021 International Consensus Guidelines for the Management of Myasthenia Gravis recommend rituximab as an early treatment option for those with MuSK+MG.[3]

Most robust response with rituximab is observed in MuSK+ patients. Studies using rituximab for MuSK+ patients achieved pharmacologic or complete sustained remission ≥1 year.[25-27] Satralizumab (humanized monoclonal antibody) that binds to interleukin 6 receptor inhibiting interleukin 6 signaling and T cell activation is under evaluation.

Daratumumab is another monoclonal antibody targeting CD38 on plasma cells and reduce antibody pathogenic to MG.

Inebilizumab is a humanized anti-CD19 monoclonal antibody that targets pre-B and mature B lymphocytes expressing the CD19 surface antigen. Upon binding, it induces antibody-dependent cellular cytotoxicity, leading to B-cell depletion. In a recent Phase 3 trial inebilizumab significantly improved function and reduced disease severity in AChR+ and MuSK+ generalized MG.[28]

CONCLUSION

Newer targeted treatment for MG is rapidly evolving instead of generalized immunosuppression. Complement blockers and FcRn inhibitors can rapidly reduce harmful antibodies, making them the ideal solution during myasthenic crises or for patients who prefer subcutaneous dosing. B-cell and plasma-cell depleters offer durable control in MuSK-positive and treatment-resistant cases.

Going forward, CD19 and CD38 antibodies, CAR-T regulatory cells, and even gene-editing hold the promise of true disease modification or cure.

REFERENCES

1. Sciancalepore F, Lombardi N, Valdiserra G, Valdiserra G, Bonaso M, Cappello E, et al. Prevalence, Incidence, and Mortality of Myasthenia Gravis and Myasthenic Syndromes: A Systematic Review. Neuroepidemiology. 2025;59(5):579-92.
2. Conti-Fine BM, Milani M, Kaminski HJ. Myasthenia gravis: past, present, and future. J Clin Invest. 2006;116(11):2843-54.
3. Narayanaswami P, Sanders DB, Wolfe G, Benatar M, Cea G, Evoli A, et al. International Consensus Guidance for Management of Myasthenia Gravis: 2020 Update. Neurology. 2021;96(3):114-122.
4. Dziadkowiak E, Baczyńska D, Waliszewska-Prosół M. MuSK Myasthenia Gravis-Potential Pathomechanisms and Treatment Directed against Specific Targets. Cells. 2024;13(6):556.
5. De Bleecker JL, Remiche G, Alonso-Jiménez A, Van Parys V, Bissay V, Delstanche S, et al. Recommendations for the management of myasthenia gravis in Belgium. Acta Neurol Belg. 2024;124(4):1371-83.
6. McConville J, Farrugia ME, Beeson D, Kishore U, Metcalfe R, Newsom-Davis J, et al. Detection and characterization of MuSK antibodies in seronegative myasthenia gravis. Ann Neurol. 2004;55(4):580-4.
7. Wolfe GI, Kaminski HJ, Aban IB, Minisman G, Kuo HC, Marx A, et al. MGTX Study Group. Randomized Trial of Thymectomy in Myasthenia Gravis. N Engl J Med. 2016;375(6):511-22.
8. Martinez Salazar A, Mokhtari S, Peguero E, Jaffer M. The Role of Complement in the Pathogenesis and Treatment of Myasthenia Gravis. Cells. 2025;14(10):739.
9. DeHart-McCoyle M, Patel S, Du X. New and emerging treatments for myasthenia gravis. BMJ Med. 2023;2(1):e000241.

10. Zhu LN, Hou HM, Wang S, Zhang S, Wang GG, Guo ZY, et al. FcRn inhibitors: a novel option for the treatment of myasthenia gravis. Neural Regen Res. 2023;18(8):1637-44.
11. Miller RG, Milner-Brown HS, Mirka A. Prednisone-induced worsening of neuromuscular function in myasthenia gravis. Neurology. 1986;36(5):729-32.
12. Pascuzzi RM, Coslett HB, Johns TR. Long-term corticosteroid treatment of myasthenia gravis: report of 116 patients. Ann Neurol. 1984;15(3):291-8.
13. Silvestri NJ, Wolfe GI. Treatment-refractory myasthenia gravis. J Clin Neuromuscul Dis. 2014;15(4):167-78.
14. Howard JF Jr, Bril V, Vu T, Karam C, Peric S, De Bleecker JL, et al. ADAPT+ Study Group. Long-term safety, tolerability, and efficacy of efgartigimod (ADAPT+): interim results from a phase 3 open-label extension study in participants with generalized myasthenia gravis. Front Neurol. 2024;14:1284444.
15. Howard JF Jr, Bresch S, Genge A, Hewamadduma C, Hinton J, Hussain Y, et al. RAISE Study Team. Safety and efficacy of zilucoplan in patients with generalised myasthenia gravis (RAISE): a randomised, double-blind, placebo-controlled, phase 3 study. Lancet Neurol. 2023;22(5):395-406.
16. Vu T, Meisel A, Mantegazza R, Annane D, Katsuno M, Aguzzi R, et al. Terminal Complement Inhibitor Ravulizumab in Generalized Myasthenia Gravis. NEJM Evid. 2022 ;1(5):EVIDoa2100066.
17. Howard JF Jr, Utsugisawa K, Benatar M, Murai H, Barohn RJ, Illa I, et al. REGAIN Study Group. Safety and efficacy of eculizumab in anti-acetylcholine receptor antibody-positive refractory generalised myasthenia gravis (REGAIN): a phase 3, randomised, double-blind, placebo-controlled, multicentre study. Lancet Neurol. 2017;16(12):976-86.
18. McNamara LA, Topaz N, Wang X, Hariri S, Fox L, MacNeil JR. High Risk for Invasive Meningococcal Disease Among Patients Receiving Eculizumab (Soliris) Despite Receipt of Meningococcal Vaccine. MMWR Morb Mortal Wkly Rep. 2017;66(27):734-7.
19. Matic A, Bril V. Rozanolixizumab for Myasthenia Gravis: a breakthrough treatment and future prospects. Immunotherapy. 2025;17(5):309-16.
20. Bril V, Drużdż A, Grosskreutz J, Habib AA, Mantegazza R, Sacconi S, et al. MycarinG, MG0004 and MG0007 study investigators. Rozanolixizumab in generalized myasthenia gravis: Pooled analysis of the Phase 3 MycarinG study and two open-label extensions. J Neuromuscul Dis. 2025;12(2):218-30.
21. Sánchez-Tejerina D, Sotoca J, Llaurado A, López-Diego V, Juntas-Morales R, Salvado M. New Targeted Agents in Myasthenia Gravis and Future Therapeutic Strategies. J Clin Med. 2022;11(21):6394.
22. Wiendl H, Abicht A, Chan A, Della Marina A, Hagenacker T, Hekmat K, et al. Guideline for the management of myasthenic syndromes. Ther Adv Neurol Disord. 2023;16:17562864231213240. Erratum in: Ther Adv Neurol Disord. 2024;17:17562864241246400.
23. Valaparambil KA, Sundaram S, Nair SS. Rituximab in Refractory Myasthenia Gravis - Challenges and Lessons Learnt. Ann Indian Acad Neurol. 2024;27(6):706-9.
24. Yang X, Zhang W, Guo J, Ma C, Li B. Efficacy and safety of low-dose rituximab in the treatment of myasthenia gravis: a systemic review and meta-analysis. Front Neurol. 2024;15:1439899.

25. Piehl F, Eriksson-Dufva A, Budzianowska A, Feresiadou A, Hansson W, Hietala MA, et al. Efficacy and Safety of Rituximab for New-Onset Generalized Myasthenia Gravis: The RINOMAX Randomized Clinical Trial. JAMA Neurol. 2022;79(11):1105-12.
26. Nowak RJ, Coffey CS, Goldstein JM, Dimachkie MM, Benatar M, Kissel JT, et al. NeuroNEXT NN103 BeatMG Study Team. Phase 2 Trial of Rituximab in Acetylcholine Receptor Antibody-Positive Generalized Myasthenia Gravis: The BeatMG Study. Neurology. 2022;98(4):e376-89.
27. Hehir MK, Hobson-Webb LD, Benatar M, Barnett C, Silvestri NJ, Howard JF Jr, et al. Rituximab as treatment for anti-MuSK myasthenia gravis: Multicenter blinded prospective review. Neurology. 2017;89(10):1069-77.
28. Nowak RJ, Benatar M, Ciafaloni E, Howard JF Jr, Leite MI, Utsugisawa K, et al. MINT Investigators. A Phase 3 Trial of Inebilizumab in Generalized Myasthenia Gravis. N Engl J Med. 2025;392(23):2309-20.

CHAPTER

Monoclonal Antibodies in Bacterial Infections in the Critically Ill

Shobhit Jadhav, Sudivya Sharma

INTRODUCTION

The alarming rise in multidrug-resistant (MDR) bacterial infections has become a critical global health concern, threatening to undermine decades of progress in infectious disease management.[1] MDR pathogens such as *Clostridioides difficile, Staphylococcus aureus, Pseudomonas aeruginosa,* and carbapenem-resistant *Enterobacteriaceae* exhibit resistance to multiple antibiotic classes through diverse mechanisms, including enzymatic drug degradation, efflux pump overexpression, alteration of drug targets, and biofilm formation.[1] The limited efficacy of conventional antibiotics against these organisms has accelerated the search for alternative therapeutic modalities.

Monoclonal antibodies (mAbs) offer a promising precision-based approach, as they can be designed to specifically target bacterial virulence factors, neutralize toxins, block pathogen adhesion to host tissues, and enhance immune-mediated clearance.[1] Unlike broad-spectrum antibiotics, mAbs exert concrete actions, potentially reducing collateral damage to the normal microbiota and limiting the selective pressures that drive resistance.

A significant clinical breakthrough in this field is bezlotoxumab, a fully human immunoglobulin G1 (IgG1) mAb targeting *C. difficile* toxin B. By neutralizing the toxin's cytotoxic effects, bezlotoxumab prevents mucosal damage and inflammation, thereby reducing the likelihood of recurrent *C. difficile* infection. Clinical trials demonstrated that a single intravenous infusion of bezlotoxumab, given alongside standard-of-care antibiotics, significantly lowered recurrence rates in high-risk patients compared to placebo.[2] Its approval by the US Food and Drug Administration in 2016 marked the first regulatory endorsement of a mAb for the prevention of a bacterial infection, setting an important precedent for future developments.[2]

These advances illustrate the potential of mAbs to complement, and in some cases enhance, existing antibiotic therapies. By focusing on pathogen-specific virulence mechanisms, mAbs may play a pivotal role in the next generation of interventions against MDR bacterial infections.[1,2]

MECHANISM OF ACTION OF MONOCLONAL ANTIBODIES[3]

Antibodies (immunoglobulins) are glycoproteins produced by B lymphocytes in response to foreign antigens such as bacteria, viruses, or toxins.

Polyclonal antibodies are a heterogeneous mixture of immunoglobulins secreted by different B-cell clones, each recognizing distinct epitopes of the same antigen. Clinically, polyclonal preparations are used as antisera for rabies, hepatitis B, and snake venom exposure.

Monoclonal antibodies are highly specific immunoglobulin molecules engineered to recognize a single epitope on an antigen. Structurally, they are Y-shaped glycoproteins composed of two identical heavy chains and two identical light chains linked by disulfide bonds. Each chain consists of variable (V) and constant (C) regions. The variable regions at the amino-terminal ends of both heavy and light chains form the antigen-binding fragment (Fab), which determines specificity through complementarity-determining regions (CDRs). The constant region of the heavy chain forms the crystallizable fragment (Fc), which mediates effector functions through interactions with fragment crystallizable gamma receptors (FcγR) on immune cells and the activation of the complement system **(Fig. 1)**.

Antitoxins are antibodies (usually polyclonal) that neutralize toxins secreted by bacteria (e.g., horse-derived diphtheria antitoxin, human tetanus immunoglobulin (HTIG), equine-derived heptavalent botulinum antitoxin (HBAT), snake and scorpion antivenoms.

MONOCLONAL ANTIBODIES IN SEPSIS: TARGETING PATHOGENS AND INFLAMMATORY MEDIATORS

Sepsis represents a dysregulated host response to infection, leading to life-threatening organ dysfunction. Conventional management relies on antibiotics and supportive therapy, but the rise of MDR organisms and the

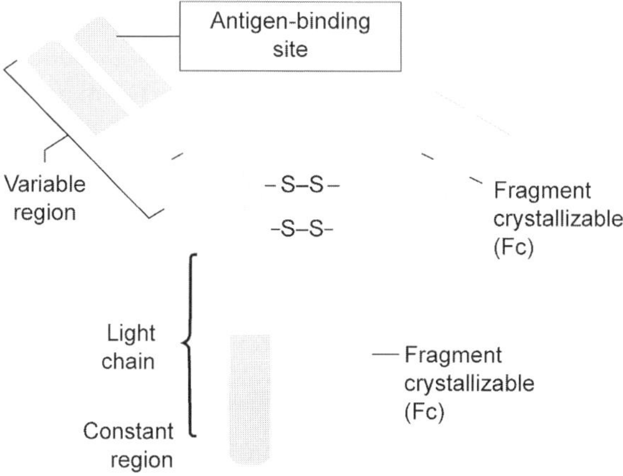

Fig. 1: Basic structure of a monoclonal antibody.

limitations of broad-spectrum antimicrobials have catalyzed interest in mAbs as targeted therapeutics. mAbs offer the potential for precision intervention through two principal strategies: (1) Directly targeting the infectious organism or its components and (2) modulating host immune responses by suppressing inflammatory mediators implicated in sepsis progression[3] role in suppressing cytokine storm.[4]

Targeting the Organism

There are several mechanisms by which mAbs can target the organism, such as neutralizing bacterial toxins, inhibiting virulence factors, blocking their adhesion, disrupting biofilms, and enhancing opsonophagocytosis. A short account is detailed underneath.

Neutralization of Bacterial Toxins and Virulence Factors

Certain mAbs are designed to bind and inactivate exotoxins or enzymes secreted by bacteria. This neutralization prevents the toxins from interacting with host cell receptors, thereby mitigating cytotoxicity and tissue damage. For example, antitoxin antibodies can block *C. difficile* toxins A and B from binding to intestinal epithelial cells, reducing disease severity.

Opsonization and Phagocytic Clearance

Through their Fc region, mAbs can facilitate opsonization, marking bacterial cells for recognition and ingestion by phagocytes, such as neutrophils and macrophages. This process enhances pathogen clearance via FcγR-mediated phagocytosis.

Complement-dependent Cytotoxicity

Monoclonal antibodies can activate the classical complement pathway upon binding to bacterial surface antigens. Complement activation leads to the formation of the membrane attack complex, resulting in bacterial cell lysis. This CDC mechanism is particularly relevant for Gram-negative bacteria with accessible outer membrane structures.

Antibody-dependent Cellular Cytotoxicity

By engaging FcγR on immune effector cells such as natural killer (NK) cells, mAbs can trigger antibody-dependent cellular cytotoxicity (ADCC). In this process, immune cells release cytotoxic granules that induce apoptosis in antibody-coated bacterial cells.

Inhibition of Bacterial Adhesion and Biofilm Formation

Some mAbs prevent the initial stages of bacterial colonization by blocking adhesins or surface molecules necessary for binding to host tissues. Others target components of the extracellular polymeric substance, thereby disrupting biofilm architecture and increasing bacterial susceptibility to antibiotics.

Immune Modulation

Beyond direct antibacterial activity, mAbs can modulate the immune system by dampening excessive inflammatory responses or enhancing antigen presentation. This immunomodulatory effect can be beneficial in severe infections where host-mediated damage contributes to morbidity.

Notable examples include:

- Raxibacumab and obiltoxaximab, both directed against the protective antigen of Bacillus anthracis, block lethal and edema factor internalization, preventing toxemia and sepsis progression.
- Bezlotoxumab, targeting *C. difficile* toxin B, reduces recurrent infection risk and prevents systemic dissemination in animal models.
- 514G3 (anti-*S. aureus* protein A) enhances opsonic killing and improves survival in MRSA sepsis models.
- Bispecific antibodies such as MEDI3902 against *P. aeruginosa* combine antivirulence and antiadhesion activities, with preclinical data showing synergism with antibiotics.
- These agents exemplify how pathogen-directed mAbs can reduce bacterial load and toxin-mediated injury, complementing antimicrobial therapy and potentially lowering mortality.[4]

Targeting Inflammatory Mediators

In parallel with antimicrobial activity, mAbs can attenuate the exaggerated immune activation driving organ injury in sepsis. This approach is grounded in the understanding that sepsis pathogenesis involves both hyperinflammation (cytokine storm) and later immunosuppression (immunoparalysis). Modulating these pathways with mAbs offers a means to restore immune balance.

Mechanisms and Key Molecules

- *ADAM17 inhibition:* MEDI3622 blocks the disintegrin and metalloproteinase ADAM17, improving neutrophil recruitment and bacterial clearance in polymicrobial sepsis models.
- *Immune checkpoint blockade:* Nivolumab, an anti-PD-1 antibody, reverses T-cell exhaustion and improves immune competence in septic patients with immunosuppression.
- *Vascular stabilization:* Adrecizumab, a non-neutralizing antiadrenomedullin antibody, reduces vascular leakage, and improves endothelial function in septic shock.

- *Complement inhibition:* Vilobelimab (anti-C5a) selectively neutralizes proinflammatory complement activity without impairing the membrane attack complex, mitigating inflammation-driven tissue damage.

Monoclonal Antibodies for Cytokine Storm Suppression in Sepsis

Cytokine storm—a hallmark of severe sepsis—is characterized by uncontrolled release of proinflammatory cytokines, such as tumor necrosis factor-alpha (TNF-α), interleukin-1 beta (IL-1β), interleukin-6 (IL-6), and interferon-gamma (IFN-γ). Several mAbs in development or early clinical use target this hyperinflammatory state:

- Anti–IL-6 receptor mAbs (e.g., tocilizumab) have been repurposed from rheumatology and COVID-19 to sepsis research, aiming to blunt IL-6-driven systemic inflammation.
- Anti–IL-1β mAbs (e.g., canakinumab) target upstream inflammatory cascades.
- TNF-α inhibitors (e.g., afelimomab) have shown mixed results historically, with benefits likely dependent on patient stratification and timing.
- Anti-C5a mAbs, as above, dampen complement-mediated cytokine release.

Current evidence suggests that optimal benefits from cytokine-targeted mAbs may depend on precision medicine strategies, with biomarker-guided selection of patients in specific immune phases of sepsis.[4,5]

ROLE OF MONOCLONAL ANTIBODIES IN VIRAL AND FUNGAL INFECTIONS

In viral infections, mAbs play a pivotal role by neutralizing viral particles, blocking cell entry, and modulating immune responses. Palivizumab, a humanized mAb against the respiratory syncytial virus (RSV) fusion protein, is a clinically approved prophylactic agent in high-risk infants.[6] Similarly, broadly neutralizing antibodies (bNAbs) targeting the human immunodeficiency virus type 1 (HIV-1) envelope glycoprotein have shown promise in both prevention and treatment settings. mAbs have also been deployed successfully against the Ebola virus, severe acute respiratory syndrome coronavirus 2 (SARS-CoV-2), and rabies, offering targeted and immediate immunity, especially in the absence of effective vaccines or during outbreaks.[7]

Fungal infections, particularly invasive mycoses caused by *Candida*, *Aspergillus*, and *Cryptococcus* species, represent a growing therapeutic challenge, especially in immunocompromised patients. mAbs targeting fungal cell wall components, such as β-glucans and mannoproteins, can disrupt fungal growth and enhance immune recognition. The mAb 18B7 against *Cryptococcus neoformans* capsular polysaccharide has shown protective effects in experimental models, while other antibodies targeting heat shock proteins and surface adhesins are under development. These strategies hold promise for adjunctive therapy alongside antifungal drugs, potentially reducing mortality in high-risk populations.[8]

Monoclonal Antibodies for Immunodetection of Amp-C[9]

The emergence of β-lactamase-mediated resistance represents one of the most critical threats in the management of gram-negative bacterial infections. Among β-lactamases, AmpC enzymes (class C β-lactamases) are widespread and confer resistance to most penicillins, broad-spectrum cephalosporins, and β-lactam/β-lactamase inhibitor combinations. Conventional phenotypic and molecular diagnostic methods often face limitations in sensitivity, specificity, and coverage of the diverse AmpC variants, which currently number over 4,000 allelic forms.

Recent research has developed broadly reactive MAbs targeting a highly conserved 17-amino acid sequence within the AmpC β-lactamase family. These MAbs demonstrated strong cross-reactivity with multiple clinically significant AmpC variants, including DHA, cephamycin-hydrolyzing (CMY), *Pseudomonas*-derived cephalosporinase (PDC), AmpC cephalosporinase type (ACT), and *Acinetobacter*-derived cephalosporinase (ADC) families, and were able to detect natural β-lactamase enzymes in clinical isolates through enzyme-linked immunosorbent assay (ELISA), Western blotting, and immunoprecipitation. Epitope mapping revealed that the majority of these antibodies recognize an 11-amino acid sequence conserved across diverse AmpC enzymes, offering a promising platform for rapid immunodetection of β-lactamase-mediated resistance in both clinical and epidemiological contexts. Their high affinity and specificity suggest potential integration into immunosensor-based diagnostic systems, thereby enabling earlier resistance detection and improved antimicrobial stewardship strategies.

Monoclonal Antibodies Against Multidrug-resistant *Pseudomonas aeruginosa*

Monoclonal antibodies against *P. aeruginosa* have focused on two major virulence targets: the exopolysaccharide Psl, which promotes biofilm formation and shields bacteria from phagocytosis, and the type III secretion system tip protein *Pseudomonas* control regulator V (PcrV), which is required for translocation of cytotoxins. A posthoc analysis of a phase IIa study of panobacumab, an immunoglobulin M (IgM) anti-LPS O11 antibody, suggested higher clinical resolution and faster time to resolution when full dosing was received in nosocomial *P. aeruginosa* pneumonia.[10] Antibody strategies against PcrV moved from a strong biological rationale to human testing: An anti-PcrV PEGylated Fab (KB001) was safe in colonized, mechanically ventilated patients and showed a numerically lower incidence of *P. aeruginosa* pneumonia versus placebo in a phase 2a trial.[11] The bispecific MEDI3902 (anti-Psl/anti-PcrV) displayed potent activity across rabbit bloodstream infection and pneumonia models,[12] but in the randomized EVADE study among colonized, mechanically ventilated adults, Gremubamab (MEDI3902) did not reduce nosocomial *P. aeruginosa* pneumonia incidence overall.[13]

In cystic fibrosis, the PEGylated anti-PcrV Fab successor KB001-A demonstrated acceptable safety and tolerability but only modest effects on clinical endpoints.[14] Together, these data support continued development of mAbs that combine anti-virulence mechanisms and broad epitope coverage while emphasizing patient selection and pharmacokinetic/pharmacodynamic alignment in trials.

Monoclonal Antibodies against *Acinetobacter baumannii*

Although *Acinetobacter baumannii* remains one of the most challenging MDR pathogens, no MAb has yet advanced to completed human clinical trials. Preclinical studies have focused on developing antibodies targeting capsular polysaccharides and other surface antigens to enhance immune-mediated clearance. Nielsen et al. developed MAb 65, a humanized IgG1 that complemented the earlier MAb C8, expanding strain coverage to 39% of clinical isolates and demonstrating potent protection in murine bacteremia and pneumonia models, particularly when combined with colistin.[15] Huang et al. generated MAbs 8E6 and 1B5, which exhibited complement-mediated bactericidal activity and in vivo protection against pan-drug-resistant strains.[16] Yang et al. reported Pse-MAB1, a mAb with direct bactericidal activity against A. baumannii, independent of complement, representing a novel therapeutic mechanism.[17] More recently, Zhu et al. identified mAb1416, a human-derived antibody targeting the KL49 capsular type, which provided complete prophylactic protection in a neonatal sepsis mouse model and is a promising candidate for future human evaluation.[18]

POLYCLONAL IMMUNOGLOBULINS IN SEPSIS (INTRAVENOUS IMMUNOGLOBULIN)

Polyclonal Immunoglobulins are derived from pooled immunoglobulins of healthy individuals, and their composition closely corresponds to that of plasma. IVIG has been used with variable success in sepsis due to mechanisms like targeting bacterial superantigens/toxins (e.g., *Staphylococcus* and *Streptococcus*), downregulation of proinflammatory cytokines (TNF-α, IL-1, IL-6), upregulation of anti-inflammatory mediators (IL-10, soluble TNF receptor), FcγR modulation (↑ inhibitory FcγRIIB, ↓ activating FcγRs), and Complement inhibition (blocking C3a, C5a deposition).[19]

While mAbs, which are always based on the IgG class, IVIG preparations contain IgG, IgM, traces of IgA, cytokines, and soluble receptors (although >90% protein components are still IgG).

Polyvalent immunoglobulin has limited role, limited only to patients with primary immunodeficiency. However, in conditions such as immunodeficiency in chronic lymphocytic leukemia (CLL), allogeneic hematopoietic stem cell transplantation (AHSCT), and solid organ transplant, they may be considered only on a case-by-case basis under a clinical trial.[20,21]

ADVERSE EFFECTS OF MONOCLONAL ANTIBODY ADMINISTRATION[22]

Monoclonal antibody administration, while offering high target specificity, is not without risk, and adverse events can arise from both immune-mediated and nonimmune-mediated mechanisms. Immune-mediated reactions include type I hypersensitivity responses, such as urticaria, angioedema, and anaphylaxis, often related to preexisting or therapy-induced antidrug antibodies; type II cytotoxic reactions; type III immune complex-mediated syndromes, including serum sickness and vasculitis; and type IV delayed-type T-cell-mediated reactions, such as Stevens–Johnson syndrome and toxic epidermal necrolysis. Infusion-related reactions are among the most frequently observed adverse events, occurring in up to 77% of patients receiving rituximab and around 40% with trastuzumab during the first infusion, and can manifest as fever, chills, hypotension, dyspnea, or more severe cytokine release syndrome (CRS). CRS, characterized by rapid-onset systemic inflammation and multiorgan dysfunction, is most often associated with T-cell-engaging antibodies or immune checkpoint inhibitors but can occur with other mAbs. Nonimmune-mediated adverse effects may result from target-related toxicity [e.g., on-target/off-tumor effects such as cardiotoxicity with human epidermal growth factor receptor 2 (HER2)-targeted agents], complement activation, or alterations in immune homeostasis. Preventive strategies, including premedication with corticosteroids, antihistamines, and acetaminophen, as well as slower infusion rates for initial doses, have been shown to mitigate the incidence and severity of these reactions **(Table 1)**.

FOOD AND DRUG ADMINISTRATION-APPROVED AND OTHER MONOCLONAL ANTIBODIES CURRENTLY UNDER HUMAN TRIALS

The following are some of the ongoing human trials involving the use of mAb in bacterial sepsis:[4]

- *TRL1068—anti-biofilm mAb (Phase I):* A first-in-human, Phase I clinical trial is assessing TRL1068, a native human mAb designed to disrupt bacterial biofilms—a mechanism that contributes to persistent infections

TABLE 1: FDA-approved or investigational mAbs.

Antibody name	*Target pathogen*	*Target antigen/ mechanism*	*Indication/use*	*Key reference*
Palivizumab	Respiratory syncytial virus (RSV)	F protein (fusion protein)	Prevention of serious RSV infection in high-risk infants	The IMPACT-RSV Study Group, 1998[6]
Ibalizumab	HIV-1	CD4 receptor (postattachment inhibitor)	Treatment of multidrug-resistant HIV-1	Emu et al., 2018[23]
Ansuvimab	Ebola virus (Zaire ebolavirus)	Viral glycoprotein	Treatment of Ebola virus disease	Corti et al., 2016[24]
Atoltivimab/ maftivimab/ odesivimab	Ebola virus (Zaire ebolavirus)	Multiple epitopes on the viral glycoprotein	Treatment of Ebola virus disease	Mulangu et al., 2019[25]
Casirivimab/ imdevimab	SARS-CoV-2 (COVID-19)	Spike protein receptor-binding domain	Treatment and post-exposure prophylaxis for COVID-19	Weinreich et al., 2021[26]
Sotrovimab	SARS-CoV-2 (COVID-19)	Conserved spike protein epitope	Treatment of mild-to-moderate COVID-19 in high-risk patients	Gupta et al., 2021[27]
MHAA4549A, CR6261, CR 8020, MEDI8852, TCN032	Influenza A	Membrane fusion inhibitors (targeting HA stem) + Fc-mediated immune functions TCN032-viral budding inhibitor + Fc-mediated immune functions	Treatment of severe influenza A infection (investigational, human trials)	Bonomini et al., 2025[28]
Raxibacumab	*Bacillus anthracis*	Protective antigen	Anthrax infection	Panteleo et al., 2022[7]
Obiltoxaximab	*Bacillus anthracis*	Protective antigen	Prevention of inhalational anthrax	Panteleo et al., 2022[7]
Bezlotoxumab	*Clostridioides difficile*	Enterotoxin B	Prevention of *C. difficile* infection recurrence	Panteleo et al., 2022[7]

(COVID-19: coronavirus disease 2019; FDA: Food and Drug Administration; HIV-1: human immunodeficiency virus type 1; IMPACT-RSV: IMpact-RSV (Respiratory Syncytial Virus) study; mAbs: monoclonal antibodies; SARS-COV-2: severe acute respiratory syndrome coronavirus 2) and sepsis. Early results have shown promising safety and potential biofilm disruption effects.

- *Vilobelimab (IFX-1)—anti-C5a mAb (Phase II):* A Phase II, multicenter, randomized, placebo-controlled trial conducted in Germany evaluated vilobelimab, a recombinant mAb targeting complement component C5a, in patients with severe sepsis or septic shock. The primary outcomes included pharmacodynamics, pharmacokinetics, and safety.

A recent 2025 review highlights that several antibacterial mAbs targeting *P. aeruginosa* (e.g., panobacumab, rivabazumab, and gremubamab) and *S. aureus* (e.g., tosatoxumab, suvratoxumab) have been evaluated in clinical trials. While many showed favorable safety profiles, clinical efficacy—especially in pneumonia or systemic infection settings—has often been inconclusive.[29]

FUTURE DIRECTIONS

The therapeutic landscape of mAbs is entering a transformative phase marked by advanced molecular engineering, novel delivery strategies, and expanded clinical applications. From their origins as laboratory curiosities to their current status as precision therapeutics, mAbs have demonstrated remarkable efficacy across oncology, infectious diseases, and autoimmune disorders. However, the next wave of innovation is poised to address persisting challenges such as precision delivery, manufacturing complexity, high costs, and limited access in resource-constrained settings.

Emerging platforms such as antibody-drug conjugates (ADCs) exemplify the progress toward enhancing target specificity while minimizing systemic toxicity, driven by breakthroughs in linker chemistry, payload optimization, and regulatory standardization.[30] In parallel, in vivo production of mAbs using synthetic nucleic acids offers a paradigm shift, potentially enabling scalable, rapid, and cost-effective deployment of antibody therapies in both therapeutic and outbreak scenarios.[31] Together, these developments represent not merely incremental advances but a redefinition of how mAbs can be designed, delivered, and deployed globally. As these technologies mature, they hold the promise of reshaping the accessibility, effectiveness, and scope of antibody-based interventions in the coming decade.

CONCLUSION

Advances in understanding immune evasion highlight the importance of aligning antibody target epitopes with mechanisms of action and optimizing delivery to the infection site. mAbs hold promise for the treatment of bacterial infections; however, current evidence remains limited and continues to evolve.

REFERENCES

1. Mallari P, Rostami LD, Alanko I, Howaili F, Ran M, Bansal KK, et al. The Next Frontier: Unveiling Novel Approaches for Combating Multidrug-Resistant Bacteria. Pharm Res. 2025;42(6):859-89.

2. Markham A. Bezlotoxumab: First Global Approval. Drugs. 2016;76(18):1793-8.
3. Lu RM, Hwang YC, Liu IJ, Lee CC, Tsai HZ, Li HJ, et al. Development of therapeutic antibodies for the treatment of diseases. J Biomed Sci. 2020;27(1):1.
4. Kharga K, Kumar L, Patel SKS. Recent advances in monoclonal antibody-based approaches in the management of bacterial sepsis. Biomedicines. 2023;11(3):765.
5. van der Poll T, Shankar-Hari M, Wiersinga WJ. The immunology of sepsis. Immunity. 2021;54(11):2450-64.
6. The IMpact-RSV Study Group. Palivizumab, a humanized respiratory syncytial virus monoclonal antibody, reduces hospitalization from respiratory syncytial virus infection in high-risk infants. The IMpact-RSV Study Group. Pediatrics. 1998;102(3 Pt 1):531-7.
7. Pantaleo G, Correia B, Fenwick C, Joo VS, Perez L. Antibodies to combat viral infections: development strategies and progress. Nat Rev Drug Discov. 2022;21(9):676-96.
8. Boniche C, Rossi SA, Kischkel B, Barbalho FV, Moura ÁND, Nosanchuk JD, et al. Immunotherapy against systemic fungal infections based on monoclonal antibodies. J Fungi (Basel). 2020;6(1):31. doi: 10.3390/jof6010031.
9. Bielskė K, Petraitytė-Burneikienė R, Avižinienė A, Dapkūnas J, Plikusienė I, Juciutė S, et al. Broadly reactive monoclonal antibodies against beta-lactamases for immunodetection of bacterial resistance to antibiotics. Sci Rep. 2025;15(1):19094.
10. Que YA, Lazar H, Wolff M, François B, Laterre PF, Mercier E, et al. Assessment of panobacumab as adjunctive immunotherapy for the treatment of nosocomial Pseudomonas aeruginosa pneumonia. Eur J Clin Microbiol Infect Dis. 2014;33(10):1861-7.
11. François B, Luyt CE, Dugard A, Wolff M, Diehl JL, Jaber S, et al. Safety and pharmacokinetics of an anti-PcrV PEGylated monoclonal antibody fragment in mechanically ventilated patients colonized with Pseudomonas aeruginosa: a randomized, double-blind, placebo-controlled trial. Crit Care Med. 2012;40(8):2320-6.
12. Le HN, Tran VG, Vu TTT, Gras E, Le VTM, Pinheiro MG, et al. Treatment efficacy of MEDI3902 in Pseudomonas aeruginosa bloodstream infection and acute pneumonia rabbit models. Antimicrob Agents Chemother. 2019;63(8):e00710-19.
13. Chastre J, François B, Bourgeois M, Komnos A, Ferrer R, Rahav G, et al. Safety, efficacy, and pharmacokinetics of gremubamab (MEDI3902), an anti-Pseudomonas aeruginosa bispecific human monoclonal antibody, in P. aeruginosa-colonised, mechanically ventilated intensive care unit patients: a randomised controlled trial. Crit Care. 2022;26(1):355.
14. Jain R, Beckett VV, Konstan MW, Accurso FJ, Burns JL, Mayer-Hamblett N, et al; KB001-A Study Group. KB001-A, a novel anti-inflammatory, found to be safe and well-tolerated in cystic fibrosis patients infected with Pseudomonas aeruginosa. J Cyst Fibros. 2018;17(4):484-91.
15. Nielsen TB, Yan J, Slarve M, Lu P, Li R, Ruiz J, et al. Monoclonal antibody therapy against Acinetobacter baumannii. Infect Immun. 2021;89(10):e00162-21.
16. Huang D, Zeng Z, Li Z, Li M, Zhai L, Lin Y, et al. Sequential Immune Acquisition of Monoclonal Antibodies Enhances Phagocytosis of Acinetobacter baumannii by Recognizing ATP Synthase. Vaccines (Basel). 2024;12(10):1120.

17. Yang X, Wei R, Liu H, Wei T, Zeng P, Cheung YC, et al. Discovery of a Monoclonal Antibody That Targets Cell-Surface Pseudaminic Acid of Acinetobacter baumannii with Direct Bactericidal Effect. ACS Cent Sci. 2024;10(2):439-46.
18. Baker S, Krishna A, Higham S, Naydenova P, O'Leary S, Scott JB, et al. Exploiting human immune repertoire transgenic mice for protective monoclonal antibodies against antimicrobial resistant Acinetobacter baumannii. Nat Commun. 2024;15(1):7979.
19. Gelfand EW. Intravenous immune globulin in autoimmune and inflammatory diseases. N Engl J Med. 2012;367(21):2015-25.
20. Pedraza-Sánchez S, Cruz-González A, Palmeros-Rojas O, Gálvez-Romero JL, Bellanti JA, Torres M. Polyvalent human immunoglobulin for infectious diseases: Potential to circumvent antimicrobial resistance. Front Immunol. 2023;13:987231.
21. Orange JS, Hossny EM, Weiler CR, Ballow M, Berger M, Bonilla FA, et al. Use of intravenous immunoglobulin in human disease: a review of evidence by members of the Primary Immunodeficiency Committee of the American Academy of Allergy, Asthma and Immunology. J Allergy Clin Immunol. 2006;117(4 Suppl):S525-53.
22. Baldo BA. Adverse events to monoclonal antibodies used for cancer therapy: Focus on hypersensitivity responses. Oncoimmunology. 2013;2(10):e26333.
23. Emu B, Fessel J, Schrader S, Kumar P, Richmond G, Win S, et al. Phase 3 study of ibalizumab for multidrug-resistant HIV-1. N Engl J Med. 2018;379(7):645-54.
24. Corti D, Misasi J, Mulangu S, Stanley DA, Kanekiyo M, Wollen S, et al. Protective monotherapy against lethal Ebola virus infection by a potently neutralizing antibody. Science. 2016;351(6279):1339-42.
25. Mulangu S, Dodd LE, Davey RT Jr, Tshiani Mbaya O, Proschan M, Mukadi D, et al. A randomized, controlled trial of Ebola virus disease therapeutics. N Engl J Med. 2019;381(24):2293-303.
26. Weinreich DM, Sivapalasingam S, Norton T, Ali S, Gao H, Bhore R, et al. REGN-COV2, a neutralizing antibody cocktail, in outpatients with Covid-19. N Engl J Med. 2021;384(3):238-51.
27. Gupta A, Gonzalez-Rojas Y, Juarez E, Crespo Casal M, Moya J, Falci DR, et al. Early treatment for Covid-19 with SARS-CoV-2 neutralizing antibody sotrovimab. N Engl J Med. 2021;385(21):1941-50.
28. Bonomini A, Mercorelli B, Loregian A. Antiviral strategies against influenza virus: an update on approved and innovative therapeutic approaches. Cell Mol. Life Sci. 82, 75 (2025).
29. Piscaglia M, Scaglione G, Genovese C, Borgonovo F, Brivio F, Rampichini F, et al. Exploring Human Use of Monoclonal Antibodies Against Critical Bacteria: A Scoping Review of Clinical Trials. Infect Dis Ther. 2025;14(8):1619-47.
30. Wang R, Hu B, Pan Z, Mo C, Zhao X, Liu G, et al. Antibody-Drug Conjugates (ADCs): current and future biopharmaceuticals. J Hematol Oncol. 2025;18(1):51.
31. Chung C, Kudchodkar SB, Chung CN, Park YK, Xu Z, Pardi N, et al. Expanding the Reach of Monoclonal Antibodies: A Review of Synthetic Nucleic Acid Delivery in Immunotherapy. Antibodies (Basel). 2023;12(3):46.

CHAPTER 17

Is Bayesian Analysis in Critical Care Trials the Way Forward for Future Research?

Anirban Som, Dalim Kumar Baidya

INTRODUCTION

Decision-making under uncertainty is the cornerstone of practicing medicine, a challenge that reaches its apex in the dynamic environment of critical care. For much of modern medicine, the frequentist school of statistical thought has been the bedrock of the research framework used to generate evidence. For more than a century, this approach, with its foundation in long-run frequencies and hypothesis testing, has been the standard for clinical trials.

However, the landscape is changing. Over the last few decades, an exponential growth in computational power has cleared the path for the reemergence of an older, yet arguably more intuitive, statistical philosophy: The Bayesian approach. While its foundational theorems were described by the Reverend Thomas Bayes in the 18th century, Bayesian inference was largely sidelined for nearly two centuries, primarily due to the intractable calculations it demanded. During this period, the frequentist paradigm rose to prominence, championed by influential statisticians like RA Fisher, because it offered tools that aligned with the scientific desire for objectivity.

It was not until the development of powerful computational algorithms like Markov Chain Monte Carlo (MCMC) in the late 20th century that the full potential of Bayesian analysis became accessible. This computational revolution has ignited a resurgence of Bayesian methods across numerous disciplines, including medicine. This revival is particularly relevant to critical care, a field that has seen a series of large, expensive, and ultimately inconclusive randomized controlled trials (RCTs). These ambiguous results often stem from the immense difficulty of studying diverse patients and complex clinical syndromes under the rigid structure of traditional trial designs.

This inherent limitation of conventional methods has fueled the development of more pragmatic approaches that leverage Bayesian methods.[1] These methods are uniquely capable of adapting to accumulating data, incorporating prior knowledge, and providing direct, probabilistic answers to the questions clinicians care about most. This shift is increasingly viewed not as a statistical novelty, but as a necessary evolution in clinical research. This chapter will demystify the core tenets of Bayesian thinking, explore the ongoing debates surrounding its use, and examine its application in critical care research.

PRINCIPLES OF BAYESIAN STATISTICS

At their heart, the frequentist and Bayesian paradigms are separated by a philosophical chasm, rooted in two fundamentally different interpretations of what probability means. The frequentist approach defines probability as the long-run frequency of an event if an experiment were repeated an infinite number of times.[2] In this framework, the true effect of a new drug or intervention is considered a single, fixed, but unknown constant. The goal is to estimate this fixed value.

The Bayesian paradigm, in contrast, interprets probability as a measure of the strength of a belief, or the confidence in a hypothesis.[3] Within this framework, an unknown parameter—such as a treatment effect—is not a fixed constant but a random variable that can be described by a probability distribution. This philosophical divide leads to a practical one: the questions they answer are different. The frequentist method calculates the probability of observing the collected data (or more extreme data) *assuming a specific hypothesis is true*, which gives rise to the familiar *p*-value. Bayesian inference, however, directly addresses the question that clinicians and patients intuitively ask: "Given the evidence we have just observed, what is the probability that this treatment is effective?"[4]

A Simple Analogy: Is the Coin Fair?

To make sense of these abstract concepts, let us consider a simple investigation: determining if a coin is fair. A *frequentist* researcher would state a "null hypothesis" that the coin is perfectly fair (i.e., the probability of heads is exactly 0.5). To test this, they might flip the coin 100 times. If they get 58 heads, they will calculate a *p*-value, which answers the convoluted question: "If we *assume* the coin is perfectly fair, what is the probability of getting a result at least as extreme as 58 heads?" The conclusion is a statement about the data, conditional on the hypothesis. It cannot assign a probability to the hypothesis itself.

A *Bayesian* researcher approaches this by updating beliefs. They start with a *prior* belief about the coin's fairness, expressed as a probability distribution. This could reflect a strong belief that the coin is fair, or it could reflect more uncertainty. Next, they conduct the experiment—flipping the coin 100 times and observing 58 heads (the *data* or *likelihood*). Finally, they use Bayes' theorem to combine the prior belief with the new data, producing a *posterior* belief—an updated probability distribution. The conclusion is a direct, probabilistic statement about the parameter: "Given the 58 heads, there is now a 90% probability that the coin's true bias toward heads lies between

0.48 and 0.67." The Bayesian conclusion is a direct statement about the likely value of the parameter, which is often what we intuitively want to know.

Probability as a Degree of Belief

The clinical mindset is, in many ways, inherently Bayesian. A physician evaluating a patient begins with a set of differential diagnoses based on the initial presentation—this is, in essence, a *prior probability*. They then gather new evidence from the patient's history, physical examination, and diagnostic tests (the *data*). This new information is used to update their initial beliefs, leading to a revised and more certain working diagnosis—a *posterior probability*. This intuitive process of updating belief in light of new evidence is precisely what Bayesian statistics formalizes.[5] For instance, a 70-year-old smoker with chest pain has a high prior probability of acute coronary syndrome. A normal ECG and negative troponin test would significantly lower this probability, leading the clinician to update their belief. The appeal of Bayesian analysis is that it mirrors this logical process and provides a direct answer to the fundamental question: "Based on this new trial data, what is the probability that this treatment is beneficial for my patient?"[1]

The Core Components: Prior, Likelihood, and Posterior Distributions

Bayes' theorem provides the mathematical engine for this process of updating beliefs, expressed further as a proportionality.

Posterior Probability $\propto$ *Likelihood* $\times$ *Prior Probability*[3]

Each component plays a critical role:

- *The prior:* A probability distribution representing all existing knowledge or belief about a parameter *before* the current study's data are considered. Priors can be *informative* (based on substantial pre-existing evidence), *noninformative* or "vague" (designed to let the data speak for itself) or designed to be *skeptical* or *enthusiastic* for sensitivity analyses.[3]
- *The likelihood:* A function containing all the information from the new data collected in the current study. It quantifies how probable the observed data are for different values of the model parameters. A key feature is that only the data that were actually observed matter.[6]
- *The posterior:* The updated probability distribution for the parameter of interest. It represents a revised state of knowledge that combines the prior beliefs with the evidence from the data. All inferences are drawn from this posterior distribution.
- *Credible intervals:* The results of a Bayesian analysis are typically summarized with credible intervals. A 95% credible interval represents a range within which there is a 95% probability that the true value of

the parameter lies, given the data and the model.[1] This interpretation is direct and clinically useful. It contrasts sharply with the frequentist 95% confidence interval, which has a much more convoluted interpretation: If one were to repeat the experiment an infinite number of times, 95% of the calculated confidence intervals would contain the true, fixed parameter value. For clinical decision-making, the direct probabilistic meaning of the credible interval is often considered more practical.

CRITIQUES AND DEBATES

Despite its intuitive appeal and growing power, the widespread adoption of Bayesian methods faces several cultural, technical, and philosophical barriers.

Barriers to Widespread Adoption

The most significant obstacle is educational; many clinicians, journal reviewers, and researchers are simply not as familiar with the Bayesian framework as they are with traditional frequentist methods, creating a substantial cultural hurdle.

Furthermore, while modern computing has made these analyses possible, the methods themselves can be complex. Techniques like MCMC require specialized expertise to implement correctly and to perform diagnostic checks that ensure the algorithms have converged to produce a reliable approximation of the true posterior distribution.[7] In the regulatory sphere, the application of Bayesian statistics is still evolving. Although agencies like the US Food and Drug Administration (FDA) have issued guidance for medical device trials,[8] there remains a degree of caution. Regulators often prefer analyses that are perceived as simpler, and they have valid concerns about controlling long-run error rates (like the Type I error), which must be addressed through careful simulation in a Bayesian context.

The Challenge of Prior Specification

The most persistent and philosophically charged criticism of Bayesian statistics revolves around the subjective nature of choosing a prior distribution. Critics argue that because different researchers could choose different priors, they could analyze the same dataset and arrive at different conclusions, undermining scientific objectivity.

Proponents of the Bayesian approach counter that this "subjectivity" is actually a form of structured transparency. The Bayesian framework forces researchers to explicitly state their assumptions and prior beliefs, laying them open for scrutiny, debate, and testing.[3] The standard method for addressing this concern is to conduct a *sensitivity analysis*, where the primary analysis is repeated with a range of different priors (e.g., neutral, skeptical, and enthusiastic) to demonstrate how much the conclusions depend on the initial assumptions. If the conclusions remain stable across a variety of reasonable priors, the findings are considered robust.

However, this leads to another debate surrounding the "many-priors" paradigm, where re-analyses of trials present a large array of posterior probabilities derived from different priors. Critics contend that this can hinder scientific consensus, as opposing parties can each select a prior that supports their preexisting beliefs, especially when the data itself is not strong enough to overwhelm the prior.[9] A proposed solution is to shift from a "many-priors" approach to an "adversarial" or "skeptical" approach. Here, the analysis is focused on a more pragmatic question: is the new evidence strong enough to convince a prespecified "reasonable skeptic?" If the data can shift the belief of a well-defined skeptic toward embracing a treatment effect, a much more robust claim for consensus can be made.[10]

CHALLENGES TO RESEARCH IN CRITICAL CARE

The intensive care unit (ICU) presents one of the most challenging environments for conducting high-quality clinical research. The confluence of patient complexity, clinical acuity, and underlying biological diversity helps explain why so many large-scale trials in this field have failed to produce definitive results.[11]

Inherent Patient Heterogeneity

Critical illnesses such as sepsis and acute respiratory distress syndrome (ARDS) are not single diseases but complex clinical syndromes with a wide array of underlying causes and pathophysiological mechanisms.[12] A 25-year-old patient with ARDS from a viral pneumonia is biologically worlds apart from a 70-year-old with ARDS secondary to severe pancreatitis, yet they are often enrolled together in the same trial. Lumping these heterogeneous patient profiles together in a traditional RCT can significantly dilute treatment effects. An intervention that is highly effective in one biological subgroup may be completely ineffective or even harmful in another. When these opposing effects are averaged across the entire trial population, the result is often a neutral or "negative" finding.[13] This heterogeneity of treatment effect (HTE) is widely recognized as one of the primary reasons for the failure to find conclusive answers in many critical care trials.

High Background Mortality and Competing Risks

The high mortality rate inherent to critical illness creates a difficult statistical problem known as *competing risks*. Death is a competing event that prevents the observation of other important, nonfatal outcomes, such as the number of ventilator-free days or long-term cognitive function.[14] For example, consider a new sedative that reduces delirium but has no effect on mortality. The benefit of this sedative on cognitive outcomes will only be observable in the patients who survive. Standard statistical analyses can be severely biased if they do not properly account for the fact that a substantial portion of the patient population was removed from the opportunity to experience the outcome. Analyzing these functional outcomes, which are "truncated by death," requires specialized statistical methods to avoid generating biased conclusions that could misrepresent a treatment's true effect on survivors.[15]

The Limitations of Traditional Approaches

The combined methodological hurdles of the ICU render traditional, fixed-design frequentist RCTs inefficient and often ineffective. Given the significant heterogeneity among patients, the sample sizes required to detect what are likely to be modest treatment effects can become exceptionally large. At the same time, ethical constraints and logistical challenges make enrolling large numbers of critically ill patients a slow and expensive endeavor. As a consequence, critical care trials are often underpowered from the start, designed with undue optimism about the potential size of the treatment effect.[11] This lack of power, combined with the diluting effect of patient heterogeneity, creates a perfect storm for producing inconclusive results. The history of sepsis research, for example, is littered with expensive trials of agents targeting single inflammatory pathways that failed to show any benefit when studied in a broad, undifferentiated population.[16] This repeating cycle of inefficiency and failure has provided a powerful motivation within the critical care research community to embrace more adaptive and sophisticated methodological approaches.[17]

A SHOWCASE OF CURRENT APPLICATIONS

Reflecting these challenges, the adoption of Bayesian methods in critical care research was limited until about 15 years ago. Since then, the number of publications using this paradigm has grown steadily, signaling a widespread recognition of its pragmatic and intuitive advantages **(Fig. 1)**.

Reanalysis of "Negative" Trials

One of the most impactful applications of Bayesian statistics has been in the re-analysis of data from frequentist trials that produced a "nonsignificant" result ($p > 0.05$). Such a result is often misinterpreted as "evidence of no effect," when in reality, it simply means the evidence was not strong enough to reject the null hypothesis. A prominent example is the Bayesian reanalysis of the *ANDROMEDA-SHOCK* trial, which compared a resuscitation strategy guided by peripheral perfusion to one guided by serum lactate levels.[18] The original frequentist analysis found an 8.5% absolute reduction in 28-day mortality

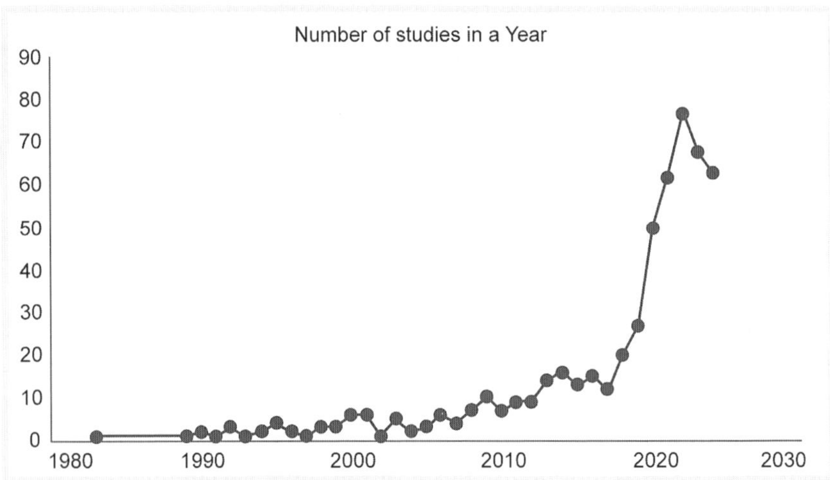

Fig. 1: The number of critical care studies with reference to Bayesian methods published each year. The PubMed search query used was ("bayes theorem" [MeSH Terms] OR ("bayes" [All Fields] AND "theorem" [All Fields]) OR "bayes theorem" [All Fields] OR ("bayesian" [All Fields] AND "analysis" [All Fields]) OR "bayesian analysis" [All Fields]) AND ("intensive care units" [MeSH Terms] OR ("intensive" [All Fields] AND "care" [All Fields] AND "units" [All Fields]) OR "intensive care units" [All Fields] OR "icu" [All Fields]).

with the peripheral perfusion strategy—a difference many clinicians would consider highly meaningful—but the result was not statistically significant ($p = 0.06$). A subsequent Bayesian reanalysis, however, demonstrated a consistently high probability (often >95%) that the perfusion-guided strategy was superior across a wide range of plausible priors.[19] This reanalysis did not change the data, but it profoundly changed the interpretation, shifting the conclusion from ambiguity to a direct, probabilistic statement about the likelihood of benefit.

Adaptive Platform Trials

Perhaps the most transformative application of Bayesian methods has been in the design and execution of *adaptive platform trials (APTs)*. An APT is an innovative research model designed to simultaneously evaluate multiple interventions against a common control within a single, perpetual trial infrastructure. Critically, this approach allows researchers to use accumulating data to adapt the trial's conduct in real time—for instance, by dropping ineffective treatments, graduating superior ones, or modifying randomization probabilities to favor more promising interventions.[17] The Bayesian framework is the natural statistical engine for these adaptations.

The premier example is the *REMAP-CAP* (Randomized Embedded Multifactorial Adaptive Platform for Community-acquired Pneumonia) trial, which was designed to study community-acquired pneumonia and became a world-leading platform for evaluating coronavirus disease 2019 (COVID-19) therapies during the pandemic.[20] By using a Bayesian adaptive design, REMAP-CAP was able to rapidly identify the survival benefit of interleukin-6 (IL-6) receptor antagonists and demonstrate the harm of other interventions in a fraction of the time and with far fewer patients than traditional, separate RCTs would have required.[21] Building on this success, a new generation of APTs is emerging to tackle long-standing questions in critical care, such as *INCEPT (Intensive Care Platform Trial),*[22] *PANTHER (Precision medicine Adaptive Network platform Trial in Hypoxaemic acutE Respiratory failure),*[23] and *TRAITS,*[24] which are designed to evaluate common interventions, test targeted therapies in specific biological subphenotypes, and randomize patients based on measurable "treatable traits," respectively.

Hierarchical Models for Phenotyping and Personalization

The ultimate goal of clinical research is to find the right treatment for the right patient. *Bayesian hierarchical models* are exceptionally well-suited for quantifying HTE by allowing subgroups to "borrow strength" from each other, leading to more robust estimates, especially for smaller subgroups. For instance, a proposed Bayesian multivariate hierarchical model helps to estimate treatment effects more accurately by borrowing information across different outcomes and patient characteristics, ultimately optimizing individualized treatment decision rules.[25]

Evidence Synthesis

Finally, the Bayesian approach offers a uniquely flexible framework for conducting meta-analyses. Bayesian hierarchical models can perform not only standard random-effects meta-analyses but also complex *network meta-analyses (NMAs).* An NMA uses a Bayesian model to combine both direct and indirect evidence to estimate the relative effectiveness of all treatments in a network. This allows for the ranking of all available treatments, creating a comprehensive evidence hierarchy that can guide clinical practice.[26] For example, NMA can help determine which vasopressor is associated with the best outcomes in septic shock when many agents have only been compared to a common standard but not to each other.[27]

A VISION FOR THE FUTURE OF CRITICAL CARE RESEARCH

The landscape of critical care research is in the midst of a profound transformation, driven by the challenges of the ICU and the development of more pragmatic statistical tools. Bayesian analysis is emerging as a framework that can enable more intuitive, efficient, and clinically relevant research.

A Pragmatic Hybrid Statistical Approach

The path forward is not about the wholesale replacement of one statistical paradigm with another, but rather about the thoughtful and complementary use of both Bayesian and frequentist methods, selecting the best tool for the research question at hand.[28] While a large, simple superiority trial in a well-defined population might be perfectly served by a traditional frequentist design, a trial in a rare disease or one requiring adaptation is a natural fit for a Bayesian approach. This pragmatic view avoids statistical dogma and focuses on using the best tool for the job.

From Broad Syndromes to Treatable Traits

By making it easier to identify and quantify HTE, Bayesian tools are helping researchers uncover distinct, biologically based patient phenotypes hidden within broad clinical syndromes. The ultimate implication of this work is that the very definitions of critical illnesses are likely to evolve. Vague, descriptive syndromes like "sepsis" or "ARDS" may gradually give way to a new taxonomy based on specific, actionable, and "*treatable traits.*"[24] In this future, a patient would no longer be treated for "sepsis," but rather for their specific profile of underlying dysfunctions, such as "endothelial barrier dysfunction and profound immunosuppression," with therapies targeted to those specific mechanisms.

Digital Twins: Simulating the Individual Patient

Perhaps the most speculative but revolutionary future role for Bayesian analysis lies in creating *digital twins*—dynamic, virtual models of an individual patient, continuously updated with real-time data. These models could use techniques like Bayesian networks to simulate a patient's likely physiological response to an intervention *before* it is administered. This would allow clinicians to test different treatment strategies—such as alternative ventilator settings or vasopressor choices—in a risk-free virtual environment to select the optimal, personalized therapy for the real patient at the bedside.[29] This represents a monumental leap beyond simple risk prediction toward true causal simulation and personalized medicine.

A Call for Improved Standards

For this vision to be realized, the research community must embrace a renewed commitment to transparency and education. The responsible and effective use of Bayesian methods requires clear and rigorous communication. Adherence to reporting standards, such as the *Bayesian Analysis Reporting Guidelines,*[30] is essential to ensure that analyses are conducted and presented with clarity and reproducibility. This must be coupled with targeted educational initiatives, including workshops, integration into curricula, and clearer explanations in high-impact publications—to build broad competence and confidence in this powerful paradigm among clinicians, researchers, and regulatory bodies alike.

CONCLUSION

The unique environment of the ICU, with its inherent patient heterogeneity and clinical urgency, has frequently exposed the limitations of traditional research methodologies. The Bayesian paradigm is not merely a statistical tool but a philosophical shift, offering a framework that naturally accommodates uncertainty and aligns with the iterative nature of clinical reasoning. By empowering researchers to design more efficient adaptive trials, synthesize evidence more robustly, and pursue a future of personalized medicine, Bayesian analysis represents the most promising path toward resolving long-standing clinical questions and truly advancing critical care.

REFERENCES

1. Yarnell CJ, Abrams D, Baldwin MR, Brodie D, Fan E, Ferguson ND, et al. Clinical trials in critical care: can a Bayesian approach enhance clinical and scientific decision making? Lancet Respir Med. 2021;9(2):207-16.
2. Greenland S, Senn SJ, Rothman KJ, Carlin JB, Poole C, Goodman SN, et al. Statistical tests, P values, confidence intervals, and power: a guide to misinterpretations. Eur J Epidemiol. 2016;31(4):337-50.
3. In: Spiegelhalter DJ, Abrams KR, Myles JP (Eds). Bayesian Approaches to Clinical Trials and Health-Care Evaluation. New Jersey: John Wiley & Sons; 2004.
4. Goodman SN. Toward evidence-based medical statistics. 1: The P value fallacy. Annals of Internal Medicine. 1999;130(12):995-1004.
5. Eddy DM. Probabilistic reasoning in clinical medicine: problems and opportunities. In: Kahneman D, Slovic P, Tversky A (Eds). Judgment under Uncertainty: Heuristics and Biases. Cambridge: Cambridge University Press; 1982. pp. 249-67.
6. Berry DA. Interim analysis in clinical trials: the role of the likelihood principle. Am Statistic. 1987;41(2):117-22.
7. In: Brooks S, Gelman A, Jones GL, Meng XL (Eds). Handbook of Markov Chain Monte Carlo. New Delhi: CRC Press; 2011.
8. U.S. Food and Drug Administration. Guidance for the Use of Bayesian Statistics in Medical Device Clinical Trials. U.S. Food and Drug Administration; 2010.
9. de Grooth HJ, Cremer CL. Bayes and the Evidence Base: Reanalyzing Trials Using Many Priors Does Not Contribute to Consensus. Am J Respir Crit Care Med. 2023;209(5):483-4.
10. Zampieri FG, Casey JD, Shankar-Hari M, Harrell FE Jr, Harhay MO. Using Bayesian Methods to Augment the Interpretation of Critical Care Trials. An Overview of Theory and Example Reanalysis of the Alveolar Recruitment for Acute Respiratory Distress Syndrome Trial. Am J Respir Crit Care Med. 2021;203(5):543-51.

11. Harhay MO, Wagner J, Ratcliffe SJ, Bronheim RS, Gopal A, Green S, et al. Outcomes and statistical power in adult critical care randomized trials. Am J Respir Crit Care Med. 2014;189(12):1469-78.
12. Seymour CW, Liu VX, Iwashyna TJ, Brunkhorst FM, Rea TD, Scherag A, et al. Assessment of Clinical Criteria for Sepsis: For the Third International Consensus Definitions for Sepsis and Septic Shock (Sepsis-3). JAMA. 2016;315(8):762-74.
13. Iwashyna TJ, Burke JF, Sussman JB, Prescott HC, Hayward RA, Angus DC. Implications of Heterogeneity of Treatment Effect for Reporting and Analysis of Randomized Trials in Critical Care. Am J Respir Crit Care Med. 2015;192(9):1045-51.
14. Zhang Z. Survival analysis in the presence of competing risks. Ann Transl Med. 2017;5(3):47.
15. Colantuoni E, Scharfstein DO, Wang C, Hashem MD, Leroux A, Needham DM, et al. Statistical methods to compare functional outcomes in randomized controlled trials with high mortality. BMJ. 2018;360:j5748.
16. Opal SM, Fisher CJ, Dhainaut JFA, Vincent JL, Brase R, Lowry SF, et al. Confirmatory interleukin-1 receptor antagonist trial in severe sepsis: a phase III, randomized, double-blind, placebo-controlled, multicenter trial. The Interleukin-1 Receptor Antagonist Sepsis Investigator Group. Critical Care Medicine. 1997;25(7):1115-24.
17. Angus DC, Huang AJ, Lewis RJ, Abernethy AP, Califf RM, Landray M, et al. The Integration of Clinical Trials With the Practice of Medicine: Repairing a House Divided. JAMA. 2024;332(2):153-62.
18. Hernández G, Ospina-Tascón GA, Damiani LP, Estenssoro E, Dubin A, Hurtado J, et al. Effect of a resuscitation strategy targeting peripheral perfusion status vs serum lactate levels on 28-day mortality among patients with septic shock: The ANDROMEDA-SHOCK randomized clinical trial. JAMA. 2019;321(7):654-64.
19. Zampieri FG, Damiani LP, Bakker J, Ospina-Tascón GA, Castro R, Cavalcanti AB, et al. Effects of a Resuscitation Strategy Targeting Peripheral Perfusion Status versus Serum Lactate Levels among Patients with Septic Shock. A Bayesian Reanalysis of the ANDROMEDA-SHOCK Trial. Am J Respir Crit Care Med. 2020;201(4):423-9.
20. Angus DC, Derde L, Al-Beidh F, Al-Beidh F, Arabi Y, van Bentum-Puijk W, others. The REMAP-CAP (Randomized Embedded Multifactorial Adaptive Platform for Community-acquired Pneumonia) Study. Rationale and Design. Ann Am Thorac Soc. 2020;17(7):879-91.
21. REMAP-CAP Investigators. Interleukin-6 Receptor Antagonists in Critically Ill Patients with Covid-19. New England Journal of Medicine. 2021;384(16):1491-502.
22. Granholm A, Møller MH, Kaas-Hansen BS, Jensen AKG, Munch MW, Kjær MN, et al. INCEPT : The Intensive Care Platform Trial-Design and protocol. Acta Anaesthesiol Scand. 2025;69(4):e70023.
23. Bos L, McAuley DF. PANTHER – Precision medicine Adaptive Network platform Trial in Hypoxemic acute respiratory failure. [Online] Available from https://www.ersnet.org/science-and-research/clinical-research-collaboration-application-programme/panther-precision-medicine-adaptive-network-platform-trial-in-hypoxemic-acute-respiratory-failure/ [Last accessed January, 2026].

24. Shankar-Hari M. (2023). TRAITS – Enabling Precision Medicine for Intensive Care. [Online] Available https://traits-trial.ed.ac.uk/ [Last accessed January, 2026].
25. Wu D, Goldfeld KS, Petkova E, Park HG. A Bayesian multivariate hierarchical model for developing a treatment benefit index using mixed types of outcomes. BMC Med Res Methodol. 2024;24(1):218.
26. Salanti G, Del Giovane C, Chaimani A, Caldwell DM, Higgins JPT. Evaluating the Quality of Evidence from a Network Meta-Analysis. Tu YK, ed. PLoS ONE. 2014;9(7):e99682.
27. Nagendran M, Maruthappu M, Gordon AC, Gurusamy KS. Comparative safety and efficacy of vasopressors for mortality in septic shock: A network meta-analysis. J Intensive Care Soc. 2016;17(2):136-45.
28. Senn S. You may believe you are a Bayesian but you are probably wrong. Rationality, Markets and Morals. 2011;2:48-66.
29. Katsoulakis E, Wang Q, Wu H, et al. Digital twins for health: a scoping review. NPJ Digit Med. 2024;7(1):77.
30. Kruschke JK. Bayesian Analysis Reporting Guidelines. Nat Hum Behav. 2021;5(10):1282-91.

CHAPTER 18

TREML4 and Immunotherapy of Sepsis

Anjali Mishra, Deven Juneja

INTRODUCTION

Sepsis is defined by the Surviving Sepsis Campaign (SSC) as a life-threatening organ dysfunction caused by a dysregulated host response to infection.[1] According to the Global Burden of Disease Study 2017, sepsis accounted for approximately 48.9 million cases and 11.0 million deaths worldwide in 2017, representing about 20% of all global fatalities.[2] The incidence of sepsis and septic shock varies significantly across continents, with a notably higher burden observed in low- and middle-income countries (LMICs). In India, studies indicate that overall sepsis-related mortality ranges from 25 to 30%, while deaths due to septic shock may reach as high as 50%.[3]

Historically, sepsis-induced organ dysfunction and mortality have been attributed to the complex interactions between the initial pro-inflammatory and the subsequent anti-inflammatory responses. The majority of the adverse outcomes of sepsis are a result of host's dysregulated immune response to systemic infection. During the early phase, systemic inflammatory response syndrome (SIRS) is predominant, causing overwhelming cytokine release, activation of coagulation and complement pathways, and necrotic cell death, resulting in multiple organ failure (MOF). As a compensatory mechanism, the host mounts an anti-inflammatory response, known as the compensatory anti-inflammatory response syndrome (CARS), which is marked by immune cell apoptosis, expansion of regulatory T cells (Tregs) and myeloid-derived suppressor cells (MDSCs), and suppression of pro-inflammatory gene transcription. This phase renders the host vulnerable to secondary infections and delayed recovery. In some patients, immune homeostasis is reestablished, resulting in clinical resolution. However, others progress to a state of persistent immune dysfunction **(Table 1)**. The severity of the immune phase is influenced by both pathogen-derived factors, e.g., virulence, and pathogen-associated molecular patterns (PAMPs) and host-specific factors such as genetic predisposition, age, comorbidities, and medication history as depicted in **Table 2**.[4,5]

SEPSIS-ASSOCIATED IMMUNOSUPPRESSION

The two major categories of the immune system, the innate and the adaptive immune cells, get activated by pathogen invasion and relocate locally to the

TABLE 1: Immune response phases and outcomes in sepsis.

Phase	*Time course*	*Key immune features*	*Clinical outcomes*
Initial hyperinflammation	Hours to days	• Excessive immune activation • Cytokine storm • Coagulation and complement activation • Necrotic cell death • Pattern recognition receptor overexpression	• Systemic inflammatory response syndrome (SIRS) • Multiple organ failure (MOF) • Early death
Compensatory anti-inflammatory response (CARS)	Days to weeks	• Immune suppression • T-cell and myeloid cell dysfunction • Anti-inflammatory cytokine release • Impaired pro-inflammatory gene expression • Expansion of Treg cells and MDSCs	• Increased infection susceptibility • Delayed recovery • Entry into immunosuppressive phase
Recovery or persistent dysregulation	Weeks to months	• Immune rebalancing (in recovery) • Or chronic immunosuppression and inflammation	• Rapid recovery in mild/moderate cases • Recurrent infections • Ongoing organ dysfunction
Persistent inflammation, immunosuppression, and catabolism syndrome (PICS)	≥14 days in ICU and beyond	• Ongoing inflammation • Metabolic dysfunction (protein catabolism, cachexia) • Organ failure • Immunosenescence	• Late deaths • Opportunistic infections • Long-term morbidity and mortality

TABLE 2: Factors contributing to severity of sepsis.

Pathogen-derived	*Host-derived*
• Microbial load • Virulence • Pathogen-associated molecular patterns (PAMPs)	• Genetic background • Age • Comorbidities • Medications • Environmental factors

target site to prevent pathogen multiplication. Innate immune cells serve as the primary defense mechanism by detecting invading pathogens or PAMPs. Simultaneously, the complement pathway is activated, contributing to the pro-inflammatory process through the generation of complements C3a and C5a. This inflammatory environment can induce the release of damage-associated molecular patterns (DAMPs), such as high mobility group box 1 (HMGB1), which are released from necrotic and apoptotic cells. These DAMPs further enhance the activation of innate immune cells, leading to further production of key pro-inflammatory cytokines such as interleukin-1 beta (IL-1β) and tumor necrosis factor-alpha (TNF-α) that activate coagulation and complement system.[6,7]

IMMUNE PARALYSIS

In sepsis, both inflammation and immunosuppression can occur simultaneously or sequentially. During early phases of SIRS, immune balance may be restored early if the immune system successfully eliminates the invading pathogens. However, inadequate or delayed elimination of pathogens may lead to dysregulated immune responses, predisposing patients to secondary infections and prolonged immunosuppression. This dysregulated state can progress to immune exhaustion, metabolic dysfunction, and muscle wasting—collectively termed as Persistent Inflammation, Immunosuppression, and Catabolism Syndrome (PICS). PICS is characterized by ongoing low-grade inflammation, muscle wasting, organ dysfunction, and immune senescence, contributing to late mortality and poor long-term outcomes.[4] PICS may be multifactorial and is also observed in critically ill patients following noninfective insults such as acute pancreatitis, major trauma, or cardiopulmonary bypass.[8] If this immunosuppression continues, there is high mortality due to immune dysfunction causing secondary infections and chronic catabolism.[9] Clinical evidence suggests that during the advanced stages of sepsis, approximately 9–18% of patients suffer with secondary infections caused by opportunistic pathogens, 13–30% develop fungal infections, and latent viral reactivation occurs in about 43% of cases.[10]

The Tregs and helper T (Th) lymphocytes secrete anti-inflammatory cytokines that suppress the immune response. This release of anti-inflammatory mediators can inhibit the Th1 immune response, thereby suppressing the pro-inflammatory activity and decreasing the production of pro-inflammatory cytokines. This causes a marked reduction in the levels of TNF-α, IL-1β, IL-6, and other cytokines typically produced by monocytes, resulting in immune paralysis in the host.[11] Sepsis also impairs the differentiation of immature myeloid cells into mature immune cells, promoting their development into MDSCs, which suppress both innate and adaptive immunity.[12] It also disrupts energy metabolism in immune cells by inhibiting oxidative phosphorylation and glycolysis, leading to reduced ATP production. This has been attributed as a key factor in sepsis-induced immune paralysis.[13]

TOLL-LIKE RECEPTORS

Toll-like receptors (TLRs) are a group of highly conserved, noncatalytic transmembrane proteins that serve as pattern recognition receptors (PRRs) involved in the innate immune response. They also play a pivotal role in linking innate and adaptive immunity.[14] Among them, TLR-4 is a type I transmembrane protein found on various cell types, including macrophages and monocytes. Studies in animal models have demonstrated that TLR-4 detects lipopolysaccharides (LPS) from gram-negative bacteria and triggers intracellular signaling cascades through pathways such as nuclear factor kappa-light-chain-enhancer of activated beta cells (NF-κB) and Jun N-terminal kinase (JNK) or stress-activated protein kinase (SAPK).[15] It has been observed that TLR-4 may enhance the inflammatory response during the early phase of sepsis. Although monoclonal antibodies directed against TLR-4 have been developed, based on this understanding, as a therapeutic strategy to control the exaggerated inflammatory reaction and cytokine storm, none have shown significant results in sepsis.[16]

TREM FAMILY

Triggering Receptors Expressed on Myeloid cells (TREMs) and TREM-like transcript (TREML) are immunoglobulins that take part in biological processes involving inflammation, coagulation, cell differentiation, and metabolism.[17] TREMs have been gaining interest as an important subject of investigation in the context of infectious and autoimmune diseases. They interact with specific ligands present on the cell membrane surface, and the intracellular domain is coupled with DNAX-activating protein of 12 kDa (DAP12). This may result in downregulation of JAK2/STAT3 (Janus kinase 2/signal transducer and activator of transcription 3) and NF-κB, which play important roles in the body's innate immune responses.[18]

A study by Christina et al. demonstrated that *TREML4* gene knockout significantly reduced thymic atrophy and apoptosis in neutrophils, macrophages, and dendritic cells in a murine model of bacterial sepsis. *TREML4*-deficient (Treml4-/-) mice demonstrated markedly lower levels of neutrophil apoptosis than wild-type mice, both during the early inflammatory phase and the subsequent secondary infection stage. Notably, no significant differences were observed in the phenotypic profiles of mature lymphocytes between Treml4-/- and wild-type mice. In Treml4-/- mice, proinflammatory signaling pathways including NF-κB and ERK/MAPK were markedly suppressed, accompanied by significantly lower levels of inflammatory mediators compared to the wild-type.[19] These findings support the hypothesis that the protective effects of *TREML4* deficiency in sepsis are likely attributable to decreased apoptosis of innate immune cells, especially neutrophils, in Treml4-/- mice.[19]

TABLE 3: Potential effects of TREML4 in sepsis management.

Mechanism	*Effect on sepsis*	*Clinical implication*
Regulation of inflammation	Modulates cytokine response and reduces hyperinflammation	May prevent early organ damage and systemic inflammatory response
Innate immune cell death control	Limits apoptosis of neutrophils and macrophages during sepsis causing innate immune modulation	Preserves immune function during immunosuppressive phase
Calcium homeostasis	Maintains intracellular calcium balance in immune cells	Supports proper cell signaling and survival
Endoplasmic reticulum stress response modulation	Reduces endoplasmic reticulum stress in immune cells	Enhances cell resilience under septic conditions
Myeloperoxidase activation	Regulates neutrophil activity and oxidative burst	Balances microbial killing with tissue protection
Improved survival in animal models	Genetic deletion of TREML4 improves survival in polymicrobial sepsis murine models	Suggests therapeutic potential for targeting TREML4

(TREML4: triggering receptors expressed on myeloid cells like 4)

Furthermore, in a secondary infection model using multidrug-resistant *Pseudomonas aeruginosa*, Treml4-/- mice showed notably higher neutrophil counts in the bloodstream, bronchoalveolar lavage fluids, and bone marrow relative to wild-type mice. Remarkably, nearly all Treml4-/- mice survived the infection, whereas all wild-type mice died within 6 days. In addition, profoundly lower levels of inflammatory cytokines were found in Treml4-/- mice than wildtype mice, coupled with less activation of NF-κB inflammatory signaling pathway.[20] These findings outline the potential of *TREML4* as an important regulator of inflammatory cytokine secretion and a potential therapeutic target for sepsis immunotherapy **(Table 3)**.[17-20]

IMMUNOMODULATORY DRUGS IN SEPSIS

Currently, immunomodulatory therapies including corticosteroids, growth factors, cytokine modifiers and complement or coagulation regulators have been tried and employed for sepsis management. Immunomodulatory agents like IL-7 and anti-programmed cell death protein 1 (anti-PD-1) have emerged as promising therapeutic options to combat immunesuppression phase of sepsis. Recently, immune-enhancing therapies such as interferon-gamma (IFN-γ), granulocyte-macrophage colony-stimulating factor

(GM-CSF) and mesenchymal stem cells (MSCs) are also being explored to reestablish immune competence in septic patients.[21,22] Some of these newer agents have been summarized in **Table 4**.

TABLE 4: Immunomodulatory drugs and mechanisms.

Drugs	*Mechanism*	*Clinical evidence*
Immunosuppressor		
Anti-TNFα inhibitor	Inhibit the pro-inflammatory response caused by TNFα	Single clinical trial showed no significant effect. Meta-analysis suggested a 28-day mortality reduction
IL-1R antagonist	Inhibit IL-1R and pro-inflammatory response	Could be effective in macrophage activation syndrome (MAS)
TLR-4 antagonist	Inhibit TLR-4 and inflammatory signaling pathway	Clinical trials showed no significant effect
Endotoxin antagonists	Neutralize endotoxin of gram-negative bacteria	Clinical trials showed no significant effect.
TREML4 suppression/ gene knockout models	Suppress NF-κB and ERK/ MAPK signaling, reduce neutrophil apoptosis, and lower cytokine release	Preclinical studies show improved survival in septic mice; no human trials yet
Immunopotentiator		
Anti-programmed cell death protein 1 (anti-PD-1)	Inhibit PD-1/PD-L1 signaling pathway and reduce apoptosis of immune cells	Organ damage, secondary infection rate, and mortality have been reduced
IL-7	Inhibit T-cell apoptosis and maintenance of diversity of T-cell receptors	Significantly improved lymphocyte count
Granulocyte–macrophage colony-stimulating factor (GM-CSF)	Promote the proliferation and maturation of granulocytes and monocytes	Promoting infection control in patients with sepsis, no reported effect on mortality
Mesenchymal stem cells (MSC)	Regulate the functions of immune cells; secrete growth factors; differentiate and mature into damaged tissue cells	Preliminary clinical safety has been established, but further evidence is lacking

(ERK: extracellular signal-regulated kinase; IL: interleukin; MAPK: mitogen-activated protein kinase; NF-κB: nuclear factor kappa-light-chain-enhancer of activated beta cells; PD-L1: programmed cell death-ligand 1; TNFα: tumor necrosis factor alpha; TLR-4: toll-like receptor-4; TREML4: triggering receptors expressed on myeloid cells like 4)

DRUGS TO SUPPRESS HYPERINFLAMMATION

Due to SIRS response in sepsis, traditionally the treatment has been focused on anti-inflammatory treatments. Drugs like anti-TNF-α therapy showed some benefit in reducing 28-day mortality in severe cases.[23] Anakinra, an IL-1 receptor antagonist, demonstrated limited overall efficacy, yet it holds potential as a treatment option for patients with macrophage activation syndrome (MAS).[24]

Lipopolysaccharide, a lethal endotoxin released during the lysis of gram-negative bacteria, plays a central role in the pathogenesis of gram-negative sepsis by activation of PAMPs.[25] Interestingly, antibiotic-related bacterial killing can also cause a significant release of LPS, further amplifying the inflammatory process. Based on this mechanism, neutralizing endotoxins has been studied as a potential treatment strategy. One such agent, AB103 (p2TA), a peptide antagonist designed to block the interaction between bacterial superantigens and the CD28 receptor on T cells was shown to reduce mortality in preclinical sepsis models. Despite the promising results in animal studies, there is still no definitive clinical evidence supporting its efficacy in human sepsis.[26]

IMMUNOPOTENTIATOR THERAPY

Programmed Cell Death Protein 1 Antagonists

Programmed cell death protein 1 and programmed cell death-ligand 1 (PD-L1) are type I transmembrane glycoprotein, which are expressed on immune cells and bind to the surface of antigen-presenting cells (APC). Expression of this glycoprotein is upregulated on T cells and APCs contributing to apoptosis of T cells and multiorgan injury.[27] In vitro studies in mice have shown that treatment with anti-PD-1 antibody anti-PD-L1 antibodies can restore immune cell function in patients with sepsis by reducing the apoptosis of T lymphocytes and neutrophils. Studies in animal models demonstrated that administering anti-PD-L1 antibodies enhanced survival rates in septic mice.[28] Though PD-1 and PD-L1 antagonists have given promising results in animal models, at present their clinical utility is limited to cancer treatment.

Interleukin-7

Interleukin 7 has been shown to prevent apoptosis of nonactivated T lymphocytes and help restore lymphocyte numbers during sepsis. Although its primary targets are lymphocytes, IL-7 also supports the proliferation of B-cell precursors, thymocytes, and mature peripheral T-cells.[29] Moreover, IL-7 enhances monocyte function by stimulating IFN-γ production and has been shown to lower mortality in animal models. Clinical trials have also reported that IL-7 therapy reasonably increased lymphocyte counts in patients with septic shock and severe lymphopenia, without causing excessive inflammatory response.[30]

Granulocyte–Macrophage Colony-stimulating Factor

Granulocyte-macrophage colony-stimulating factor, which has traditionally been used to manage leukopenia, is an immunomodulatory agent that acts on hematopoietic progenitor cells to stimulate their proliferation and differentiation. It promotes the maturation of granulocytes and mononuclear macrophages and facilitates their release into peripheral circulation. Findings from 12 randomized controlled trials (RCTs) suggest that GM-CSF may play a role in infection control among sepsis patients; however, these studies did not report outcomes related to patient mortality.[31,32] A Phase 3 clinical trial (NCT0261528) is currently ongoing to assess the impact of GM-CSF on secondary infections and 28-day survival rates in sepsis patients admitted to ICU.

Mesenchymal Stem Cells

Mesenchymal stem cells are pluripotent stem cell with self-renewal properties. They possess anti-inflammatory and immunomodulatory properties, making them a potential therapeutic option for sepsis. Preclinical studies have demonstrated that MSCs can significantly improve survival in animal models and offer protective effects for various organs, including the heart, liver, kidneys, and lungs. These effects are largely attributed to their ability to modulate immune responses and suppress both specific and nonspecific immunity. They also secrete several growth factors, such as fibroblast growth factor (FGF) and transforming growth factor (TGF), which help with tissue repair.[33,34]

There is emerging clinical data to seek the potential of MSCs in sepsis treatment. A phase I RCT conducted in Canada by Ahn et al. in 2017 used a dose-escalation approach to evaluate MSC therapy in nine pediatric patients with septic shock. The findings revealed that except one child (a 6-month-old who succumbed to *Enterobacter cloacae* infection), rest all recovered following a single MSC infusion.[35] In another study, Perlee et al. induced sepsis in 32 healthy volunteers via LPS injection and administered MSCs at varying doses. The study indicated that MSCs possess broad immunoregulatory potential without causing significant adverse effects.[36] Although these early findings are encouraging, further clinical research is required to validate the safety and effectiveness of MSC-based therapies for sepsis.

CHALLENGES AND LIMITATIONS

Although immunotherapy is a rapidly evolving field with foreseeable benefits, it also carries challenges due to its potential adverse effects. These therapies including, monoclonal antibodies and immunomodulators, may cause systemic toxicities affecting different organ systems, including cardiovascular, endocrine, dermatologic, gastrointestinal, neurologic, and pulmonary systems.[37] Commonly observed adverse effects like flulike symptoms, local injection-site reactions, and infusion-related and immune reactions (acute anaphylaxis and cytokine release syndrome) necessitate cautious administration and vigilant monitoring of these therapies.[38]

The heterogeneity of patients with sepsis poses a huge challenge that impedes the development of precise and effective treatments. Complex and heterogeneous nature of sepsis is another limitation, with patients showing significant differences in clinical features, disease progression, and therapeutic responses. The variability is influenced by multiple factors, including age, sex, genetic makeup, underlying health conditions, infection type, immune response, and extent of organ dysfunction. This makes it difficult to identify a protocolized regimen to achieve therapeutic targets and mandates patient-specific and stratified treatment plans.[39,40]

Furthermore, timing of intervention is critical; the immune response in sepsis transitions from a hyperinflammatory to an immunosuppressive phase, and inappropriate timing of immunomodulatory agents can worsen outcomes.[41] Another limitation is the lack of reliable biomarkers to differentiate hyperinflammation from immunosuppression, which makes the process of patient selection and response prediction difficult. There are additional safety concerns that immunomodulating therapies may increase the risk of secondary infections or autoimmune complications in already vulnerable patients. Furthermore, there are regulatory and ethical challenges in trial designs, especially in critically ill patients that further complicate clinical translation process.[4] Hence, it requires precise patient stratification, biomarker-guided approaches, and better understanding of immune trajectories in sepsis to achieve clinical success with immunomodulatory therapies.

CONCLUSION

Despite advances in critical care, effective treatment remains difficult because the immune system can be both, hyperinflamed and suppressed during different phases of the illness. Most therapies have focused on reducing inflammation, but majority have not improved survival significantly. Therefore, managing the exaggerated inflammatory response alongside correcting immune suppression may be the most optimum therapeutic strategies for immunoregulatory management in sepsis. TREML4 is a promising target in this area. It plays a role in regulating inflammation and immune cell death. Studies in animals have shown that blocking TREML4 reduces inflammation, decreases neutrophil apoptosis, and improves survival. However, further research and robust clinical trials are needed before clinical implementation. To address challenges such as heterogeneous patient profiles, optimal treatment timing, and potential side effects, and enhance sepsis outcomes, future treatments must prioritize personalized approaches that consider individual immune status.

REFERENCES

1. Singer M, Deutschman CS, Seymour CW, Shankar-Hari M, Annane D, Bauer M, et al. The Third International Consensus Definitions for Sepsis and Septic Shock (Sepsis-3). JAMA. 2016;315(8):801-10.
2. Rudd KE, Johnson SC, Agesa KM, Shackelford KA, Tsoi D, Kievlan DR, et al. Global, regional, and national sepsis incidence and mortality, 1990-2017: Analysis for the Global Burden of Disease Study. Lancet. 2020;395:200-11.
3. Todi S, Mehta Y, Zirpe K, et al. Other contributors to SEPSIS Registry. A multicentre prospective registry of one thousand sepsis patients admitted in Indian ICUs: (SEPSIS INDIA) study. Crit Care. 2024;28(1):375.
4. Hotchkiss RS, Monneret G, Payen D. Sepsis-induced immunosuppression: From cellular dysfunctions to immunotherapy. Nat Rev Immunol. 2013;13(12):862-74.
5. Delano MJ, Ward PA. Sepsis-induced immune dysfunction: can immune therapies reduce mortality? J Clin Invest. 2016;126(1):23-31.
6. Foley NM, Wang J, Redmond HP, Wang JH. Current knowledge and future directions of TLR and NOD signaling in sepsis. Mil Med Res. 2015;2:1.
7. Kang R, Chen R, Zhang Q, Hou W, Wu S, Cao L, et al. HMGB1 in health and disease. Mol Asp Med. 2014;40:1-116.
8. Pandharipande PP, Girard TD, Ely EW. Long-term cognitive impairment after critical illness. N Engl J Med. 2014;370(2):185-6.
9. Cao M, Wang G, Xie J. Immune dysregulation in sepsis: experiences, lessons and perspectives. Cell Death Discov. 2023;9:465.
10. Huang SJ, Ai T, Hu H, Wang J, Wang JL. Immunotherapy for sepsis induced by infections: clinical evidence and potential targets. Discov Med. 2022;34(172):83-95.
11. Gruda MC, Ruggeberg KG, O'Sullivan P, Guliashvili T, Scheirer AR, Golobish TD, et al. Broad adsorption of sepsis-related PAMP and DAMP molecules, mycotoxins, and cytokines from whole blood using CytoSorb® sorbent porous polymer beads. PLoS One. 2018;13(1):e0191676.
12. Darden DB, Bacher R, Brusko MA, Knight P, Hawkins RB, Cox MC, et al. Single-Cell RNA-seq of Human Myeloid-Derived Suppressor Cells in Late Sepsis Reveals Multiple Subsets With Unique Transcriptional Responses: A Pilot Study. Shock. 2021;55(5):587-95.
13. Schluter J, Peled JU, Taylor BP, Markey KA, Smith M, Taur Y, et al. The gut microbiota is associated with immune cell dynamics in humans. Nature. 2020;588(7837):303-7.
14. Huang SJ, Li ZL, Ma XL, Du B, Wang JL. TREML4: a potential target for immunotherapy of sepsis. Discov Med. 2021;32(166):87-92.
15. Ryu JK, Kim SJ, Rah SH, Kang JI, Jung HE, Lee D, et al. Reconstruction of LPS transfer cascade reveals structural determinants within LBP, CD14, and TLR4-MD2 for efficient LPS recognition and transfer. Immunity. 2017;46:38-50.

16. Kalil AC, LaRosa SP, Gogate J, Lynn M, Opal SM; Eritoran Sepsis Study Group. Influence of severity of illness on the effects of eritoran tetrasodium (E5564) and on other therapies for severe sepsis. Shock. 2011;36(4):327-31.
17. Allcock RJ, Barrow AD, Forbes S, Beck S, Trowsdale J. The human TREM gene cluster at 6p21.1 encodes both activating and inhibitory single IgV domain receptors and includes NKp44. Eur J Immunol. 2003;33(2):567-77.
18. Amatngalim GD, Nijnik A, Hiemstra PS, Hancock RE. Cathelicidin peptide LL-37 modulates TREM-1 expression and inflammatory responses to microbial compounds. Inflammation. 2011;34(5):412-25.
19. Nedeva C, Menassa J, Duan M, Liu C, Doerflinger M, Kueh AJ, et al. TREML4 receptor regulates inflammation and innate immune cell death during polymicrobial sepsis. Nat Immunol. 2020;21(12):1585-96.
20. Menassa J, Nedeva C, Pollock C, Puthalakath H. TLR4: The fall guy in sepsis? Cell Stress. 2020;4(12):270-2.
21. Ono S, Tsujimoto H, Hiraki S, Aosasa S. Mechanisms of sepsis-induced immunosuppression and immunological modification therapies for sepsis. Ann Gastroenterol Surg. 2018;2:351-8.
22. Vincent JL, Sun Q, Dubois MJ. Clinical trials of immunomodulatory therapies in severe sepsis and septic shock. Clin Infect Dis. 2002;34:1084-93.
23. Lv S, Han M, Yi R, Kwon S, Dai C, Wang R. Anti-TNF-α therapy for patients with sepsis: a systematic meta-analysis. Int J Clin Pract. 2014;68(4):520-8.
24. Karakike E, Giamarellos-Bourboulis EJ. Macrophage Activation-Like Syndrome: A Distinct Entity Leading to Early Death in Sepsis. Front Immunol. 2019;10:55.
25. Cecconi M, Evans L, Levy M, Rhodes A. Sepsis and septic shock. Lancet. 2018;392(10141):75-87.
26. Bulger EM, Maier RV, Sperry J, Joshi M, Henry S, Moore FA, et al. A Novel Drug for Treatment of Necrotizing Soft-Tissue Infections: A Randomized Clinical Trial. JAMA Surg. 2014;149(6):528-36.
27. Hotchkiss RS, Monneret G, Payen D. Immunosuppression in sepsis: A novel understanding of the disorder and a new therapeutic approach. Lancet Infect Dis. 2013;13(3):260-8.
28. Patera AC, Drewry AM, Chang K, Beiter ER, Osborne D, Hotchkiss RS. Frontline Science: Defects in immune function in patients with sepsis are associated with PD-1 or PD-L1 expression and can be restored by antibodies targeting PD-1 or PD-L1. J Leukoc Biol. 2016;100(6):1239-54.
29. Levy Y, Sereti I, Tambussi G, Routy JP, Lelièvre JD, Delfraissy JF, et al. Effects of recombinant human interleukin 7 on T-cell recovery and thymic output in HIV-infected patients receiving antiretroviral therapy: results of a phase I/IIa randomized, placebo controlled, multicenter study. Clin Infect Dis. 2012;55:291-300.
30. Francois B, Jeannet R, Daix T, Walton AH, Shotwell MS, Unsinger J, et al. Interleukin-7 restores lymphocytes in septic shock: the IRIS-7 randomized clinical trial. JCI Insight. 2018;3(5):e98960.
31. Bo L, Wang F, Zhu J, Li J, Deng X. Granulocyte-colony stimulating factor (G-CSF) and granulocyte-macrophage colony stimulating factor (GM-CSF) for sepsis: a meta-analysis. Crit Care. 2011;15:R58.
32. Mathias B, Szpila BE, Moore FA, Efron PA, Moldawer LL. A review of GMCSF therapy in sepsis. Medicine (Baltimore). 2015;94:e2044.

33. Kingsley SM, Bhat BV. Could stem cells be the future therapy for sepsis? Blood Rev. 2016;30:439-52.
34. Luo CJ, Zhang FJ, Zhang L, Geng YQ, Li QG, Hong Q, et al. Mesenchymal stem cells ameliorate sepsis-associated acute kidney injury in mice. Shock 2014;41(2):123-9.
35. Ahn SY, Chang YS, Kim JH, Sung SI, Park WS. Two-year follow-up outcomes of premature infants enrolled in the phase I trial of mesenchymal stem cells transplantation for bronchopulmonary dysplasia. J Pediatr. 2017;185:49-54.e2.
36. Perlee D, van Vught LA, Scicluna BP, Maag A, Lutter R, Kemper EM, et al. Intravenous Infusion of Human Adipose Mesenchymal Stem Cells Modifies the Host Response to Lipopolysaccharide in Humans: A Randomized, Single-Blind, Parallel Group, Placebo Controlled Trial. Stem Cells. 2018;36(11):1778-88.
37. Kichloo A, Albosta M, Dahiya D, Guidi JC, Aljadah M, Singh J, et al. Systemic adverse effects and toxicities associated with immunotherapy: a review. World J Clin Oncol. 2021;12:150-63.
38. Hansel TT, Kropshofer H, Singer T, Mitchell JA, George AJ. The safety and side effects of monoclonal antibodies. Nat Rev Drug Discov. 2010;9:325-38.
39. Kwok AJ, Mentzer A, Knight JC. Host genetics and infectious disease: new tools, insights and translational opportunities. Nat Rev Genet. 2021;22:137-53.
40. Davenport EE, Burnham KL, Radhakrishnan J, Humburg P, Hutton P, Mills TC, et al. Genomic landscape of the individual host response and outcomes in sepsis: a prospective cohort study. Lancet Respir Med. 2016;4(4):259-71.
41. Van der Poll T, van de Veerdonk FL, Scicluna BP, Netea MG. The immunopathology of sepsis and potential therapeutic targets. Nat Rev Immunol. 2017;17(7):407-20.

CHAPTER 19

Application of Omics in the Critically Ill

Sahil Kataria, Ruchi Gupta, Sumit Ray

INTRODUCTION

Critically ill patients suffer from life-threatening conditions such as acute kidney injury (AKI), acute respiratory distress syndrome (ARDS), and sepsis, for which current guidelines provide broad, one-size-fits-all management recommendations.[1,2] While standardized protocols have improved overall care, mortality in critical illness remains unacceptably high.[1,3] One major challenge is the tremendous heterogeneity among patients who share the same clinical syndrome. Even when diagnosed with the same condition, patients may follow divergent trajectories and respond differently to therapies.[4]

This recognition has spurred interest in personalized medicine (or precision medicine) in critical care, which aims to tailor therapies to the biological profile of each patient rather than treating all patients identically. Omics technologies offer a unique opportunity to dissect patient heterogeneity at a molecular level. By capturing high-dimensional biological data, omics can identify endotypes (biologically distinct subgroups) within syndromes that appear clinically similar; tailoring diagnosis, prognosis, and therapy to a patient's biological profile rather than treating all patients with the same label identically.[5,6] This chapter outlines the principal omics domains and the biological layers they interrogate, and subsequently examines key clinical questions in critical care, illustrating how these layers advance precision medicine.

BIOLOGICAL LAYERS INTERROGATED BY OMICS

Omics technologies provide complementary perspectives on the biological complexity of critical illness by interrogating distinct layers of molecular and cellular organization **(Fig. 1)**. Genomics captures inherited predispositions, transcriptomics reflects dynamic immune activation or suppression, proteomics quantifies effector molecules, metabolomics highlights bioenergetic and biochemical shifts, and microbiomics characterizes host-microbe interactions.[6] Collectively, these domains provide the foundation for precision medicine strategies in the ICU **(Table 1)**.

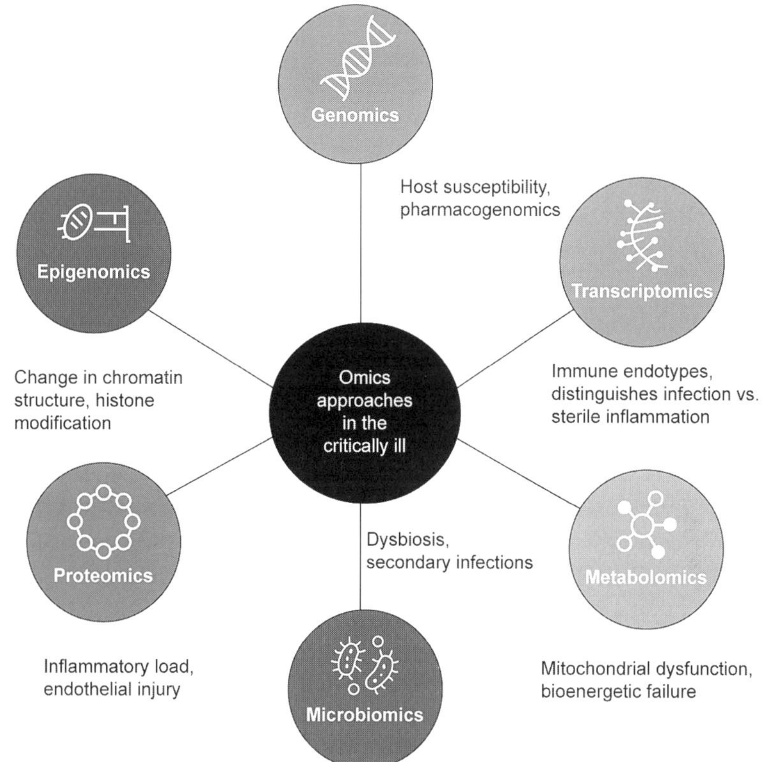

Fig. 1: Omics approaches in critical care.

TABLE 1: An overview of omics types, their biological targets, and sample requirements.

Omics type	*What it measures*	*Sample(s)*	*ICU relevance*
Genomics	DNA sequence, SNPs, structural variants	Blood, tissue	Host susceptibility, pharmacogenomics
Transcriptomics	mRNA, microRNA, non-coding RNA	Whole blood, BAL	Defines immune endotypes, infection vs. sterile inflammation
Proteomics	Protein abundance, cytokines, signaling mediators	Plasma, BAL, urine	Inflammatory load, endothelial dysfunction, prognosis
Metabolomics	Small metabolites (amino acids, lipids, organic acids)	Plasma, urine, exhaled breath	Reflects mitochondrial dysfunction, prognosis
Microbiomics	Microbial composition/diversity	Stool, BAL, oral swabs	Dysbiosis linked to secondary infection risk and outcomes

(DNA: deoxyribonucleic acid; BAL: bronchoalveolar lavage; mRNA: messenger ribonucleic acid; SNP: single nucleotide polymorphism)

CLINICAL QUESTION 1: IS THIS INFECTION? WHAT PATHOGEN IS RESPONSIBLE?

The Diagnostic Challenge

Early recognition of sepsis is life-saving: each hour of delay in antimicrobial therapy increases mortality by 7–8% in septic shock.[7] Yet, clinical signs are nonspecific, and conventional microbiology is slow: cultures take 24–72 hours and are negative in up to 40% of cases.[8] Distinguishing infectious from noninfectious systemic inflammatory response is equally difficult. Omics-based diagnostics aim to accelerate diagnosis, enhance pathogen detection, and characterize host response in parallel **(Table 2)**.

Genomics: Metagenomic next-generation sequencing (mNGS) enables culture-independent detection of microbial DNA and RNA in clinical

TABLE 2: Selected studies of omics approaches for infection diagnosis in the ICU.[6]

Omics type	*Representative studies*	*Population/ sample*	*Key findings*	*Remarks*
Genomics (mNGS)	Blood mNGS vs. culture	ICU sepsis patients, whole blood	Pathogen yield ~88% vs. 26% with culture	Higher yield even after antibiotics; contamination is a concern
	BAL mNGS in pneumonia	Ventilated patients with pneumonia	Detection 92% vs. 76% with culture	Identifies viruses and fastidious bacteria
Transcriptomics	7-gene classifier	Sepsis vs. sterile SIRS, blood RNA	AUC ~0.87 for sepsis vs. sterile	Validated across multiple cohorts
	Viral vs. bacterial classifier	Mixed acute infections, blood RNA	AUC ~0.96 for viral vs. bacterial	Prospective ED/ ICU data
	Rapid PCR cartridge-based formats	ICU pilot, whole blood	Same-day turnaround feasible	Prospective validation still needed
Dual host–pathogen	Integrated RNA + microbial sequencing	Suspected sepsis, whole blood	High sensitivity in confirmed cases; detected infection in culture-negative patients	Host signal contextualizes microbial DNA

Contd...

Contd...

Omics type	*Representative studies*	*Population/ sample*	*Key findings*	*Remarks*
Proteomics	Serum proteomic index	ICU sepsis vs. nonsepsis, serum	APOC3 and related proteins discriminated sepsis with AUC 0.772	Composite signature of lipid metabolism + inflammation
	BAL 3-protein panel (S100A8, lactotransferrin, actinin-1)	Ventilator-associated pneumonia, BAL	>90% sensitivity and specificity	Pilot-level data; BAL sampling limits feasibility
Metabolomics	10-metabolite panel	Sepsis vs. ICU controls, plasma/urine	AUC = 1.0 (internal validation)	Risk of overfitting; needs multicenter validation
Microbiomics	Gut microbiome studies	Critically ill patients, stool	Reduced diversity, pathogen overgrowth correlated with mortality and infection risk	Confounded by antibiotic exposure
	Respiratory microbiome in ARDS/VAP	Ventilated ICU patients, BAL/ oropharyngeal samples	Community shifts correlated with VAP/ ARDS phenotypes	Sampling variability and contamination are challenges

(ARDS: acute respiratory distress syndrome; BAL: bronchoalveolar lavage; mNGS: metagenomic next-generation sequencing; PCR: polymerase chain reaction; SIRS: systemic inflammatory response syndrome; VAP: ventilator-associated pneumonia)

samples, thereby overcoming many of the limitations of conventional microbiology. In a prospective study of 50 patients with sepsis, paired blood and bronchoalveolar lavage fluid (BALF) specimens were tested by both mNGS and culture across bacterial, fungal, and viral domains. The diagnostic yield of mNGS was markedly superior: pathogens were identified in 88% of blood samples compared with only 26% by culture ($p < 0.001$), and in 92% of BALF samples compared with 76% by culture ($p = 0.054$).[8] Importantly, RNA-based sequencing improved the detection of several clinically relevant bacteria, fungi, and viruses, although performance remained limited for *Mycobacterium* species and *Toxoplasma gondii.*[8] However, challenges include differentiating true pathogens from colonizers or contaminants. Integrating genomic data with host-response signatures may contextualize microbial findings and improve clinical interpretation.

Transcriptomics: Host response as diagnostic tool transcriptomic profiling targets host immune signatures rather than pathogens. During sepsis, leukocyte RNA expression changes rapidly and reproducibly. A seven-gene signature distinguished sepsis from noninfectious systemic inflammatory response syndrome (SIRS) with an area under the curve (AUC) of 0.87.[9] Other panels differentiate viral from bacterial infection with very high accuracy (AUC: 0.96).[6] These tools may reduce unnecessary antibiotics by confirming viral sepsis or support treatment when bacterial infection is present despite negative cultures. Advances in cartridge-based polymerase chain reaction (PCR) are reducing turnaround times from days to hours, enabling potential real-time ICU application. Still, clinical use requires further validation and cost-effectiveness studies.

Dual host–pathogen profiling: A novel approach integrates transcriptomics with mNGS, acknowledging that microbial DNA alone may not prove infection. By simultaneously measuring host immune response, dual profiling helps distinguish true infection from incidental microbial reads. In ICU patients with suspected lower respiratory tract infection, Langelier et al. showed that integrating host transcriptomic signatures with metagenomic sequencing achieved high sensitivity for confirmed infections and revealed pathogens in many culture-negative cases, underscoring the added value of dual host–pathogen profiling.[10] Though still early in development, this represents a paradigm shift from "organism-only" diagnostics to assays capturing both pathogen and host biology. Large-scale validation is needed to confirm reproducibility and feasibility.

Proteomics and metabolomics: Proteomic and metabolomic platforms add further depth in sepsis diagnosis. A serum panel combining ApoC3, vascular cell adhesion molecule 1 (VCAM-1), β2-microglobulin, ApoE, C-reactive protein (CRP), and procalcitonin differentiated sepsis from nonsepsis with an AUC of 0.772—superior to any single marker.[11] In ventilator-associated pneumonia, bronchoalveolar lavage (BAL) proteomics identified a three-protein panel (S100A8, lactotransferrin, and actinin-1) that correctly classified 27/30 patients in a discovery cohort, with ELISA validation.[12] Metabolomics, reflecting deranged host metabolism, also shows promise: one pilot plasma/urine metabolite panel achieved near-perfect discrimination (AUC = 1.0),[6] though likely overfitted. These tools highlight the potential of multiparametric signatures but require multicenter validation for clinical translation.

Microbiomics: Critical illness profoundly alters the host microbiome due to disease, antibiotics, altered nutrition, and devices. High-throughput sequencing reveals reduced diversity and overgrowth of pathogens such as *Enterococcus* and *Candida*. Stool studies link loss of flora with secondary infections, organ dysfunction, and mortality.[13] Respiratory tract microbiome shifts also correlate with ventilator-associated pneumonia and ARDS phenotypes. Microbiome monitoring may aid stewardship by guiding de-escalation or flagging high-risk patients. However, distinguishing causal from associative changes, standardizing sampling, and adjusting for antibiotic exposure remain challenges.

Thus, omics technologies offer complementary strategies for infection diagnosis in the critically ill—spanning rapid pathogen detection, host-response profiling, proteomics, metabolomics, and microbiome analysis. Together, they promise earlier and more precise diagnosis, potentially improving outcomes and supporting antimicrobial stewardship. Future work must focus on multicenter validation, integration into real-time clinical workflows, and demonstration of cost-effectiveness before widespread adoption.

CLINICAL QUESTION 2: WHO WILL DETERIORATE?

Why Prognosis Matters in Critical Illness?

One of the most pressing tasks in the ICU is prognostication: deciding which patients are likely to recover, which are at risk of deterioration, and which may not benefit from escalation. Current scoring systems such as SOFA and APACHE provide population-level mortality estimates but lack biological specificity. Omics-derived markers offer refinement by capturing pathways of injury, defining endotypes, and predicting complications more accurately **(Table 3)**.

Acute Respiratory Distress Syndrome: Prognostic Omics

- *Endotypes and heterogeneity*: Acute respiratory distress syndrome is well recognized as a heterogeneous syndrome. Traditional severity scores based on oxygenation or compliance often fail to capture the biological variability that influences outcomes. Latent class analyses have identified hyperinflammatory and hypoinflammatory ARDS phenotypes.[14] The hyperinflammatory endotype is characterized by markedly elevated plasma cytokines such as interleukin-6 (IL-6), IL-8, and soluble tumor necrosis factor (TNF) receptors, metabolic acidosis with low bicarbonate, and a higher requirement for vasopressors. Patients in this group demonstrate mortality rates of 45–50%. In contrast, the hypoinflammatory phenotype shows lower systemic cytokine levels, relative metabolic stability, and reduced vasopressor dependence, with mortality rates closer

TABLE 3: Prognostic omics markers in critical illness.

Syndrome	*Omics type*	*Key marker/signature*	*Prognostic implication*
ARDS	Inflammatory endotypes	Hyperinflammatory vs. hypoinflammatory	Higher mortality (~45–50% vs. 20–25%); differential response to fluids/PEEP[14,15]
	Transcriptomics (miRNAs)	miR-122 ↑, miR-887 ↑	Predicts 30-day mortality, ARDS progression[6,16]
	Proteomics	Endothelial injury, Ang-2 ↑, thrombomodulin ↑	Associated with severity and mortality; identifies patients at risk of vascular leak; potential enrichment for fluid-conservative/vasopressor strategies
	Proteomics	sRAGE ↑, SP-D ↑	Associated with alveolar epithelial damage and mortality; candidate enrichment for epithelial-protective interventions
	Proteomics	IL-10 >89 pg/mL, IGFBP7 ↑	Predicted mortality in ECMO-supported ARDS[17]
	Metabolomics	Phenylalanine ↑	Associated with mortality; worsened injury in animals[18]
Sepsis	Genomics	*FER* SNP (rs4957796)	Improved 28-day survival[19]
	Transcriptomics	SRS1 vs. SRS2 endotypes	Higher vs. lower mortality; different steroid response[20]
	Transcriptomics (miRNAs)	miR-103/107 ↓	Associated with ARDS progression and mortality[21]
	Proteomics	Endothelial vs. inflammatory clusters	Ratio predicted 28-day mortality or intubation (AUC 0.90)[22]
	Metabolomics	5-metabolite panel + vitals	Predicted 28-day mortality (AUC ~0.88)[23]
	Metabolomics (NMR)	Phosphocreatine ↑, phenylalanine ↑	Predicted death in ICU cohorts[6]
Sepsis (COVID-19)	Multiomics	Neutrophil hyperactivation, arginine depletion, tryptophan metabolites	Correlated with critical illness and T-cell dysfunction[24]

Contd…

Contd...

Syndrome	*Omics type*	*Key marker/signature*	*Prognostic implication*
AKI	Transcriptomics	43-gene panel	Predicted persistent vs. transient AKI (AUC 0.95)[25]
	Proteomics	PARK7, CDH16	Early markers of sepsis-AKI (AUC 0.90)[6]
	Proteomics (commercial)	TIMP-2/IGFBP7 (NephroCheck)	Predicts AKI progression (cell-cycle arrest)[26]
	Metabolomics	Urinary kynurenic acid (tryptophan–kynurenine pathway)	Predicted poor renal recovery and 30-day mortality[27]

(AKI: acute kidney injury; ARDS: acute respiratory distress syndrome; PEEP: positive end-expiratory pressure; ECMO: extracorporeal membrane oxygenation)

to 20–25%. Crucially, these subgroups exhibit differential responses to therapy: strategies such as high positive end-expiratory pressure (PEEP) ventilation and conservative fluid management conferred survival benefit in the hyperinflammatory but not in the hypoinflammatory endotype.[15]

- *Transcriptomics and microRNAs*: Transcriptomic studies provide additional prognostic resolution by linking gene-expression profiles and microRNAs with outcomes. For instance, elevated plasma miR-122, a liver-enriched microRNA, has been associated with 30-day mortality and concomitant acute liver dysfunction in ARDS.[16] Similarly, miR-887 has been found upregulated in septic patients who later progressed to ARDS, suggesting a role in endothelial activation and injury.[6] These markers highlight the ability of transcriptomics not only to predict outcomes but also to reveal mechanistic insights into organ cross-talk and endothelial dysfunction.
- *Proteomics and metabolomics*: In ARDS patients on extracorporeal membrane oxygenation (ECMO), elevated IL-10 early after ECMO initiation has been linked to increased mortality and organ dysfunction, although specific prognostic thresholds remain to be validated in larger cohorts.[17] Similarly, Dong et al. showed that higher plasma IGFBP7 increases 28-day mortality risk, and platelet count appears to mediate part of this effect, suggesting platelet dysfunction is in the causal pathway. Metabolomic studies have further emphasized the prognostic role of amino acid metabolism. Elevated plasma phenylalanine has been consistently associated with increased mortality (AUC ~0.80).[18] Together, these findings underscore how multiomics approaches can stratify ARDS patients and guide precision therapies.

Sepsis: Prognostic Omics

Sepsis is characterized by profound inter-individual heterogeneity, which makes prognosis particularly challenging. Omics technologies have begun to uncover predictors that have refined prognostication and identify therapeutic opportunities.

- *Genomics and transcriptomics*: A landmark genome-wide association study of pneumonia–sepsis patients identified a variant in the *FER* gene (rs4957796) that conferred improved 28-day survival, implicating endothelial and neutrophil signaling pathways in disease resilience.[19] Transcriptomic profiling has further stratified patients into distinct immune response subtypes. The Sepsis Response Signature (SRS) framework distinguishes SRS1, marked by immunosuppression, T-cell exhaustion, and downregulation of HLA-DR, from SRS2, which demonstrates preserved immune activation. SRS1 patients consistently show higher mortality and respond differently to corticosteroids, providing an example of how transcriptomic endotyping can guide therapy.[20]
- *MicroRNAs and proteomics*: Specific microRNAs have also been linked to prognosis. Lower circulating levels of miR-103 and miR-107 are associated with greater inflammatory responses, higher SOFA scores, and increased risk of ARDS development or death.[21] At the proteomic level, sepsis severity correlates strongly with endothelial and microvascular integrity. Rovas et al. identified proteomic clusters enriched in endothelial-protective proteins (Angpt-1, ADAMTS13) versus inflammatory cytokines, correlating with disease severity. In COVID-19 patients, composite biomarkers derived from these signatures predicted 28-day mortality or intubation with an AUC of 0.90.[22]
- *Metabolomics and integrative omics*: Metabolomic profiling has identified shifts in indole derivatives, fatty acids, creatine, choline, and amino acids such as phenylalanine as predictors of poor outcome. In a prospective cohort of 188 sepsis patients, a seven-metabolite panel predicted 28-day mortality with an AUROC of 0.88 [95% confidence interval (CI): 0.78–0.97].[23] Nuclear magnetic resonance (NMR)-based studies further linked elevated phosphocreatine and phenylalanine to adverse outcomes. Multiomics studies in COVID-19 have revealed that critically ill patients exhibit neutrophil hyperactivation, arginine depletion, and accumulation of immunosuppressive tryptophan metabolites correlating with T-cell dysfunction, in contrast to milder cases characterized by robust interferon responses.[24] These results underscore how omics can reveal shared prognostic pathways across diverse sepsis etiologies.

Acute Kidney Injury: Prognostic Omics

Acute kidney injury remains a common and devastating complication of critical illness. Traditional markers such as serum creatinine and urine output detect kidney injury only after significant functional decline, limiting prognostic value. Omics profiling provides opportunities to distinguish patients with transient, reversible AKI from those who will progress to persistent injury, dialysis dependence, or death.

- *Transcriptomics:* Transcriptomic analyses have generated promising prognostic classifiers. A 43-gene expression panel developed in septic AKI patients distinguished transient from persistent AKI with remarkable accuracy (AUC: 0.95), far outperforming a 58-variable clinical model (AUC: 0.74).[25] This highlights the ability of transcriptomics to provide mechanistic insights into pathways of renal recovery versus maladaptation, with direct implications for triage and clinical trial stratification.
- *Proteomics*: Urinary proteomic studies have identified PARK7 (DJ-1) and CDH16 (cadherin-16) as early markers of sepsis-associated AKI, with AUCs of 0.90 and 0.89, respectively.[6] These proteins reflect oxidative stress and tubular injury, respectively. The commercial NephroCheck assay [(TIMP-2)·(IGFBP7)]—reflecting G1 cell-cycle arrest—predicted AKI progression with an AUC of 0.80, significantly outperforming prior biomarkers (all <0.72).[26] Such proteomic tools not only forecast prognosis but may also suggest therapeutic targets, for instance modulation of cell-cycle arrest pathways.
- *Metabolomics*: Urinary metabolomic profiling further complements these approaches. Urinary kynurenic acid, a tryptophan-kynurenine metabolite, predicted poor renal recovery and higher mortality in septic AKI, findings supported by experimental models linking tryptophan/purine shifts to mitochondrial dysfunction.[27] Beyond prognostication, these findings may inform therapeutic interventions, such as antioxidants or mitochondrial protectants, to improve outcomes.

CLINICAL QUESTION 3: WHICH THERAPY WILL WORK?

Why Treatment Stratification Matters?

A central challenge in critical care is that therapies often fail in clinical trials despite biological plausibility. This is largely because heterogeneous patient populations obscure subgroup-specific treatment effects. Omics approaches allow identification of biologically distinct endotypes, enabling stratification of therapy to those most likely to benefit.[6] Such precision could reduce neutral trial outcomes and improve bedside care.

Acute Respiratory Distress Syndrome: Omics to Guide Therapy

Traditional severity definitions of ARDS cannot capture the heterogeneity of inflammatory responses. Omics-guided analyses have identified hyperinflammatory and hypoinflammatory phenotypes.[14,15] The hyperinflammatory group demonstrates higher mortality but also appears to benefit from strategies such as higher PEEP and conservative fluid balance. In contrast, hypoinflammatory patients do not gain the same benefit, suggesting that identical therapies can have opposite effects depending on endotype. A recent study by Nishikimi et al. (2024) using latent class analysis in

544 patients with severe ARDS on VV-ECMO identified three sub-phenotypes ("Dry", "Wet", and "Fibrotic"). The "Wet" phenotype showed a significant reduction in 90-day mortality when treated with higher PEEP ($\geq$10 cmH_2O) in the early phase of ECMO, whereas "Dry" and "Fibrotic" types did not show such benefit.[28] Elevated angiopoietin-2 and thrombomodulin reflect endothelial dysfunction, suggesting potential benefit from vascular-stabilizing strategies (e.g., fluid-conservative management, vasopressor selection, and drugs targeting endothelial permeability pathways). Similarly, increased sRAGE and SP-D highlight epithelial injury, pointing to epithelial-protective interventions such as surfactant therapies, epithelial repair enhancers, or approaches to reduce ventilator-induced epithelial stretch. While not yet validated in prospective randomized controlled trials (RCTs), these biomarkers provide a biological rationale for precision therapy trials in ARDS. Dual host–pathogen profiling further distinguishes sterile inflammation from infection, guiding both antibiotic and immunomodulatory use. Transcriptomic studies add further layers by linking gene-expression programs and microRNAs to inflammation and immune modulation, potentially serving as markers for tailoring immunotherapies.

Sepsis: Precision Immunomodulation

In sepsis, transcriptomic profiling defines immune response signatures with prognostic and therapeutic implications. The SRS1 endotype is immunosuppressed and has higher mortality, while SRS2 shows preserved immune function and lower mortality.[20] Secondary analyses suggest that corticosteroids may help SRS2 patients but not SRS1, illustrating the importance of endotype-specific therapy. Similar logic applies to newer immunomodulators: patients with profound immune suppression, identified by omics markers, might benefit from granulocyte-macrophage colony-stimulating factor (GM-CSF) or checkpoint inhibitors, while others could be harmed.

Acute Kidney Injury: Predicting who Benefits from Renal Replacement Therapy

For AKI, timing of renal replacement therapy (RRT) remains debated. Omics profiling, particularly transcriptomics, distinguishes transient from persistent AKI with high accuracy.[25] Persistent AKI patients may require early RRT, while transient cases might recover with supportive care alone. Proteomic and metabolomic markers of tubular stress and mitochondrial dysfunction could also guide nephroprotective strategies and trial design.[26]

Hence, these findings suggest that treatment stratification using omics can refine both trial design and clinical decisions. Instead of uniform therapy, patients can be selected for interventions such as corticosteroids, immunomodulators, or RRT based on biological endotypes, moving critical care closer to precision medicine **(Table 4)**.

TABLE 4: Omics-guided treatment stratification in critical illness.

Syndrome	*Omics type*	*Marker/signature*	*Predicted therapeutic response*
ARDS	Inflammatory endotypes (cytokine/proteomic clustering)	Hyper- vs. hypoinflammatory phenotypes	Higher PEEP and conservative fluid balance benefit for hyperinflammatory subgroup (validated in ARDS trials)
	Transcriptomics	Gene-expression, miRNAs	Linked to differential immunotherapy response
	Lactylation-based transcriptomics phenotypes	Low vs. high-lactylation phenotypes (ALDOB, CCT5, EP300, PFKP, PPIA, SIRT1)	High-lactylation phenotype associated with higher mortality; potential for tailoring treatment intensity/immunomodulatory therapy
	Subphenotypes in ECMO ARDS	"Dry", "Wet", "Fibrotic" classes (AR-ECMO)	"Wet" phenotype shows improved survival with higher PEEP during ECMO; others less responsive[28]
Sepsis	Transcriptomic endotypes (SRS1 vs. SRS2)	SRS1: immunosuppressed; SRS2: preserved immunity	SRS2 may benefit more from corticosteroids; SRS1 less so
	Multiomics	Immune suppression signatures	Guide use of GM-CSF or checkpoint inhibitors
AKI	Transcriptomics	43-gene classifier	Persistent AKI → early RRT; transient AKI → supportive care[25]
	Clinical/biomarker models	TIMP-2 × IGFBP7 (NephroCheck)	Elevated cell-cycle arrest markers predict AKI progression; early detection so treatment can adapt

(AKI: acute kidney injury; ARDS: acute respiratory distress syndrome; ECMO: extracorporeal membrane oxygenation; GM-CSF: granulocyte-macrophage colony-stimulating factor; RRT: renal replacement therapy)

CLINICAL QUESTION 4: WHAT COMPLICATIONS WILL DEVELOP?

Why Complication Prediction Matters?

Intensive care unit patients frequently develop secondary complications such as ventilator-associated pneumonia (VAP), multiorgan dysfunction, delirium, and coagulopathy. Predicting these events before clinical manifestation could allow preventive strategies, shorten ICU stay, and improve outcomes. Omics approaches provide sensitive tools to detect biological changes preceding complications.

Microbiome and Infection Risk

Microbiome sequencing demonstrates that critical illness disrupts microbial communities, reducing diversity and allowing pathogen overgrowth.[13] Shifts in the respiratory microbiome precede VAP, while gut dysbiosis predicts secondary sepsis. These signatures may allow pre-emptive antimicrobial stewardship or targeted decontamination.

Organ Dysfunction and Systemic Complications

Metabolomics highlights metabolic derangements preceding multiple organ dysfunction syndrome (MODS). Elevated indole derivatives, altered fatty acids, and oxidative stress metabolites correlate with liver and cardiac dysfunction.[23] Proteomic analyses reveal endothelial and coagulation signatures predicting thrombotic complications, potentially allowing earlier recognition of disseminated intravascular coagulation (DIC).[22]

Neurological Outcomes

Delirium and long-term cognitive decline remain difficult to predict. Proteins such as tau and neurofilament light chain, combined with transcriptomic signatures of synaptic dysfunction, have been associated with higher delirium risk and worse outcomes. Early detection may guide preventive strategies such as sedation minimization or neuroprotective therapy.

Thus, by anticipating complications, omics-driven prediction shifts ICU care from reactive to proactive. Identifying high-risk patients for VAP, MODS, or delirium could prompt preventive interventions and resource prioritization, potentially improving survival and quality of life after critical illness **(Table 5)**.

CLINICAL QUESTION 5: HOW SHOULD WE MONITOR RESPONSE?

Why Dynamic Monitoring Matters?

Critical illness evolves over time, yet most clinical biomarkers are static. Serial omics profiling offers real-time insight into whether a patient is recovering

TABLE 5: Omics-based predictors of ICU complications.

Complication	*Omics type*	*Marker/signature*	*Predictive implication*
VAP/secondary sepsis	Microbiomics	Gut dysbiosis; respiratory microbiome shifts	Predicts infection risk; informs stewardship[13]
Multiorgan failure (MODS)	Metabolomics	Indole/tryptophan derivatives; fatty-acid alterations	Predicts MODS and organ dysfunction[23]
Thrombosis/DIC	Proteomics	Endothelial/ coagulation protein clusters (e.g., Angpt-1, ADAMTS13 vs. cytokine-rich cluster)	Early signal of coagulopathy/ microvascular injury[22]

(DIC: disseminated intravascular coagulation; MODS: multiple organ dysfunction syndrome; VAP: ventilator-associated pneumonia)

or deteriorating. This dynamic approach could guide decisions such as escalation, de-escalation, or withdrawal of therapies.

Immune Response Trajectories

Transcriptomic monitoring reveals immune recovery versus exhaustion. Patients who re-express HLA-DR and restore T-cell activation pathways are more likely to recover, while those with persistent immune suppression develop secondary infections and have worse outcomes. These patterns allow clinicians to track the biological impact of therapies.[20]

Vascular and Metabolic Recovery

Proteomic panels measuring angiopoietins and adhesion molecules can indicate endothelial stabilization or ongoing vascular leak.[22] Similarly, metabolomics can track normalization of amino acid and lipid metabolism.[23] Persistent accumulation of oxidative stress metabolites signals poor prognosis and ongoing injury despite therapy.

Microbiome Resilience

Recovery of gut microbial diversity correlates with improved outcomes.[13] Patients whose microbiota rebound after critical illness show lower infection rates and mortality, while persistent dysbiosis predicts complications. Monitoring microbiome recovery may, therefore, complement traditional labs in assessing treatment response.

Dynamic omics monitoring enables timely decision-making: whether to continue or stop antibiotics, escalate immunotherapy, or withdraw futile

TABLE 6: Omics-based dynamic monitoring of treatment response.

Domain	*Omics type*	*Dynamic marker*	*Monitoring implication*
Immune recovery	Transcriptomics	Serial HLA-DR/T-cell activation signatures	Distinguish recovery vs. immune exhaustion[20]
Endothelial function	Proteomics	Angiopoietins, adhesion molecules; endothelial vs. inflammatory cluster balance	Track vascular stabilization vs. leak[22]
Metabolic recovery	Metabolomics	Normalization of amino acid/lipid metabolites	Identify recovery vs. persistent metabolic stress[23]
Host resilience	Microbiomics	Restoration of gut microbial diversity	Fewer infections; improved survival[13]

treatments. It represents a step toward real-time, personalized ICU care **(Table 6)**.

CLINICAL QUESTION 6: HOW TO IMPLEMENT OMICS IN TODAY'S ICU?

Current Limitations

Despite their promise, omics approaches face practical barriers to daily ICU use. Sequencing and mass spectrometry still require >24 hours, too slow for time-critical interventions such as antibiotic initiation. Costs remain high, especially for whole-genome sequencing and proteomics, limiting access outside specialized centers. Just as importantly, the vast datasets produced are not easily interpretable—clinicians need actionable reports, not raw molecular profiles.[6]

Practical Solutions

Practical solutions are emerging. Rather than deploying full-scale platforms, small validated biomarker panels can be implemented as rapid cartridge assays, similar to troponin or procalcitonin. Embedding omics signals into familiar systems such as SOFA or APACHE can also enhance prognostic value without disrupting workflows. Artificial intelligence may help integrate multiomics data, into algorithms for diagnosis, prognosis and helping tease out the heterogeneity of treatment effects (HTEs). These algorithms will be clinically useful only if they remain transparent and explainable if they are to gain clinician trust.[29]

Bioinformatics offers potential solutions. Advanced computational pipelines and machine-learning models can integrate multiomics datasets with clinical variables to deliver rapid, clinically actionable phenotyping. The COMBAT consortium, developed during COVID-19, demonstrated how open multiomics databases can accelerate discovery and reproducibility.[30] Similar multinational efforts in sepsis, ARDS, and AKI would enable cross-validation and reduce duplication.

Beyond its immediate practical role for the clinician at the bedside, one of the most exciting element of "omics" data interpretation utilizing bioinformatics is the potential to tease out the HTE on different sub-groups or sub-endotype of patients with ARDS, sepsis, AKI, and other disease syndromes, which will help identify potential target treatments for different subgroups and enhance precision medicine.

One of the major challenges in translating omics into routine clinical practice is ensuring representation of diverse global populations in study design, evaluation, and early access to research outputs and emerging therapies. This would be critical to avoid inequities in delivery of healthcare as precision medicine evolves. As platforms become cheaper and more automated, bioinformatics-driven workflows may bridge the current translational gap, enabling precision therapies at the bedside. Alongside these advances, ethical considerations—equity, privacy, and avoidance of deterministic prognostication must remain central.

CONCLUSION

Omics technologies are redefining critical care by answering fundamental clinical questions: diagnosing infection earlier, identifying patients at risk of deterioration, predicting therapeutic response, anticipating organ failure, and enabling dynamic monitoring. These insights move ICU practice beyond one-size-fits-all syndromic care toward individualized, biology-based decision-making. Translation, however, must be pragmatic. The most immediate gains will likely come from rapid biomarker panels, integration of omics signals into existing scores, and expansion of collaborative repositories. Over time, multiomics integration and single-cell technologies will provide richer mechanistic understanding, while AI will help translate complex datasets into usable bedside tools.

The ICU of the future will remain grounded in clinical judgment, but enriched by molecular precision. By embedding omics into structured frameworks, critical care can evolve from treating syndromes to treating patients as unique biological individuals—ushering in a new era of personalized intensive care.

REFERENCES

1. Angus DC, van der Poll T. Severe sepsis and septic shock. N Engl J Med. 2013;369(9):840-51.

2. Bellomo R, Kellum JA, Ronco C. Acute kidney injury. Lancet. 2012;380(9843):756-66.
3. Prescott HC, Calfee CS, Thompson BT, Angus DC, Liu VX. Toward Smarter Lumping and Smarter Splitting: Rethinking Strategies for Sepsis and Acute Respiratory Distress Syndrome Clinical Trial Design. Am J Respir Crit Care Med. 2016;194(2):147-55.
4. Seymour CW, Gomez H, Chang CH, Clermont G, Kellum JA, Kennedy J, et al. Precision medicine for all? Challenges and opportunities for a precision medicine approach to critical illness. Crit Care. 2017;21(1):257.
5. Pickkers P, Kox M. Towards precision medicine for sepsis patients. Crit Care. 2017;21(1):11.
6. See KC. Personalizing Care for Critically Ill Adults Using Omics: A Concise Review of Potential Clinical Applications. Cells. 2023;12(4):541.
7. Kumar A, Roberts D, Wood KE, Light B, Parrillo JE, Sharma S, et al. Duration of hypotension before initiation of effective antimicrobial therapy is the critical determinant of survival in human septic shock. Crit Care Med. 2006;34(6):1589-96.
8. Chien JY, Yu CJ, Hsueh PR. Utility of Metagenomic Next-Generation Sequencing for Etiological Diagnosis of Patients with Sepsis in Intensive Care Units. Microbiol Spectr. 2022;10(4):e0074622.
9. Sweeney TE, Shidham A, Wong HR, Khatri P. A comprehensive time-course-based multicohort analysis of sepsis and sterile inflammation reveals a robust diagnostic gene set. Sci Transl Med. 2015;7(287):287ra71.
10. Langelier C, Kalantar KL, Moazed F, Wilson MR, Crawford ED, Deiss T, et al. Integrating host response and unbiased microbe detection for lower respiratory tract infection diagnosis. Nat Microbiol. 2018;3:1329-39.
11. Li M, Ren R, Yan M, Chen S, Chen C, Yan J. Identification of novel biomarkers for sepsis diagnosis via serum proteomic analysis using iTRAQ-2D-LC-MS/MS. J Clin Lab Anal. 2022;36(1):e24142.
12. Nguyen EV, Gharib SA, Palazzo SJ, Chow YH, Goodlett DR, Schnapp LM. Proteomic profiling of bronchoalveolar lavage fluid in critically ill patients with ventilator-associated pneumonia. PLoS One. 2013;8(3):e58782.
13. Zaborin A, Smith D, Garfield K, Quensen J, Shakhsheer B, Kade M, et al. Membership and behavior of ultra-low-diversity pathogen communities present in the gut of humans during prolonged critical illness. mBio. 2014;5(5):e01361-14.
14. Calfee CS, Delucchi K, Parsons PE, Thompson BT, Ware LB, Matthay MA; NHLBI ARDS Network. Subphenotypes in acute respiratory distress syndrome: latent class analysis of data from two randomised controlled trials. Lancet Respir Med. 2014;2(8):611-20.
15. Famous KR, Delucchi K, Ware LB, Kangelaris KN, Liu KD, Thompson BT, et al.; ARDS Network. Acute Respiratory Distress Syndrome Subphenotypes Respond Differently to Randomized Fluid Management Strategy. Am J Respir Crit Care Med. 2017;195(3):331-8. Erratum in: Am J Respir Crit Care Med. 2018;198(12):1590. Erratum in: Am J Respir Crit Care Med. 2019;200(5):649.
16. Rahmel T, Rump K, Adamzik M, Peters J, Frey UH. Increased circulating microRNA-122 is associated with mortality and acute liver injury in the acute respiratory distress syndrome. BMC Anesthesiol. 2018;18(1):75.
17. Liu CH, Kuo SW, Ko WJ, Tsai PR, Wu SW, Lai CH, et al. Early measurement of IL-10 predicts the outcomes of patients with acute respiratory distress syndrome receiving extracorporeal membrane oxygenation. Sci Rep. 2017;7(1):1021.

18. Xu J, Pan T, Qi X, Tan R, Wang X, Liu Z, et al. Increased mortality of acute respiratory distress syndrome was associated with high levels of plasma phenylalanine. Respir Res. 2020;21(1):99.
19. Rautanen A, Mills TC, Gordon AC, Hutton P, Steffens M, Nuamah R, et al. Genome-wide association study of survival from sepsis due to pneumonia: FER gene implicated. Lancet Respir Med. 2015;3:53-60.
20. Davenport EE, Burnham KL, Radhakrishnan J, Humburg P, Hutton P, Mills TC, et al. Genomic landscape of the individual host response and outcomes in sepsis: a prospective cohort study. Lancet Respir Med. 2016;4(4):259-71.
21. Wang Q, Feng Q, Zhang Y, Zhou S, Chen H. Decreased microRNA 103 and microRNA 107 predict increased risks of acute respiratory distress syndrome and 28-day mortality in sepsis patients. Medicine (Baltimore). 2020;99(25):e20729.
22. Rovas A, Buscher K, Osiaevi I, Drost CC, Sackarnd J, Tepasse PR, et al. Microvascular and proteomic signatures overlap in COVID-19 and bacterial sepsis: the MICROCODE study. Angiogenesis. 2022;25(4):503-15.
23. Wang J, Sun Y, Teng S, Li K. Prediction of sepsis mortality using metabolite biomarkers in the blood: a meta-analysis of death-related pathways and prospective validation. BMC Med. 2020;18:83.
24. Wu P, Chen D, Ding W, Wu P, Hou H, Bai Y, et al. The trans-omics landscape of COVID-19. Nat Commun. 2021;12(1):4543.
25. Zhang Z, Chen L, Liu H, Sun Y, Shui P, Gao J, et al.; CMAISE Consortium. Gene signature for the prediction of the trajectories of sepsis-induced acute kidney injury. Crit Care. 2022;26(1):398.
26. Kashani K, Al-Khafaji A, Ardiles T, Artigas A, Bagshaw SM, Bell M, et al. Discovery and validation of cell cycle arrest biomarkers in human acute kidney injury. Crit Care. 2013;17(1):R25.
27. Aregger F, Uehlinger DE, Fusch G, Bahonjic A, Pschowski R, Walter M, et al. Increased urinary excretion of kynurenic acid is associated with non-recovery from acute kidney injury in critically ill patients. BMC Nephrol. 2018;19(1):44.
28. Nishikimi M, Ohshimo S, Bellani G, Fukumoto W, Anzai T, Liu K, et al.; J-CARVE Registry Group. Identification of novel sub-phenotypes of severe ARDS requiring ECMO using latent class analysis. Crit Care. 2024;28(1):343.
29. Topol EJ. High-performance medicine: the convergence of human and artificial intelligence. Nat Med. 2019;25(1):44-56.
30. Overmyer KA, Shishkova E, Miller IJ, Balnis J, Bernstein MN, Peters-Clarke TM, et al. Large-Scale Multi-omic Analysis of COVID-19 Severity. Cell Syst. 2021;12(1):23-40.e7.

CHAPTER 20

Block Chain in Critical Care

Srinivas Samavedam, Tejasree Rajoli

INTRODUCTION

Critical care units (ICUs) are among the most technologically advanced and resource-intensive areas in healthcare. They provide continuous monitoring and life-sustaining interventions for critically ill patients, who are often highly unstable and require rapid decision-making. In these settings, vast amounts of data are generated every second from ventilators, infusion pumps, hemodynamic monitors, imaging devices, and laboratory systems. The challenge lies not only in collecting this data but also in integrating, securing, and interpreting it in real-time to guide clinical decisions.[1]

Traditional electronic health record (EHR) systems and centralized hospital databases often struggle with issues such as interoperability and vulnerability to cyberattacks. Furthermore, patients' privacy and consent management remain pressing concerns, especially as healthcare data becomes a prime target for intruders. In this context, block chain technology has emerged as a potential game-changer. By providing a decentralized, transparent, and tamper-proof ledger for transactions and data exchange, block chain can address many of the structural challenges in critical care medicine. Beyond data storage, block chain's integration with smart contracts, artificial intelligence (AI), and the Internet of Medical Things (IoMT) may transform ICU workflows, improve medication safety, and enhance patient outcomes.

This chapter explores the fundamentals of block chain technology, its applications in critical care medicine, current pilot projects, existing challenges, and future directions for integrating block chain into ICU practice.

FUNDAMENTALS OF BLOCK CHAIN TECHNOLOGY

Block chain is essentially a distributed ledger technology (DLT) that records transactions across a decentralized network of nodes. Each block in the chain contains a set of records, a timestamp, and a cryptographic hash of the previous block, ensuring immutability and transparency. Unlike traditional centralized systems where a single server controls access, block chain distributes copies of the ledger across participants. This design eliminates single points of failure and enhances trust among stakeholders **(Fig. 1)**.

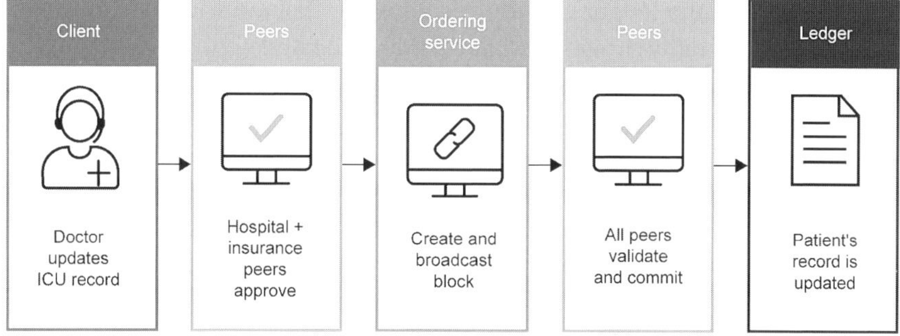

Fig. 1: Example of basic structure of block chain in healthcare.

The key features of block chain relevant to critical care medicine include:

- *Decentralization:* Data is stored across multiple nodes, preventing reliance on a single authority.
- *Immutability:* Once recorded, data cannot be altered without consensus, ensuring reliability.
- *Transparency and auditability:* Transactions are visible to authorized participants, enabling traceability.
- *Smart contracts:* Self-executing contracts programmed with predefined rules, useful for automating processes such as consent verification or triggering alerts.

Types of block chain:

- *Public (permissionless) block chains*: Open to anyone but less suited for healthcare due to privacy concerns
- *Private (permissioned) block chains:* Controlled access networks such as Hyperledger Fabric, ideal for ICU environments
- *Hybrid or consortium block chains:* Combine features of public and private models, balancing transparency with confidentiality.

Consensus mechanisms such as Proof of Work (PoW), Proof of Stake (PoS), and Practical Byzantine Fault Tolerance (PBFT—the basic stage of the IBM Hyperledger) determine how participants agree on valid transactions. In healthcare, energy-efficient methods like PBFT or Proof of Authority (PoA—used for the types of algorithms that guarantee access to data) are preferred, since they provide scalability without the heavy computational costs of PoW.

APPLICATIONS IN CRITICAL CARE MEDICINE

The ICU environment presents unique challenges where block chain technology can add value:

- *Data security and cybersecurity:* Healthcare data breaches are increasingly frequent, with ICUs being prime targets due to the high value of sensitive patient data.[1] Block chain enhances cybersecurity by ensuring that data recorded on the ledger cannot be altered or deleted without detection. This immutability provides an auditable trail of all actions, reducing the risk of tampering. Cryptographic encryption further safeguards patient confidentiality.

- *Interoperability and real-time data sharing:* ICUs rely on multiple devices from different vendors, often resulting in fragmented data silos. Block chain enables secure, standardized data sharing across systems. For example, a patient's ventilator data, laboratory results, and medication records can be integrated on a block chain, ensuring clinicians access unified, real-time information. This interoperability is critical during emergencies, interhospital transfers, or multidisciplinary consultations.[2]
- *Medication safety and supply chain integrity:* Medication errors and counterfeit drugs are serious threats in critical care. Block chain allows end-to-end tracking of pharmaceuticals from manufacturer to bedside. Clinicians can verify the authenticity, storage conditions, and chain of custody of medications, reducing risks of counterfeit or expired drugs reaching patients.[1]
- *Consent management and ethical decision-making:* Critical care often involves high-stakes decisions about life support, resuscitation, and end-of-life care. Block chain can securely record patient or family consent, ensuring decisions are immutable and legally valid. This is especially valuable in disputes or medicolegal cases.[1]
- *Integration with AI and IoMT:* Block chain can integrate continuous physiologic data from IoMT devices, such as wearable monitors and smart infusion pumps. Smart contracts can trigger automated responses, such as alerting clinicians if a patient's oxygen saturation drops below a threshold. When combined with AI algorithms, block chain ensures the data feeding predictive models is authentic and tamper-proof.[1]
- *Resource and workflow optimization:* Block chain-based systems can track ICU bed availability, ventilator usage, and staffing resources in real time. Transparent and auditable records help hospital administrators allocate scarce resources efficiently, a feature especially relevant during pandemics or mass casualty incidents.

CASE STUDIES AND PILOT PROJECTS

- *ICU data management platforms:* Research using Hyperledger Fabric has demonstrated how permissioned block chains can securely store ICU sensor data, ensuring immutability and controlled access while supporting decision-making tools[2]
- *Emergency and critical care transfers:* Block chain has been tested in emergency medicine to facilitate seamless data transfer between ambulances, emergency departments, and ICUs. This reduces delays in care by providing clinicians with immediate access to accurate medical histories.[3]

- *Pharmaceutical supply chains:* Pilot programs have used block chain to track the ICU drug supply chain, verifying authenticity and ensuring that temperature-sensitive medications such as biologics are transported under optimal conditions.[4]
- *Clinical trials in critical care:* Block chain can store trial data transparently, preventing manipulation and ensuring patient safety. In ICUs, where trial enrollment and consent are often complex, block chain simplifies consent tracking and compliance auditing.

CHALLENGES AND LIMITATIONS

Despite its promise, block chain implementation in ICUs faces several barriers:

- *Scalability:* ICUs generate massive data streams. Storing all data directly on a block chain may be impractical. Hybrid models combining block chain with distributed databases or cloud storage are being explored.
- *Regulatory compliance:* Laws like GDPR (General Data Protection Regulation) and HIPAA (Health Insurance Portability and Accountability Act) require patient data privacy, yet block chain's immutability conflicts with the "right to be forgotten". Solutions such as off-chain storage and zero-knowledge proofs are under investigation.
- *Implementation costs:* Deploying block chain requires investment in infrastructure, training, and integration with legacy systems.
- *Governance models:* Multistakeholder environments, such as hospitals, insurers, and regulators, must agree on governance structures, permissions, and dispute mechanisms.
- *Cultural and institutional resistance:* Healthcare institutions may be slow to adopt block chain due to unfamiliarity and concerns about disruption of existing systems.[5]

FUTURE DIRECTIONS

Several emerging trends suggest block chain's role in critical care will expand:

- *Hybrid architectures*: Combining block chain with cloud and distributed storage to balance scalability with security
- *Federated learning models*: Block chain can coordinate AI training across multiple hospitals without centralizing patient data, protecting privacy while enhancing predictive analytics.
- *Smart ICU ecosystems*: Integration of block chain with IoMT devices, AI decision support, and robotic process automation to create intelligent ICU environments
- *Global standardization*: Development of international guidelines for block chain interoperability, data sharing, and security in healthcare

- *Pandemic preparedness*: Block chain-enabled systems could track ICU resources, patient outcomes, and vaccine distribution during future health crises.

CONCLUSION

Block chain technology has the potential to transform critical care medicine by addressing long-standing challenges of data security, interoperability, medication safety, and consent management. While technical, regulatory, and institutional barriers remain, ongoing pilot projects demonstrate the feasibility and benefits of block chain-enabled ICUs. Future integration with AI, IoMT, and hybrid cloud architectures could usher in a new era of secure, efficient, and patient-centered critical care. To realize this vision, collaboration between clinicians, technologists, policymakers, and patients is essential.

REFERENCES

1. Gondode P, Dass C, Kumar S, Malviya A, Ashwin M, Khanna P. Blockchain in Critical Care. Indian J Crit Care Med. 2025;29(6):525-30.
2. Guimarães T, Moreira A, Peixoto H, Santos M. ICU Data Management—A Permissioned Blockchain Approach. Procedia Comput Sci. 2020;177:546-51.
3. Wu TC, Ho CTB. Blockchain Revolutionizing in Emergency Medicine: A Scoping Review of Patient Journey through the ED. Healthcare (Basel). 2023;11(18):2497.
4. Haleem A, Javaid M, Singh RP, Suman R, Rab S. Blockchain technology applications in healthcare: An overview. Int J Intell Netw. 2021;2:130-9.
5. Ghosh PK, Chakraborty A, Hasan M, Rashid K, Siddique AH. Blockchain Application in Healthcare Systems: A Review. Systems. 2023;11(1):38.

CHAPTER 21

The Physiologically Difficult Airway

Sheila Nainan Myatra, Nishanth Baliga

INTRODUCTION

Airway management—particularly tracheal intubation—is a cornerstone of care for critically ill patients. Difficult airway management has always revolved around anatomical challenges such as mask ventilation, laryngoscopy, and intubation. While technological advances (videolaryngoscopes, supraglottic airway devices, etc.) have mitigated many anatomical challenges, acute physiological derangements can independently provoke peri-intubation complications, including refractory hypoxemia, cardiovascular collapse, and cardiac arrest. The recognition of the physiologically difficult airway demands an updated, nuanced approach to airway assessment and intervention in high-risk populations.

DEFINITION AND RELEVANCE

A physiologically difficult airway is defined as one where severe physiologic derangement (e.g., hypoxemia, shock, acidosis, and right heart failure) increase the risk of cardiovascular instability, hypoxia-induced injury, or cardiac arrest during intubation, even when no anatomical difficulty exists.[1] Critically ill patients often exemplify this scenario, but the same risk profile is observed in patients with obesity, pregnancy, pediatric age, and certain acute comorbidities.

EPIDEMIOLOGY AND CLINICAL IMPACT

Large observational studies, such as the INTUBE and NAP4 audits, have quantified the incremental risk: Major peri-intubation adverse events (cardiovascular instability, severe hypoxemia, and cardiac arrest) occur in upward of 30–45% of intensive care unit (ICU) intubations versus 5–10% in elective surgical settings. Cardiovascular instability is the most common (up to 43%), followed by severe hypoxemia and cardiac arrest. These adverse events independently increase ICU mortality.[2-4]

PATIENT PHENOTYPES AND PATHOPHYSIOLOGY

Critically Ill Adults

Hypoxemia

Patients require intubation and mechanical ventilation due to hypoxia from diseases such as pneumonia, pulmonary edema, acute respiratory distress syndrome (ARDS), and asthma. Patients who are hypoxic prior to intubation are at increased risk of cardiopulmonary complications such as desaturation, cardiac dysfunction, arrythmias, hypoxic brain injury, and cardiac arrest as there may be rapid desaturation during attempts of intubation. The mechanisms of hypoxia in critically ill patients are due to shunt and ventilation-perfusion (V/Q) mismatch. Increasing fraction of inspired oxygen (FiO_2) may not be helpful in these patients as shunt pathology in these patients prevent oxygen delivery to the capillaries. Hence, these patients are at increased risk of rapid desaturation during attempts of intubation. Standard methods (non-rebreathing mask) are often insufficient. Advanced preoxygenation techniques such as noninvasive ventilation (NIV) and high-flow nasal oxygen (HFNO) have been found to be beneficial. Though efficacy of these techniques has been found to be superior but they may not completely prevent desaturation in severe disease.[5-10]

Hypotension

Critically ill patients develop hypotension which can lead to bradycardia and cardiac arrest in significant number of patients during endotracheal intubation. Patients with pre-existing hypotension are at increased risk of cardiovascular collapse and death. The causes of hypotension in these patients include hypovolemia, decreased peripheral vascular resistance, capillary leak as well as institution of positive pressure ventilation postintubation. Some predictors of hemodynamic instability post-intubation are preexisting hypotension and shock index, i.e., heart rate/systolic blood pressure >0.8 mm Hg. High shock index suggests compensatory mechanisms which keep blood pressure within normal limits. However, induction of anesthesia during intubation and institution of positive pressure ventilation tend to suppress these compensatory mechanisms leading to hypotension and shock.

Due to the high incidence of hypotension and cardiovascular instability post-intubation, it is prudent to implement measures to prevent hypotension with early use of fluids or vasopressors. Patients with hypovolemia need fluid resuscitation prior to intubation unless contraindicated due to poor cardiac reserve. Patients with decreased peripheral vascular resistance and capillary leak may need vasopressors. Drugs used for intubation such as propofol and thiopentone can cause hypotension and precipitate cardiac arrest in those who are already hypotensive. Cardio-stable drugs such as etomidate and ketamine should be used for intubation. Hemodynamic monitoring post-intubation is important to detect hypotension early so that appropriate measures can be instituted.[11-13]

Right Ventricular Failure

The right ventricle (RV) under physiological conditions functions as a low-pressure, highly compliant, and flow-dependent chamber responsible for propelling systemic venous return into the pulmonary circulation. Increases in RV afterload may occur secondary to chronic pulmonary hypertension from lung or left ventricular pathology, pulmonary arterial hypertension, or acute pulmonary embolism. The RV adapts to the increase in afterload by enhancing contractility and preload.

Clinically, it is essential to differentiate between RV dysfunction and RV failure. RV dysfunction denotes a state in which compensatory mechanisms preserve partial pump function despite increased load. In contrast, RV failure reflects the inability of the ventricle to sustain forward flow, resulting in progressive dilation, retrograde venous congestion, impaired coronary perfusion, systemic hypotension, and ultimately cardiovascular collapse. Patients with RV failure tolerate increase in afterload poorly. Hence, in these patients, intubation is associated with complications. Hypoxia and hypercarbia during and post-intubation can increase afterload. Increasing airway and intrathoracic pressures from positive pressure ventilation further overload the failing RV, leading to global circulatory collapse.

Bedside point-of-care echocardiography can be used to assess right ventricular function to differentiate RV dysfunction and failure. If patient has some contractile reserve as in RV dysfunction, judicious fluid resuscitation should be performed. Preoxygenation is important though difficult due to intracardiac shunt and V/Q mismatch. During attempts of intubation, apneic oxygenation using HFNO can be used. Vasopressors such as noradrenaline can be used in patients with hypotension as it increases systemic vascular resistance without increase in pulmonary venous pressure. The goals of mechanical ventilation include maintenance of a low mean airway pressure and avoidance of hypoxemia, atelectasis, and hypercapnia, which increase RV afterload.[14,15]

Neurological Injury

In patients with neurological injury, it is important to maintain cerebral perfusion pressure and avoid secondary injuries such as hypoxia and hypercarbia. Patients with increased intracranial pressure (ICP) due to neurological injury are at risk of worsening ICP due to induction of anesthesia and laryngoscopy. Episodes of hypoxia or hypercarbia during endotracheal intubation can lead to secondary injuries. Hence, patients with neurological injury when they need intubation and mechanical ventilation, hemodynamically stable drugs such as etomidate and ketamine should be used. Other measures to reduce ICP such as lignocaine, fentanyl, and esmolol can be used. Laryngoscopy time should be minimized as much as possible as it is a potent stimulator to increase ICP. Hypoxia and hypercarbia should be avoided as it can worsen neurological injury. Hypotension which can occur post-intubation can compromise cerebral perfusion pressure and needs to be aggressively managed.[16,17]

Obese Patients

Obesity increases both anatomical and physiological difficulty. These patients have a high metabolic demand, oxygen consumption as well as cardiac output. In these patients there is persistent pressure and volume overload which leads to structural and functional changes in the heart. Due to this, left ventricular compliance may reduce placing them at risk of left ventricular failure. Obese patients are also at risk of pulmonary complications due to physiological derangements such as diminished lung capacity, vital capacity, and chest wall compliance. These along with increased intra-abdominal pressure reduces functional residual capacity (FRC) as well as closing capacity. Brief periods of apnea in these patients during intubation can lead to rapid desaturation. Hence, when these patients require intubation and mechanical ventilation, measures such as NIV for preoxygenation, prolonged preoxygenation, ramp position, PEEP application during preoxygenation, use of videolaryngoscopy (VL), apneic oxygenation, and experienced senior airway operator should be employed to reduce complications. These patients also are at risk of aspiration due to delayed gastric emptying. Hence, measures to reduce aspiration like soluble antacids prior to intubation, rapid sequence intubation using short-acting neuromuscular blockers should be employed.[18]

Obstetric and Pregnant Patients

Pregnancy reduces FRC, increases oxygen consumption, and heightens aspiration risk due to delayed gastric emptying and acid reflux. Maternal physiologic changes compound the risk of hypoxemia and aspiration during intubation. Obstetric intubations are generally associated with increased risk of complications and failed intubation. Hence, obstetric airway should be handled only in times of emergency related to mother or fetus, critical illness to the mother.

Measures recommended to mitigate these complications are soluble antacids, prokinetics prior to intubation, senior experienced airway operator, preoxygenation with NIV, rapid sequence intubation, avoidance of positive pressure prior to intubation, use of airway adjuncts such as bougie or stylet, and confirmation of endotracheal placement using capnography.[19,20]

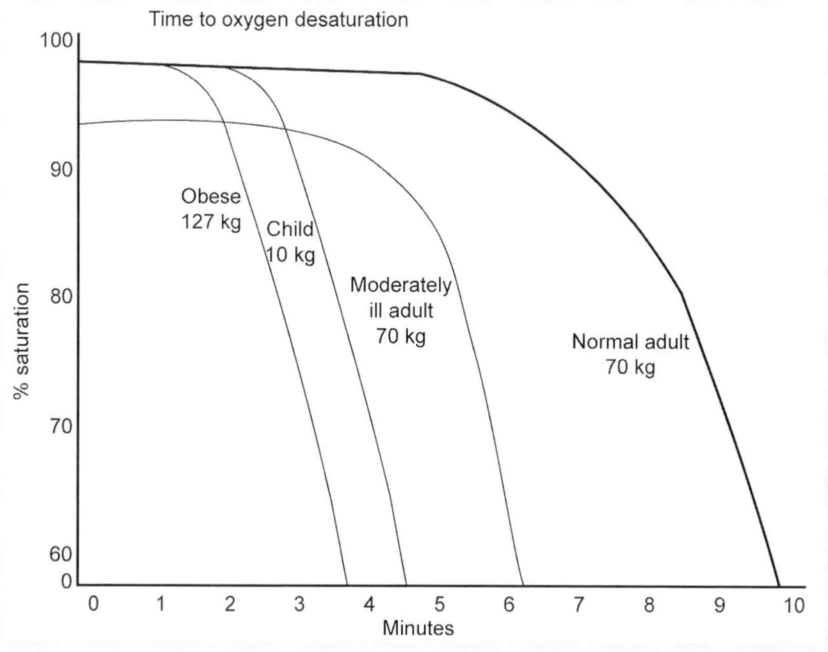

Fig. 1: Benioff curve comparing the difference in the apnea time in a normal healthy adult, a moderately ill adult, an obese patient and a child. Note the significant difference in the safe apnea time noticed between a healthy adult and an obese individual.

Pediatric Patients

Children have high oxygen consumption, low FRC, and are exquisitely susceptible to hypoxemia with brief apnea. The risk is highest in infants and neonates, and further increased in those who are acutely ill. Safe apnea time is significantly lower in pediatrics and they rapidly desaturate. Hence, in these patient's adequate preoxygenation, experienced airway handling, peri-intubation oxygenation, and minimal apnea time are some of the measures which can be employed to reduce complications **(Fig. 1)**.[21,22]

At-risk for Aspiration

Patients with delayed gastric emptying (trauma, bowel obstruction, diabetes, pregnancy, and obesity) are at risk for vomiting and aspiration with catastrophic respiratory and hemodynamic consequences during intubation. Some measures which can be employed in these patients are rapid sequence intubation (RSI) with pre-determined doses of induction agent and muscle relaxant, avoidance of bag and mask ventilation, short duration of laryngoscopy, and inflation of the tracheal cuff.

TABLE 1: MACOCHA score calculation worksheet.

Factors	*Points*
Factors related to patient Mallampati score III or IV	5
Obstructive sleep apnea syndrome	2
Reduced mobility of cervical spine	1
Limited mouth opening <3 cm	1
Factors related to pathology Coma	1
Severe hypoxemia (<80%)	1
Factors related to operator Nonanesthesiologist	1
Total	12

TABLE 2: Hypotension prediction score (HYPS).

HYPS	*Expected risk of PIH*
≤1.5	Low (≤19%)
2–10.5	Moderate (20–39%)
11–18.5	High (40–59%)
≥19	Very high (≥60%)

(PIH: postintubation hypotension)

ASSESSMENT TOOLS AND RISK PREDICTION

The MACOCHA score integrates both anatomic and physiologic variables (Mallampati III/IV, sleep apnea, reduced mouth opening, cervical immobility, coma, hypoxemia, and nonanesthesiologists operator) to risk-stratify ICU intubations. The score has a maximum of 12 points, with 0 points predicting an easy intubation and 12 points predicting a very difficult one. However, even advanced scores cannot entirely predict adverse events, highlighting the need for clinical vigilance and scenario planning[23] **(Table 1)**.

Hemodynamic instability post-intubation in patients with patent ductus arteriosus (PDA) is common. The hypotension prediction score (HYPS) **(Table 2)** is a tool that was recently proposed for the prediction of post-intubation hypotension (PIH) in the critically ill.[24]

MANAGEMENT STRATEGIES

Preprocedural Optimization

- *Team preparation:* At least two skilled operators, clear role assignment, predefined backup plans, and equipment checks are essential.

- *Positioning:* Head-up/ramped positioning optimizes preoxygenation, FRC, and reduces aspiration risk.[25]
- *Hemodynamic optimization:* Judicious fluid administration (for shock or hypovolemia), vasopressor support, and avoidance of agents with strong myocardial depressant effects are recommended. Routine pre-intubation large bolus fluids are not consistently beneficial and should be individualized.
- *Induction agents:* Ketamine and etomidate are preferred for unstable patients. Propofol is commonly associated with higher rates of peri-intubation hypotension and should be avoided in unstable patients when possible.
- *Muscle relaxants:* Succinylcholine or rocuronium are the preferred neuromuscular blocking agents during intubation. Succinylcholine is avoided in conditions such as skeletal muscle myopathies, hyperkalemia, burns post 48 hours, known allergy, or history of malignant hyperthermia.

Advanced Oxygenation

- *Preoxygenation:* A recent systematic review of randomized trials comparing preoxygenation strategies for intubation of critically ill patients showed preoxygenation with NIV or HFNO compared to facemask oxygen might prevent hypoxemia during tracheal intubation of adults who are critically ill. Compared with HFNO, NIV probably decreases the incidence of hypoxemia during intubation. Therefore, for moderate-to-severe hypoxemia, NIV should be preferred.[26] Both NIV and HFNO reduce but do not eliminate the risk of desaturation; combination therapy may offer incremental benefit.[6,8]
- *Apneic oxygenation:* Oxygen delivered via nasal cannula at 15 L/min or HFNO should be continued throughout apnea, especially in those at risk for rapid desaturation.[9]

Rapid Sequence Intubation

- A modified RSI technique which consists of titrated administration of rapid-onset sedative hypnotic and a rapid-acting neuromuscular blocking agent, and/or gentle mask ventilation should be considered in patients with a physiologically difficult airway to prevent peri-intubation complications. Use of cricoid pressure is debatable. In case of difficulty in visualization of vocal cords during intubation, cricoid pressure should be released.
- *Mask ventilation during RSI:* Gentle positive-pressure ventilation between induction and laryngoscopy is increasingly supported, with data indicating a lower risk of hypoxemia and no increase in aspiration compared to apneic oxygenation alone.[27]

- *Delayed sequence intubation:* In uncooperative patients in whom preoxygenation may not be possible due to their mental status, a low dissociative dose of ketamine to facilitate preoxygenation can be given. It has been found to reduce peri-intubation hypoxia compared to standard RSI in this subset of patients.[28]

Airway Device Choices and Adjuncts

- VL enhances glottic view, increases first-pass success, and is favored in critically ill patients as aids in supervision and assistance of the airway operator by providing a shared view of the glottis. A stylet or bougie should be ready for use, as adjuncts improve tube passage success.[29-31]
- Checklists and bundles (e.g., Montpellier protocol) incorporating preoxygenation, vasopressor readiness, and backup plans may improve adherence to best practices, but clinical evidence for outcome benefit is mixed.[32]

Postintubation Considerations

- *Confirmation of tracheal tube placement*: Immediate confirmation of endotracheal tube placement using waveform capnography, rapid transition to protective ventilation settings, and ongoing hemodynamic and oxygenation monitoring are crucial.[33]
- Ventilation with lung protective strategy including tidal volume of 6–8 mL/kg of predicted body weight (PBW), positive-end expiratory pressure (PEEP) of >5 cmH_2O, plateau pressure <30 cm of H_2O, and FiO_2 titrated to a target SpO_2 between 92 and 95% should be adopted in most patients.
- Fluid responsiveness needs to be evaluated using dynamic indices before fluid administration in patients with PDA, especially who develop persistent hypotension post-intubation. Bedside point-of-care ultrasound (POCUS) can provide real-time hemodynamic and respiratory assessment and can be used to guide resuscitation and physiological optimization in these patients.[34]
- Sedation infusions need to be started post-intubation with opioids such as fentanyl, remifentanil with or without muscle relaxant infusions to ensure tube tolerance and patient-ventilator synchrony.

AWAKE INTUBATION

In select high-risk scenarios (refractory hypoxemia, severe metabolic acidosis, and RV failure), maintaining spontaneous breathing and performing an awake intubation (using VL or flexible bronchoscope) may be safer than standard RSI. This may help prevent hypotension occurring due to the use of induction agents and hypoxia following the use of neuromuscular blockade. However, performing an awake intubation is challenging in the critically ill, often due to lack of patient co-operation and the clinical condition of the patient. Ketamine may be used in sedative doses to facilitate preoxygenation and tracheal intubation (delayed sequence intubation).[28]

CONCLUSION

The physiologically difficult airway encompasses scenarios where patient physiology drives risk of catastrophic events during airway management. Recognizing at-risk patients, thoroughly optimizing hemodynamics and oxygenation, individualizing drug/induction and device choice, and employing team-based approaches are essential to reduce morbidity and mortality. Despite advanced interventions, a substantial subset remains at elevated risk, underscoring the importance of ongoing research, guideline refinement, and simulation-based preparation. A "physiology-first" mindset is imperative in airway management in the ICU and emergency settings.

REFERENCES

1. Mosier JM, Joshi R, Hypes C, Pacheco G, Valenzuela T, Sakles JC, et al. The physiologically difficult airway. West J Emerg Med. 2015;16:1109-17.
2. Cook TM, Woodall N, Frerk C; Fourth National Audit Project. Major complications of airway management in the UK: results of the Fourth National Audit Project of the Royal College of Anaesthetists and the Difficult Airway Society. Part 1: anaesthesia. Br J Anaesth. 2011;106:617-31.
3. Heffner AC, Swords DS, Neale MN, Jones AE. Incidence and factors associated with cardiac arrest complicating emergency airway management. Resuscitation. 2013;84:1500-4.
4. De Jong A, Rolle A, Molinari N, Paugam-Burtz C, Constantin J-M, Lefrant J-Y, et al. Cardiac Arrest and Mortality Related to Intubation Procedure in Critically Ill Adult Patients: A Multicenter Cohort Study. Crit Care Med. 2018;46:532-9.
5. Baillard C, Fosse JP, Sebbane M, Chanques G, Vincent F, Courouble P, et al. Noninvasive ventilation improves preoxygenation before intubation of hypoxic patients. Am J Respir Crit Care Med. 2006;174:171-7.
6. De Jong A, Jung B, Jaber S. Intubation in the ICU: we could improve our practice. Crit Care. 2014;18:209.
7. Miguel-Montanes R, Hajage D, Messika J, Bertrand F, Gaudry S, Rafat C, et al. Use of high-flow nasal cannula oxygen therapy to prevent desaturation during tracheal intubation of intensive care patients with mild-to-moderate hypoxemia. Crit Care Med. 2015;43:574-83.
8. Guitton C, Ehrmann S, Volteau C, Colin G, Maamar A, Jean-Michel V, et al. Nasal high-flow preoxygenation for endotracheal intubation in the critically ill patient: a randomized clinical trial. Intensive Care Med. 2019;45:447-58.
9. Frat JP, Ricard JD, Quenot JP, Pichon N, Demoule A, Forel JM, et al. Non-invasive ventilation versus high-flow nasal cannula oxygen therapy with apnoeic oxygenation for preoxygenation before intubation of patients with acute hypoxaemic respiratory failure: a randomised, multicentre, open-label trial. Lancet Respir Med. 2019;7:303-12.

10. Myatra SN, Divatia JV, Brewster DJ. The physiologically difficult airway: an emerging concept. Curr Opin Anaesthesiol. 2022;35(2):115-21.
11. Perbet S, De Jong A, Delmas J, Futier E, Pereira B, Jaber S, et al. Incidence of and risk factors for severe cardiovascular collapse after endotracheal intubation in the ICU: a multicenter observational study. Crit Care. 2015;19:257.
12. Heffner AC, Swords DS, Nussbaum ML, Kline JA, Jones AE. Predictors of the complication of postintubation hypotension during emergency airway management. J Crit Care. 2012;27:587-9.
13. Jabre P, Combes X, Lapostolle F, Dhaouadi M, Ricard-Hibon A, Vivien B, et al. Etomidate versus ketamine for rapid sequence intubation in acutely ill patients: a multicentre randomised controlled trial. Lancet. 2009;374(9686):293-300.
14. Grignola JC, Domingo E. Acute right ventricular dysfunction in intensive care unit. Biomed Res Int. 2017;2017:8217105.
15. Ventetuolo CE, Klinger JR. Management of acute right ventricular failure in the intensive care unit. Ann Am Thorac Soc. 2014;11:811-22.
16. Perkins ZB, Wittenberg MD, Nevin D, Lockey DJ, O'Brien B. The relationship between head injury severity and hemodynamic response to tracheal intubation. J Trauma Acute Care Surg. 2013;74:1074-80.
17. Bucher J, Koyfman A. Intubation of the neurologically injured patient. J Emerg Med. 2015;49:920-7.
18. Parameswaran K, Todd DC, Soth M. Altered respiratory physiology in obesity. Can Respir J. 2006;13:203-10.
19. Quinn AC, Milne D, Columb M, Gorton H, Knight M. Failed tracheal intubation in obstetric anaesthesia: 2 yr national case-control study in the UK. Br J Anaesth. 2013;110:74-80.
20. Munnur U, de Boisblanc B, Suresh MS. Airway problems in pregnancy. Crit Care Med. 2005;33:S259-68.
21. Harless J, Ramaiah R, Bhananker SM. Pediatric airway management. Int J Crit Illn Inj Sci. 2014;4:65-70.
22. Huang AS, Hajduk J, Rim C, Coffield S, Jagannathan N. Focused review on management of the difficult paediatric airway. Indian J Anaesth. 2019;63:428-36.
23. De Jong A, Molinari N, Terzi N, Mongardon N, Arnal JM, Guitton C, et al. Early identification of patients at risk for difficult intubation in the intensive care unit: Development and validation of the MACOCHA score in a multicenter cohort study. Am J Respir Crit Care Med. 2013;187:832-9.
24. Smischney NJ, Surani SR, Montgomery A, Franco PM, Callahan C, Demiralp G, et al. Hypotension Prediction Score for Endotracheal Intubation in Critically Ill Patients: A Post Hoc Analysis of the HEMAIR Study. J Intensive Care Med. 2022;37(11):1467-79.
25. Khandelwal N, Khorsand S, Mitchell SH, Joffe AM. Head-Elevated Patient Positioning decreases Complications of Emergent Tracheal Intubation in the Ward and Intensive Care Unit. Anesth Analg. 2016;122:1101-7.
26. Pitre T, Liu W, Zeraatkar D, Casey JD, Dionne JC, Gibbs KW, et al. Preoxygenation strategies for intubation of patients who are critically ill: a systematic review and network meta-analysis of randomised trials. Lancet Respir Med. 2025;13(7):585-96.
27. Casey JD, Rice TW, Semler MW. Bag-Mask Ventilation during Tracheal Intubation of Critically Ill Adults. Reply. N Engl J Med. 2019;380(25):2482.

28. Bandyopadhyay A, Kumar P, Jafra A, Thakur H, Yaddanapudi LN, Jain K. Peri-Intubation Hypoxia After Delayed Versus Rapid Sequence Intubation in Critically Injured Patients on Arrival to Trauma Triage: A Randomized Controlled Trial. Anesth Analg. 2023;136(5):913-9.
29. Gao YX, Song YB, Gu ZJ, Zhang JS, Chen XF, Sun H, et al. Video versus direct laryngoscopy on successful first-pass endotracheal intubation in ICU patients. World J Emerg Med. 2018;9:99-104.
30. Kory P, Guevarra K, Mathew JP, Hegde A, Mayo PH. The impact of video laryngoscopy use during urgent endotracheal intubation in the critically ill. Anesth Analg. 2013;117:144-9.
31. Jaber S, Rollé A, Godet T, Terzi N, Riu B, Asfar P, et al. Effect of the use of an endotracheal tube and stylet versus an endotracheal tube alone on first-attempt intubation success: a multicentre, randomised clinical trial in 999 patients. Intensive Care Med. 2021;47(6):653-64.
32. Corl KA, Dado C, Agarwal A, Azab N, Amass T, Marks SJ, et al. A modified Montpellier protocol for intubating intensive care unit patients is associated with an increase in first-pass intubation success and fewer complications. J Crit Care. 2018;44:191-5.
33. Karamchandani K, Nasa P, Jarzebowski M, Brewster DJ, De Jong A, et al. Tracheal intubation in critically ill adults with a physiologically difficult airway. An international Delphi study. Intensive Care Med. 2024;50(10):1563-79.
34. Khorsand S, Chin J, Rice J, Bughrara N, Myatra SN, Karamchandani K. Role of Point-of-Care Ultrasound in Emergency Airway Management Outside the Operating Room. Anesth Analg. 2023;137(1):124-36.

CHAPTER

3D Bioprinting in Critical Care Medicine: A Potential Gamechanger

Prashant Saxena, Prabhat Kumar

INTRODUCTION

Critical care medicine is defined by urgency, precision, and the constant need for innovative solutions to address complex, life-threatening conditions.[1,2] In this high-stakes environment, the demand for personalized and timely interventions often exceeds the capabilities of conventional medical tools. 3D bioprinting is a transformative technology that merges biology, engineering, and materials science to fabricate complex, patient-specific tissues, and structures with unprecedented accuracy.[3,4]

Originally developed for research and prototyping, 3D bioprinting has rapidly evolved to address critical challenges in regenerative medicine, organ transplantation, and therapeutic delivery.[5] In critical care settings, where rapid tissue repair, organ support, and tailored therapeutic devices can mean the difference between life and death, the applications of bioprinting are both compelling and urgent.[6] From custom airway stents for pediatric patients to vascular grafts for trauma victims, and even organ-on-a-chip systems for real-time drug testing, 3D bioprinting offers a frontier of solutions aligned with the personalized and dynamic nature of critical care.[7,8]

This chapter explores the current and emerging applications of 3D bioprinting within critical care medicine. It will examine the technologies that enable biofabrication, the materials and cells used, regulatory and ethical considerations, and the challenges that must be overcome to translate laboratory successes into bedside realities.[9,10] With growing clinical interest and interdisciplinary collaboration, 3D bioprinting stands poised to redefine the boundaries of what is possible in saving lives and restoring function in the intensive care unit (ICU) and beyond.

PRINCIPLES OF 3D BIOPRINTING

The 3D bioprinting combines principles of engineering, biomaterials science, and cell biology.

Stages

The bioprinting process generally involves three stages:[1,2]

1. *Pre-bioprinting:* Medical imaging (CT/MRI) and 3D computer-aided design (CAD) are used to generate patient-specific models.

Bioinks—hydrogels containing cells and biomaterials—are selected based on mechanical and biological requirements.[3,4]

2. *Bioprinting:* Layer-by-layer deposition is performed using technologies such as inkjet, extrusion, laser-assisted, or stereolithography-based bioprinters.[5-7]
3. *Post-bioprinting:* Constructs undergo cross-linking, maturation in bioreactors, and functional testing to ensure viability and performance before clinical use.[8]

Bioinks and Biomaterials

Bioinks are central to bioprinting technology. They are formulated using a combination of biomaterials and living cells, and their development has undergone significant evolution. Effective bioinks are biocompatible, mechanically stable, and support cell growth.[3,4]

- *Natural bioinks:* Alginate, gelatin, collagen, and hyaluronic acid provide biological cues for cell adhesion and proliferation.[8,9]
- *Synthetic polymers:* Polyethylene glycol (PEG), polycaprolactone (PCL), and poly(lactic-co-glycolic acid) (PLGA) offer tunable mechanical properties and controlled degradation.[5,8]
- *Decellularized extracellular matrix (dECM):* Preserves native organ-specific microarchitecture and signaling molecules.[8]
- *Advanced bioinks:* Incorporate growth factors, antimicrobial agents, or oxygen carriers to enhance construct functionality.[10]

Engineering Living Constructs

Creating functional tissues involves more than simply printing layers of cells. Engineers must replicate the cellular organization, mechanical properties, and vascular networks of natural tissues.[5,6]

- *Scaffold architecture:* Optimal porosity and surface chemistry promote vascular ingrowth and integration.[7,11]
- *Bioreactors:* Perfusion systems mimic physiological conditions to enhance maturation.[12,13]
- *Chemical and mechanical cues:* Guide cell differentiation and tissue-specific functionality.[8,14]

Collectively, these engineering strategies aim to improve the viability, longevity, and functionality of printed tissues.

Current Modalities in Bioprinting

Bioprinting encompasses several different techniques, each with its advantages and limitations:[5,7]

- *Inkjet bioprinting:* High-speed, cost-effective deposition of low-viscosity bioinks; best suited for thin tissues.[15]

- *Extrusion bioprinting:* Most common technique; supports high cell density and complex geometries, but lower resolution.[16]
- *Laser-assisted bioprinting:* Enables precise, noncontact deposition of microstructures and delicate cells.[15]
- *Stereolithography:* Photopolymerization produces highly detailed, mechanically robust scaffolds for organoids and implants.[7]

POTENTIAL APPLICATIONS IN CRITICAL CARE

Critical care medicine faces many challenges that require innovative solutions.[1,5] Organ failure, especially involving the lungs, liver, kidneys, and heart, remains a leading cause of ICU admissions and death.[2] Unfortunately, organ donation rates are too low to meet increasing needs.[6] Severe burns and major trauma cause large areas of skin and soft tissue loss, requiring quick and effective reconstruction.[4] Sepsis, a systemic inflammatory response to infection, often causes tissue damage and death due to a lack of blood flow.[17] The limitations of current treatments—including immune rejection, infection risks, and surgical complexity—highlight the need for rapid, biocompatible, and patient-specific therapies that can be applied quickly.[3,6] 3D bioprinting helps close these gaps by creating customizable tissue structures and possibly saving lives.[7,9]

Organotypic Tissue Grafts

One of the most immediate uses of bioprinting in critical care involves skin, cartilage, and bone grafts. Burn victims, especially those with full-thickness injuries, benefit from bioprinted skin that replicates both dermal and epidermal layers.[4,9] These grafts, often derived from a patient's cells, reduce the risk of rejection and speed up healing. Similarly, bone scaffolds enriched with osteogenic cells and bioactive molecules can replace segments lost due to trauma,[5] while cartilage bioprinting is being explored for facial and orthopedic reconstruction. These constructs can be printed to exact anatomical specifications, enhancing functional and cosmetic outcomes.[15]

Functional Organ Patches and Organoids

In cases of acute organ failure, full transplantation may not be immediately feasible. Bioprinted organ patches or organoids act as bridge therapies.[18] For example, printed hepatic lobules can temporarily support detoxification in liver failure. Renal organoids mimicking nephron structures can assist in filtration and waste removal during acute kidney injury.[6] Pulmonary tissue constructs that replicate alveolar structures offer potential support for gas exchange in acute respiratory distress syndrome (ARDS) or post-coronavirus disease (COVID) lung damage.[19] These miniature organ units could be integrated into extracorporeal support devices or implanted directly.

Customized Implants and Biostructures

In critical care settings, rapid access to customized implants can save lives. 3D bioprinting enables the design of patient-specific tracheal stents, vascular grafts, and nerve conduits.[7,20] These structures can be preloaded with anti-inflammatory agents or stem cells to promote regeneration.[21] For instance, personalized tracheal scaffolds can be printed for patients with airway collapse or stenosis.[22] Spinal scaffolds embedded with neurotrophic factors offer new possibilities for treating traumatic spinal injuries.[23] For pediatric tracheomalacia, biodegradable and bioprinted tracheal splints have been used to provide temporary structural support.[24] In trauma or decompressive surgeries, personalized cranial patches reduce complications and improve cosmetic outcomes.[25]

Drug Testing and Personalized Medicine

Organ-on-chip systems bioprinted with human cells can replicate physiological responses.[26]

- *Rapid drug screening:* For sepsis, ARDS, or cardiac dysfunction, in vitro testing on bioprinted heart or lung tissue helps identify the safest and most effective drug.[27]
- *Personalized therapies:* Cells from the patient can be used to model disease and predict individual responses to interventions.[28]

Biosensors and Diagnostic Platforms

Bioprinted biosensors embedded with living cells can be used in:

- *Real-time monitoring:* Sensors capable of detecting changes in pH, lactate, or cytokine levels provide real-time feedback on patient condition.[29]
- *Point-of-care diagnostics:* Small, bioprinted organoids could be used to evaluate immune or metabolic responses to treatments in ICU.[30]

Burn Care

Bioprinted skin grafts can be prepared using the patient's keratinocytes and fibroblasts.[4,9] This autologous approach minimizes rejection and improves integration.[31] Some systems are capable of printing skin directly onto wounds, offering real-time, and in situ grafting for extensive burns.[32]

Liver and Kidney Support

Miniaturized constructs such as hepatic spheroids and nephron-mimicking units can provide partial organ function while the patient awaits transplantation or recovery.[6,33] These units may be connected to extracorporeal devices for enhanced filtration and detoxification.[34]

ARDS and COVID-19

The ARDS and COVID-19 may lead to extensive lung damage.[19] Bioprinted alveolar structures could be implanted or used in lung-assist devices to improve gas exchange and reduce dependency on ventilators or extracorporeal membrane oxygenation (ECMO).[35]

Ischemic Limb Salvage

In cases of critical limb ischemia due to sepsis or trauma, bioprinted vascularized tissue patches infused with angiogenic factors can restore perfusion and promote healing,[36] potentially avoiding amputation.[37]

Case Studies and Real-world Progress

Institutions such as the Wake Forest Institute for Regenerative Medicine have demonstrated successful preclinical applications of bioprinted skin and cartilage.[38] Companies such as Organovo and CELLINK are leading the commercial development of liver and kidney tissues.[39] Clinical trials are underway to assess the efficacy of bioprinted constructs for orthopedic and reconstructive surgery.[40] Hybrid laboratories within hospitals are now being established to integrate bioprinting with surgical and ICU services, marking a significant step toward clinical translation.[41]

While regulatory approval remains a challenge, several preclinical and early clinical examples demonstrate the promise of bioprinting. Skin bioprinting systems have shown success in porcine burn models, reducing healing time and scar formation.[32] Cartilage implants have been used to treat focal defects in animal joints with encouraging results.[42] Liver and kidney organoids have demonstrated partial functionality in rodent models of organ failure.[33] These case studies underscore the potential for translating research into practical ICU solutions.[43]

ADVANTAGES OVER TRADITIONAL APPROACHES

3D bioprinting offers several advantages that align closely with the needs of critical care medicine. Its capacity for customization enables patient-specific treatments, reducing immune rejection and improving efficacy.[3,6] The ability to produce tissues rapidly at the bedside may dramatically cut treatment delays.[7] Compared to traditional donor-based transplantation, bioprinted constructs can be standardized, reducing variability and enhancing predictability.[10] Furthermore, incorporating angiogenic or antimicrobial agents into the constructs can accelerate healing and minimize complications.[8,20] By decreasing dependence on organ donors and improving access to tailored treatments, 3D bioprinting could reshape the clinical landscape of intensive care.[1,8]

TECHNICAL AND TRANSLATIONAL CHALLENGES

Vascularization

The biggest challenge in printing functional, thick tissues is achieving effective vascularization.[5,7] Without blood vessels, cells in the interior of a construct die due to a lack of oxygen and nutrients.[44] Approaches being tested include embedding microchannels in scaffolds, printing endothelial cell layers, and using proangiogenic growth factors such as vascular endothelial growth factor (VEGF).[5] Researchers are also experimenting with sacrificial bioinks that create voids for vessel formation.[18]

Cell Sourcing and Immunogenicity

Obtaining a sufficient quantity of cells, particularly autologous stem cells, remains a major obstacle.[6] While induced pluripotent stem cells (iPSCs) offer scalability, they come with regulatory and differentiation challenges.[45] Allogeneic sources are more readily available but raise concerns about immune rejection and ethical acceptability.[7,12]

Infrastructure and Sterility

Printing biological tissues in a critical care environment requires equipment that is sterile, portable, and user-friendly.[46] Printers must be integrated into clean rooms or controlled ICU environments. Additionally, bioinks and cell cultures must be stored, handled, and transported under strict conditions to maintain viability.[47]

Regulatory and Ethical Barriers

The regulatory framework for bioprinting is still evolving.[10,11] The Food and Drug Administration (FDA) and European Medicines Agency (EMA) require rigorous testing for safety, reproducibility, and functionality.[48] Ethical concerns include the creation of human tissues for nontherapeutic use, consent for emergency applications, and equitable access.[12,17] Developing universal standards for bioprinted tissues will be essential to ensure safe deployment.

Economics, Logistics, and Healthcare Integration

While the upfront costs of bioprinters and infrastructure are high, long-term savings from reduced hospitalization, lower rejection rates, and improved outcomes may offset these expenses.[49] Supply chains for bioinks and cells need to be robust and standardized. Clinical staff must be trained to operate bioprinters and manage constructs.[50] Deployment models could include centralized manufacturing hubs or mobile units for field hospitals and rural care.[13,14]

Risks, Limitations, and Failure Modes

Despite the promise, several risks remain. These include construct failure due to poor integration, infection risks from nonsterile components, or unanticipated immune responses.[8,46] Long-term studies on bioprinted implants are scarce, and the potential for oncogenesis or chronic inflammation remains.[51] Manufacturing inconsistencies, data privacy concerns, and the misuse of bioprinting technologies for unethical purposes also warrant caution.[17]

VISION FOR THE FUTURE

The future of 3D bioprinting in critical care is bright. Advances in artificial intelligence (AI) could allow for the optimization of construct design, improving both function and manufacturability.[52] Researchers aim to print entire organs such as hearts or kidneys, which could eventually be transplanted.[53] Portable bioprinters for military and disaster zones are also in development, promising rapid care in austere environments.[54] Global collaboration and equitable access will be key to realizing this potential.

Future prospective areas for bioprinting can be summarized under a few headings:

- Emergency tissue patching
- Hybrid machines in ICUs
- Biofabrication of full organs
- AI-driven bioprinting.[1-9]

CONCLUSION

3D bioprinting, with its capacity for personalized, on-demand, and scalable tissue fabrication, represents a ground-breaking development in critical care medicine. Although many barriers remain, particularly around vascularization, regulation, and infrastructure but the potential to reduce mortality, morbidity, and healthcare costs is enormous. With continued interdisciplinary collaboration, 3D bioprinting could fundamentally reshape how we treat critically ill patients.

REFERENCES

1. Murphy SV, Atala A. 3D bioprinting of tissues and organs. Nat Biotechnol. 2014;32(8):773-85.
2. Ozbolat IT. Bioprinting scale-up tissue and organ constructs for transplantation. Trends Biotechnol. 2015;33(7):395-400.
3. Kang HW, Lee SJ, Ko IK, Kengla C, Yoo JJ, Atala A, et al. A 3D bioprinting system to produce humanscale tissue constructs with structural integrity. Nat Biotechnol. 2016;34(3):312-9.

4. Skardal A. Bioprinting of in situ skin grafts using autologous dermal and epidermal cells. J Tissue Eng Regen Med. 2017;11(6):1574-87.
5. Kolesky DB, Truby RL, Gladman AS, Busbee TA, Homan KA, Lewis JA. 3D bioprinting of vascularized, heterogeneous cell-laden tissue constructs. Adv Mater. 2014;26(19):3124-30.
6. Takahashi K, Yamanaka S. Induced pluripotent stem cells in medicine and biology. Development. 2013;140(12):2457-61.
7. Deuse T. Immunogenicity and tolerance of allogeneic induced pluripotent stem cells. Circ Res. 2019;124(8):1164-80.
8. Badylak SF. Immunologic and regenerative aspects of extracellular matrix scaffolds. Transl Res. 2014;163(4):268-85.
9. Albanna M, Binder KW, Murphy SV, Kim J, Qasem SA, Zhao W, et al. In situ bioprinting of autologous skin cells accelerates wound healing of extensive excisional full-thickness wounds. Sci Transl Med. 2019;9(1):1856.
10. Ventola CL. Medical applications for 3D printing: the FDA perspective. P T. 2014;39(10):704-11.
11. Morrison RJ, Kashlan KN, Flanangan CL, Wright JK, Green GE, Hollister SJ, et al. Regulatory considerations in the design and manufacturing of implantable 3D-printed medical devices. Clin Transl Sci. 2015;8(5):594-600.
12. Samuel G. Ethical and regulatory issues for bioprinting in medicine. Sci Eng Ethics. 2020;26(1):351-68.
13. Mertz L. Dream it, design it, print it in 3D: what can 3D printing do for you? IEEE Pulse. 2013;4(6):15-21.
14. Skardal A. Bioprinting for high-throughput screening. J Lab Autom. 2015;20(3):275-81.
15. Jungebluth P. Tracheobronchial transplantation: a new era. Lancet. 2011;378(9808):18179.
16. Bajaj P. Patterning the differentiation of embryonic stem cells. Biotechnol J. 2010;5(9):1005-19.
17. Parry B. Ethical considerations in 3D bioprinting. Regen Med. 2022;17(4):249-60.
18. Grigoryan B, Paulsen SJ, Corbett DC, Sazer DW, Fortin CL, Zaita AJ, et al. Multivascular networks and functional intravascular topologies within biocompatible hydrogels. Science. 2019;364(6439):458-64.
19. Nichols JE, Niles J, Riddle M, Vargas G, Schilagard T, Ma L, et al. Production and assessment of decellularized pig and human lung scaffolds. Tissue Eng Part A. 2013;19(1718):2045-62.
20. Melchiorri AJ. 3D printing in biomedical engineering. Annu Rev Biomed Eng. 2020;22:285-310.
21. Place ES, George JH, Williamsc CK, Stevens MM. Synthetic polymer scaffolds for tissue engineering. Chem Soc Rev. 2009;38(4):1139-51.
22. Zopf DA, Hollister SJ, Nelson ME, Ohye RG, Green GE. A Bioresorbable airway splint created with a three-dimensional printer. N Engl J Med. 2013;368(21):2043-5.
23. Koffler J, Zhu W, Qu X, Platoshyn O, Dulin JN, Brock J, et al. Biomimetic 3D-printed scaffolds for spinal cord injury repair. Nat Med. 2019;25(2):263-9.
24. Morrison RJ. 3D-printed biodegradable airway splints for severe tracheobronchomalacia. JAMA Otolaryngol Head Neck Surg. 2015;141(10): 946-50.

25. Wilcox B. Patient-specific cranial reconstruction using 3D printing. J Craniofac Surg. 2016;27(4):943-9.
26. Huh D, Torisawa YS, Hamilton GA, Kim HJ, Ingber DE. Microengineered physiological biomimicry: organs-on-chips. Lab Chip. 2012;12(12):2156-64.
27. Bhatia SN, Ingber DE. Microfluidic organs-on-chips. Nat Biotechnol. 2014;32(8):760-72.
28. Esch EW, Bahinski A, Huh D. Organs-on-chips at the frontiers of drug discovery. Nat Rev Drug Discov. 2015;14(4):248-60.
29. Wang X. 3D bioprinting for implantable and microfluidic devices. Biofabrication. 2015;7(3):33001.
30. Wang Z. Engineered organoids for in vitro disease modeling and drug screening. Adv Drug Deliv Rev. 2021;169:121.
31. Jorgensen AM. Direct 3D bioprinting of skin constructs onto burn wounds. Biofabrication. 2020;12(4):4500-6.
32. Albanna M. In situ bioprinting of skin for wound coverage. Adv Healthc Mater. 2019;8(12):e19001-67.
33. Wu D. Engineering of liver tissues for drug screening and transplantation. Hepatology. 2019;69(5):2246-54.
34. Li J, Wu S, Kim E, Yan K, Liu H, Liu C, et al. Electrobiofabrication: electrically based fabrication with biologically derived materials. Biofabrication. 2019;11(3):032002.
35. Nichols JE. Pulmonary tissue bioengineering. J Cell Physiol. 2018;233(6):421-7.
36. Kwon SH. 3D bioprinting of vascularized tissues for ischemic diseases. Adv Drug Deliv Rev. 2018;132:235-49.
37. Leu SY. Biofabrication of perfusable vascular networks for tissue engineering. Acta Biomater. 2018;78:119.
38. Xu T, Binder KW, Albanna MZ, Dice D, Zhao W, Yoo JJ, et al. Hybrid printing of mechanically and biologically improved constructs for cartilage tissue engineering applications. Biofabrication. 2013;5(1):015001.
39. Ma J, Wang Y, Liu J. Bioprinting of 3D tissues/organs combined with microfluidics. RSC Adv. 2018;8(39):21712-27.
40. Dababneh AB, Ozbolat IT. Bioprinting technology: a current state-of-the-art review. J Manuf Sci Eng. 2014;136(6):061016.
41. Vijayavenkataraman S, Yan WC, Lu WF, Wang CH, Fuh JYH. 3D bioprinting of tissues and organs for regenerative medicine. Adv Drug Deliv Rev. 2018;132:296-332.
42. Daly AC. 3D bioprinting of cartilage for orthopaedic applications. Acta Biomater. 2017;61:120.
43. Takebe T, Sekine K, Enomura M, Koike H, Kimura M, Ogaeri T, et al. Vascularized and functional human liver from an iPSC-derived organ bud transplant. Nature. 2013;499(7459):481-4.
44. Novosel EC, Kleinhans C, Kluger PJ. Vascularization is the key challenge in tissue engineering. Adv Drug Deliv Rev. 2011;63(45):300-11.
45. Mandai M, Watanabe A, Kurimoto Y, Hirami Y, Morinaga C, Daimon T, et al. Autologous induced stem cell-derived retinal cells for macular degeneration. N Engl J Med. 2017;376(11):1038-46.
46. Zhao Y. Bioprinting of vascularized tissues for tissue engineering applications. Acta Biomater. 2020;111:117.

47. Lee V, Singh G, Trasatti JP, Bjornsson C, Xu X, Tran TN, et al. Design and fabrication of human skin by three-dimensional bioprinting. Tissue Eng Part C Methods. 2014;20(6):473-84.
48. Food and Drug Administration. Technical Considerations for Additive-manufactured Medical Devices: Guidance for Industry and Food and Drug Administration Staff. Silver Spring: Food and Drug Administration; 2017.
49. Attaran M. The rise of 3D printing: the advantages of additive manufacturing over traditional manufacturing. Bus Horiz. 2017;60(5):677-88.
50. Murphy SV, De Coppi P, Atala A. Opportunities and challenges of translational 3D bioprinting. Nat Biomed Eng. 2020;4(4):370-80.
51. Fehling HJ. Long-term risks of tissue engineering and regenerative medicine. Nat Rev Mater. 2022;7(9):701-18.
52. Zhang B. 3D bioprinting: an emerging technology full of opportunities and challenges. BioDesign Manuf. 2020;3:939.
53. Noor N, Shapira A, Edri R, Gal I, Wertheim L, Dvir T. 3D printing of personalized thick and perfusable cardiac patches and hearts. Adv Sci (Weinh). 2019;6(11):1900344.
54. Kang J. Portable 3D bioprinting system for in situ wound healing. Biofabrication. 2021;13(3):035040.

Index

Page numbers followed by *f* refer to figure *t* refer to table

B

C

D

N

Q

R

S